Statistical Analysis
of Epidemiologic Data

MONOGRAPHS IN EPIDEMIOLOGY AND BIOSTATISTICS

Edited by Jennifer L. Kelsey, Michael G. Marmot,
Paul D. Stolley, Martin P. Vessey

Monographs in Epidemiology and Biostatistics

Volume 25

Statistical Analysis of Epidemiologic Data

SECOND EDITION

Steve Selvin, Ph.D.

University of California, Berkeley

New York   Oxford
OXFORD UNIVERSITY PRESS
1996

Oxford University Press

Oxford   New York
Athens   Auckland   Bangkok   Bombay
Calcutta   Cape Town   Dar es Salaam
Delhi   Florence   Hong Kong   Istanbul
Karachi   Kuala Lumpur   Madras   Madrid
Melbourne   Mexico City   Nairobi   Paris
Singapore   Taipei   Tokyo   Toronto

and associated companies in
Berlin   Ibadan

Library of Congress Cataloging-in-Publication Data
Selvin, S.
Statistical Analysis of Epidemiologic Data/
Steve Selvin.—2nd ed.
p. cm.—(Monographs in Epidemiology and biostatistics; v. 25)
Includes bibliographical references and index.
ISBN 0-19-509760-2
1. Epidemiology—Statistical methods.
I. Title. II. Series.
RA652.2.2.M3S45 1995 614.4'072—dc20 95-14012

9 8 7 6 5 4 3 2 1

Printed in the United States of America
on acid-free paper

for Liz

Preface

Differences among the fields of statistics, biostatistics, vital statistics and epidemiology are often emphasized. This text makes no real distinction among these disciplines and draws material from all four areas to examine the analysis of data collected to study human disease. A number of statistical methods are surveyed in a way that should be useful to researchers concerned with the application of statistics to epidemiologic data. Additionally, these methods are chosen to illustrate general principles. For example, "jackknife" estimation (Chapter 5) is an excellent way to estimate specific parameters from collected data but, at the same time, illustrates the application of a "computer-intensive" estimation method to epidemiology. Statistical procedures useful in epidemiologic analysis are scattered throughout the statistical literature, and the explanations of their properties are often presented in rather theoretical language. The aim of this textbook is to develop a clear understanding of issues important to epidemiologic data analysis without depending on sophisticated mathematics or advanced statistical theory. Running throughout the text is a "casebook theme" where real data are used to address questions surrounding the analysis of epidemiologic questions. Extensive use is made, for example, of a data set that relates the risk of coronary heart disease to behavior. The use of actual data exhibits both the strengths and the weaknesses of an analytic approach in the ultimate understanding of a disease process. With one exception, data are fully presented and therefore available to the reader to verify calculations or to try different approaches for purposes of comparison.

The level of this text is beyond introductory but short of advanced. Knowledge of elementary statistical methods, like that gained from a one-semester statistics course, is assumed and an introductory course in epidemiology is also likely to be useful background. Statistical methods based on the normal and t-distributions are reviewed briefly while other basic techniques (e.g., correlation, simple linear regression and chi-square analysis) are used but not described in detail. This text was developed from a semester course taught during the second year of a master's degree program in epidemiology and biostatistics. A number of common statistical topics in epidemiology such as measures of association and study design are purposely left to other texts so that the reader can focus on additional material particularly useful for the analysis of disease data (e.g., the analysis of cohort data, Chapter 4; spatial data analysis, Chapter 5; and the study of survival from follow up data, Chapters 11 and 12).

The calculations needed to achieve estimates or summaries with the techniques described in this text vary from easy to hard. In an age of powerful computers with "user-friendly" programs, however, the hard calculations should present no major problems. The multi-variable techniques (e.g., logistic and proportional hazard regressions) usually must be implemented with a computer program. The parameters of the logistic and the proportional hazards models were estimated by use of a specialized system named EGRET. Other computer programs that are useful for implementing the methods discussed are relatively simple and can be created on a case-by-case basis or found in popular package systems (e.g., SAS or STATA). A set of problems is found in the appendix. These problems explore a few mathematical details that are ignored in the text and are not part of the mainstream development. The exercises are not opportunities to use the methods under discussion on other "data" sets, because data manipulations problems would then become more an issue of getting the computer program to do the "right thing"—a process necessary for analyzing data but not very enlightening. The emphasis of the material presented is on the principles underlying the application of statistical methods to data common in epidemiologic research.

All statistical techniques involve attributing to the sampled population some sort of mathematical structure. This structure is frequently referred to as a "statistical model." Even the simplest t-test depends on the validity of a statistical model. This text makes explicit the models underlying specific analytic approaches. These statistical structures are useful for understanding the principles underlying a particular technique, and in many cases they make it possible to study the consequences of bias. Throughout this text the mathematical investigation of these models is presented simply as possible with some loss of rigor, and rarely are derivations presented in full generality. Readers interested in pursuing any topic in more depth will find references to relevant textbooks and journal articles.

The Second Edition

A second edition presents the opportunity to make "mid-course" corrections to improve the overall presentation of the material and to add new topics and more current illustrations. A new chapter (9) on analyzing matched data covers both discrete and continuous outcomes. The classic analytic approach to matched data is followed by the parallel application of the conditional estimation applied to the logistic regression model. Consistent with the rest of the text, this new chapter deals with the complicated conditional logistic model on an intuitive level supplemented with examples of data analysis. Chapter 4 has been reorganized and includes two new sections on contingency table data. Several new sections have also been added to Chapter 2, including one on misclassification and another on the concept of additive models underlying tabular data. In fact, all the chapters have new sections and new applications. For example, the proportional hazards model is applied to a current set of HIV/AIDS data (Chapter 12). In addition, errors and ambiguities found in the first edition have been removed and replaced with what I hope to be a clearer and more useful description of the way statistical tools are used to analyze epidemiologic data.

Berkeley   S. S.
May 1995

Acknowledgments

I would like to acknowledge the many years of support from colleagues Richard J. Brand and Nicholas P. Jewell who patiently answered many questions and engaged in numerous lunchtime conversations that resulted in a large number of contributions to the material in this text. This work was substantially improved by Mary Castle White and David F. Selvin who read the complete manuscript and also made valuable contributions. I am also especially grateful to Patricia Charley who drew the technical illustrations. I would also like to acknowledge the Department of Energy, Office of Health and Environmental Research, which funded part of this project. Finally, I wish to thank Nancy, my wife, who has contributed to this volume in a variety of ways.

Contents

12. A Model for Survival Data: Proportional Hazards Model, 391

Appendixes, 423

Statistical Analysis
of Epidemiologic Data

1 Measures of Risk: Rates and Probabilities

A rate calculated from epidemiologic data reflects risk. Probability is another widely used measure of risk that is distinct from a rate but plays a similar role in epidemiologic analysis. A rigorous definition of these quantities clarifies the similarities and differences between these two fundamental measures.

A variety of measures of risk are used in epidemiology that originate from the formal definition of a rate. Some examples of these "rates" in different settings are:

(i)

$$\text{fetal death rate} = \frac{\text{Number of fetal deaths}}{\text{Number of fetal deaths plus live births}},$$

(ii)

food-specific attack rate

$$= \frac{\text{Number of persons who ate a specific food and became ill}}{\text{Total number of persons who ate the specific food}},$$

(iii)

$$\text{generic rate} = \frac{\text{Number of events in a specific period}}{\text{Population at risk for these events in a specified period}} \times \text{base},$$

(iv)

life table mortality rate

$$= \frac{\text{Number of individuals dying in the age interval } (x_i, x_{i+1})}{\text{Number of years lived in } (x_i, x_{i+1}) \text{ by those alive at age } x_i} \times \text{base},$$

(v)

annual death rate from all causes

$$= \frac{\text{Total number of deaths during a specific year}}{\text{Number of persons in the population at midyear}} \times \text{base}.$$

The five expressions are referred to as rates but none has all the properties of a rate when the term is precisely and unambiguously defined. The fetal death rate (i) and the food-specific attack rate (ii) are proportions; the individuals in the numerator are found in the denominator, and time plays no direct role in the calculation. Both quantities are unitless. The generic rate (iii) is more like a proportion. The life table mortality rate (iv) defines the population at risk in terms of person-years and is an estimate of an average rate. The annual rate (v), under certain circumstances, is also an approximate rate, but none of these quantities should be viewed as a definition of a rate.

Rates

The word rate generally describes change associated with a phenomenon. More precisely, a rate is an instantaneous measure of change per unit of time. A familiar example of a rate is the speed of a car, measured "instantaneously" in miles per hour by the speedometer. Instantaneous change is a theoretical quantity borrowed from physics and requires special mathematics for its exact definition. Isaac Newton explored the measurement of instantaneous change three centuries ago and created some of the basic tools of calculus to develop the concept of a rate.

In symbols, the change in a continuous measure y per unit change in time t is

$$\frac{\text{change in } y}{\text{change in time}} = \frac{\delta y}{\delta t}. \tag{1.1}$$

Since y is a function of t, denoted $y(t)$, the term δy represents the difference in y at two different times or, in symbols, $\delta y = y(t + \delta t) - y(t)$. An instantaneous rate is the value of $\delta y / \delta t$ as the time interval becomes small, or formally, as δt approaches 0. The notation of calculus describes a rate as dy/dt, which represents the derivative of the function $y(t)$ with respect to t. An exact value of a rate can be calculated only when the form of the function $y(t)$ is known.

A richer definition of a rate emerges if dy/dt is measured relative to the value $y(t)$. Such a rate becomes

$$\text{rate} = \frac{dy/dt}{y(t)}. \tag{1.2}$$

Dividing by $y(t)$ yields a measure of change in the quantity represented by y relative to the magnitude of y at specific time t. This relative rate finds applications in many fields (e.g., chemistry and economics) and is particularly useful for describing the occurrence of mortality and disease in human populations. For example, a rate of 10 cases of disease per month is more meaningfully expressed as a function of the size of the population—the quantity 10 cases per month among 1,000 persons is different from 10 cases per month among a population of 100,000. Making a rate relative to population size at a specific time more strongly emphasizes a change in a small group over the same change in a larger group, producing a numeric value that reflects risk, the central purpose of a mortality or disease rate.

A mortality or disease rate is almost always defined in terms of units of time. Time is so intrinsic to the calculation that it is often considered part of the definition. This view is overly restrictive. Other types of rates exist; for example, the amount of charge or payment with reference to a base (e.g., cost of insurance per unit coverage). Or, in terms of price, rates can be cost per unit of quantity (e.g., a postage rate in dollars perpound). Dollars are certainly the most meaningful unit for insurance or sales. Airplane accidents are frequently measured per number of take-offs. For automobile accidents, risk of death should be measured as a function of miles traveled. For counts of deaths or cases of illness, however, the natural units and certainly the traditional units of measurement, are time lived or time free of a disease. Again, this choice is made so that a mortality or disease rate reflects risk.

Average Rate

Another measure of risk is an average rate. An average rate results from "averaging" instantaneous rates over a period of time. Using a calculus argument, the average rate becomes

$$\text{average rate} = \frac{\delta y}{\int_{t}^{t+\delta t} y(u)\,du}. \tag{1.3}$$

The integral in expression (1.3) is easily interpreted geometrically. It represents the area under the curve defined by $y(t)$ between times t and $t + \delta t$. An average rate measures the total change in $y(t)$, the numerator, relative to the magnitude of $y(t)$ integrated ("summed") over a period of time (δt), the denominator. Rather than an instantaneous value, the average rate is a measure of the general level of risk from time t to time $t + \delta t$. The average mortality or disease rate is again a theoretical quantity reflecting risk, but over a specified period of time. Like an instantaneous rate, an average rate can be exactly calculated only when the functional form of $y(t)$ is known.

To be concrete, suppose that $y(x)$ represents the number of individuals alive at age x in some defined population. A more common notation for describing rates in human population is

$$y(x) = l_x \quad \text{and the change in } y \text{ is} \quad \delta y = l_x - l_{x+\delta x} = d_x, \qquad (1.4)$$

where d_x is the number of deaths or cases of disease occurring among the l_x individuals in the interval x to $x + \delta x$. In this context, the denominator of the expression for the average rate [expression (1.3)] is the total time at risk accumulated by the l_x individuals alive at age x.

When the exact form of $y(x)$ is not known, an approximation is achieved by considering $y(x)$ to be a straight line (Figure 1–1). This linear approximation works best over short intervals so that a curve and a straight line do not dramatically differ. The area under the curve described by $y(x)$, in person-time units, is the cumulative time spent alive by those who survived the entire interval (x to $x + \delta x$) plus the total time lived by those persons who died during the interval before they died. If $y(x)$ is approximated by a straight line, the total time spent by those who died, on the average, is half the interval length, giving

$$\text{total time} = \text{area} = \int_{x}^{x+\delta x} y(u) \, du \approx \delta x \, l_{x+\delta x} + 0.5 \, \delta x \, (l_x - l_{x+\delta x})$$
$$= \delta x \, (l_x - 0.5 d_x). \qquad (1.5)$$

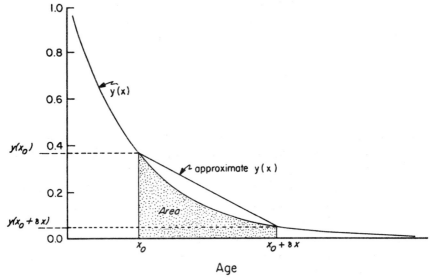

Figure 1–1. Survival curve and linear approximation over the period x_0 to $x_0 + \delta x$

Often the interval studied is one year $(\delta x = 1)$. Then, area $\approx$ $l_x - 0.5d_x \approx P_x$, where P_x represents the midyear population of the specific group under study. That is, the midyear population is a readily available estimate of the person-years of risk for a 1-year interval and, therefore, often serves as an estimate of the area under the curve. Since the midyear population P_x is commonly used as a denominator, rates are frequently stated as deaths or cases per number of individuals at risk (e.g., per 100,000 persons) which, for intervals of 1 year, is equivalent to person-years of risk. The accuracy of P_x as an estimate of the person-years of risk also depends on the assumption that $y(x)$ is at least approximately a straight line.

Generically an average rate is

$$\text{average rate} = \frac{\delta y}{\text{area}}, \tag{1.6}$$

which in applied situations often translates to

$$\text{average rate} = \frac{\text{events}}{\text{time at risk}}. \tag{1.7}$$

For example, an approximate average mortality rate is

$$\text{average mortality rate} = R_x \approx \frac{d_x}{\delta x \, (l_x - 0.5d_x)}, \tag{1.8}$$

when $\delta x = 1$ year,

$$\text{average mortality rate} = R_x \approx \frac{d_x}{P_x}. \tag{1.9}$$

Rates are usually multiplied by a base value (e.g., 100,000) to produce a number greater than one, strictly for aesthetic reasons.

A principal function of a rate is to provide a measure of risk that can be directly compared among a series of causes or among a series of groups. Rates from U.S. mortality data for a few selected causes are illustrated in Table 1–1 for males and females.

Probabilities

The probability of an event can be defined as the number of equally likely ways an event occurs divided by the total number of all possible equally likely outcomes. Other definitions exist. The theory and philosophy surrounding the study of probabilities is subtle and complex, but this simple definition serves the present purpose. Again using mortality as an example, the probability of death is estimated by the number of deaths in a specific time interval divided by the

Table 1–1. Mortality rates* for selected causes for white males and females (United States, 1986)

Disease	Male	Female
All causes	954.4	840.7
Malignant neoplasms	218.8	185.6
Malignant neoplasms of breast	0.2	34.6
Malignant neoplasms of lung	77.8	35.9
Leukemias	8.7	6.7
Cardiovascular diseases	422.0	418.7
Ischemic heart disease	251.6	214.6
Cerebrovascular diseases	50.5	76.2
Pneumonia	29.3	30.0
Appendicitis	0.2	0.2
All accidents	55.0	24.4
Suicide	22.3	5.9
Homicide	8.6	3.0

*Average rates per 100,000 person-years at risk.

number of individuals who could have died (alive at the start of the interval) or

$$P(\text{death in the interval } x \text{ to } x + \delta x) = q_x = \frac{d_x}{l_x}. \qquad (1.10)$$

A probability does not incorporate a direct reference to time, whereas a rate is a measure of change per unit of time. A probability is a unitless value always between 0 and 1. Nevertheless, these two risk measures are related, because

$$\text{rate} = R_x = \frac{d_x}{\delta x \, (l_x - 0.5d_x)} = \frac{q_x}{\delta x \, (1 - 0.5q_x)}; \quad \text{then} \quad q_x = \frac{\delta x \, R_x}{1 + 0.5 \, \delta x \, R_x}. \qquad (1.11)$$

In most cases of death or disease, the rate R_x is small, so that

$$q_x \approx \delta x \, R_x. \qquad (1.12)$$

Expression (1.12) clearly shows that the difference between a rate and a probability concerns primarily the role of time (δx). Confusion between the two arises because for many applications rates are small and based on a time interval of 1 unit (e.g., $\delta x = 1$ year) so that the values for a rate and a probability are more or less indistinguishable ($q_x \approx R_x$). Even for a relatively large mortality rate, a rate and a probability are similar. If 10 deaths in a year produce an average mortality rate of $0.01 = 1$ death per 100 person-years, then the hardly different probability of death is 0.00995. In addition, ratio measures of risk are common, and the difference between a ratio of probabilities and a ratio of rates is typically inconsequential when applied to the same time period, since

$$\text{risk ratio} = \frac{q_x}{q'_x} \approx \frac{\delta x\, R_x}{\delta x\, R'_x} = \frac{R_x}{R'_x} = \text{rate ratio.} \tag{1.13}$$

In generally unrealistic situations, a rate and a probability can be rather different. For example, if all but one person die in a population of 100 individuals during the first week over a period of 1 year, then

$$q = \frac{99}{100} = 0.99 \quad \text{but} \quad R = \frac{99}{1 + 0.5\,\dfrac{99}{52}} = 50.719 \quad \text{deaths per person-years.} \tag{1.14}$$

A rate can also be expressed as the probability of an event relative to the average time at risk. For mortality,

$$\text{average mortality rate} = \frac{\text{deaths}}{\text{total time at risk}} \approx \frac{d}{\displaystyle\sum_{i=1}^{l} t_i} = \frac{q}{\bar{t}} = \frac{\text{probability of death}}{\text{average time at risk}}, \tag{1.15}$$

where t_i represents the time observed for the ith person ($\sum t_i$ is the total observed time at risk for l individuals, making $\bar{t} = (1/l) \sum t_i$ the average time at risk for these individuals where $q = d/l$). Expression (1.15) is essentially another version of the previous expression (1.12) relating a rate and a probability. An occasionally useful view of a rate comes from noting that a rate can be expressed as a probability per unit time.

Incidence and Prevalence

Two epidemiologic measures, often expressed as rates, reflect the incidence and prevalence of a disease.

Incidence is measured in two ways:

1. Incidence rate: The number of new cases of illness over a period of time divided by the person time at risk; or more commonly,
2. Incidence proportion: The number of new cases of illness over a period of time divided by the number of persons at risk at the beginning of the time period.

A disease incidence rate is measured in person-years (time accumulated) such as the number of new lung cancer cases in 1992 divided by the number of person-years of risk during that year. The more common incidence proportion is a unitless measure of risk, where the number of newly affected individuals are counted and divided by the number of disease-free individuals who could have become affected. Incidence proportion refers to a period of time. For example, the number of coronary events in the first six years of a study divided by the number of individuals under observation is an incidence proportion. An incidence rate, like all rates, explicitly incorporates the element of time as part of the calculation.

A prevalence proportion (often erroneously called a prevalence "rate") is the number of affected individuals in a population at a specific point in time divided by the size of the population under consideration. For example, the point prevalence proportion of congenital heart defects among children under 10 years of age in a specific county is the number of existing cases divided by the number of children under 10 years of age residing in the county on a specified date. This measure of disease frequency is not a rate. Such a prevalence measure does depend on time in the sense that the cases are counted at a specific time, but it does not result in a value expressed per unit time. A point prevalence proportion, like all proportions, is unitless.

One final measure of prevalence is a period prevalence proportion (also sometimes called a "rate") which is the total number of affected individuals in a population plus a count of new cases over a defined period of time divided by the size of the population at risk under consideration. This measure is not commonly used because it combines both incidence and prevalence cases into a single not very meaningful number.

To symbolically represent prevalence and incidence measures of disease, let

l_0 = the number of disease-free individuals at time t_0,

d_0 = the number of individuals with the disease at time t_0,

l_1 = the number of disease-free individuals at time t_1 $(t_0 < t_1)$, and

c_1 = the number of disease-free individuals at time t_0 who acquired the disease between time t_0 and time t_0 plus 1 year $(t_1 = t_0 + 1)$.

The relationships between the quantities are given in Table 1–2.

Prevalence and incidence are related. If the incidence proportion is 10 new cases each month per 10,000 individuals and the duration of the disease is 5 months, then the prevalence in this population is 50 cases per 10,000 individuals. This simple relationship—that prevalence equals incidence multiplied by duration—holds under rather strict requirements called *steady-state* conditions. The concept of a steady-state population is discussed in more detail in Chapter 10. These steady-state conditions rarely occur in realistic situations, because

Table 1–2. Measures of prevalence and incidence

Type	Measure
Point prevalence proportion at time 0	$\dfrac{d_0}{l_0 + d_0}$
Point prevalence proportion at time 1	$\dfrac{d_0 + c_1}{l_1 + d_0 + c_1}$
Prevalence rate for 1 year starting at time 0	$\dfrac{d_0 + c_1}{l_1 + \frac{1}{2}c_1}$
Incidence proportion at time 1	$\dfrac{c_1}{l_0}$
Incidence rate for 1 year starting at time 0	$\dfrac{c_1}{l_1 + \frac{1}{2}c_1}$

generally diseases have complex incidence/prevalence dynamics involving such factors as race, age, and medical care. Expressions relating incidence and prevalence are discussed in detail elsewhere [1]. It is important, however, to note that for diseases of short duration, prevalence and incidence proportions are roughly equal; conversely, for conditions with long duration, prevalence and incidence measures likely provide information on different aspects of a disease.

Mortality is related to disease incidence through a measure called the case fatality proportion (sometimes called a case fatality "rate" or "ratio"). A case fatality proportion is the number of cases of a disease that ends in death from a specific cause divided by the total number of cases of that disease within a defined population. Case fatality expresses mortality risk among those with a disease. A mortality rate is a function of the number of new cases of disease that arise (incidence) in a population and the proportion of diseased individuals who die (case fatality). Like prevalence, when the case fatality proportion of a disease is near 1 (such as for pancreatic cancer), mortality and disease incidence measures are similar, and if the case fatality rate is low (such as for some kinds of skin cancer), incidence and mortality rates differ and probably measure different dimensions of the disease process (more discussion is found in [1]).

It is occasionally desirable to estimate the duration of a disease; a sometimes deceptively difficult task. Under ideal conditions, duration is estimated by identifying and following every new case until the end of the disease period. The total amount of time ill, divided by the number of persons observed, is an estimate of expected disease duration. However, complete follow-up is expensive, time consuming, and often impossible. An alternative strategy is to identify a group of existing cases at a specific point in time and ascertain the amount of time each patient was ill. Another approach is to identify and follow a number of patients with the disease for a specific period and record the observed duration of illness for each individual. Although these two types of data collection patterns are efficient ways to collect duration data, the directly calculated mean duration is length-biased. These sampling schemes yield direct estimates of duration that are probably too small, because short-lasting cases are likely to be overrepresented in the sample (see Figure 1–2), and a number of long-lasting episodes are not entirely included (they are said to be censored—a future topic).

To illustrate a length-biased estimate, consider the following data collected from a skilled nursing facility over a 4-month period (x denotes the length of stay recorded in complete months, which is the measure of duration of "illness"). The patients were observed for a maximum of 4 months, and the amount of time in the facility was recorded for each individual, including both patients who were present at the beginning of the period and patients who arrived during the

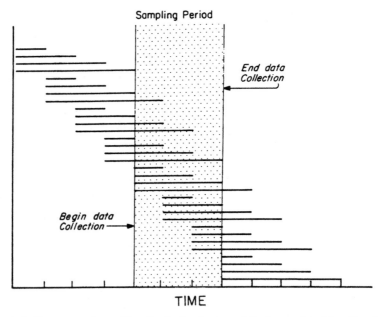

Figure 1–2. Representations of longitudinal cohorts and their associated lengths of stay for data collected over a specific time period

Table 1–3. Number of patients completing *x* months of stay during a 4-month interval

Month	$x = 0$	$x = 1$	$x = 2$	$x = 3$	$x \geq 4$	Total
Patient	39	37	24	11	5	116

period of observation (see Figure 1–2). The data are shown in Table 1–3.

The fact that lengths of stay in the facility of more than 4 months are recorded as four ($x = 4$) is one reason for bias, and the likely overrepresentation of short stays is another source of bias making it probable that $\bar{x}$ is an underestimate of the true length of stay. The mean value calculated directly from these data is $\bar{x} = 1.190$ months. This length-biased mean can be adjusted by postulating a specific statistical structure [2] and, with some algebra, yields

$$\text{estimated mean duration} = \bar{x}\,[\text{correction factor}] = \bar{x}\left[\frac{1}{1 - (1 + \bar{x})/k}\right], \quad (1.16)$$

where k is the length of maximum possible observation ($k = 4$ for the nursing home data). The adjusted value of $\bar{x}$ gives an unbiased estimated mean duration of stay $= 1.190(2.210) = 2.630$ months. For other sampling schemes, other corrections are possible (e.g., examples in [2]). The central point is that a directly calculated mean duration is often length-biased when complete follow-up is not possible but an improved estimate of duration can be found. Correction for bias, a recurring issue in statistical analysis, is described in the following chapters, particularly Chapters 11 and 12, for a specific type of length-biased data.

Survival Probability and Hazard Rate

Two specialized measures of mortality or disease based on the concepts of probabilities and rates are a survival probability and a hazard rate. Both play fundamental roles in describing data collected to study disease. These two related quantities reflect different aspects of survival.

A survival probability is simply the probability that an individual survives or is disease-free from one time to another. For example, the survival probability, symbolized by $S(t)$, is the probability that a person alive at time 0 will survive to at least time t. That is,

$$P\,(\text{surviving from time} = 0 \text{ until time} = t) = S(t)$$

or, equivalently

$$P\,(\text{surviving beyond time } t) = S(t).$$

A survival curve describes the relationship between the probability of survival and time.

A hazard rate is another frequently used measure of risk, sometimes called the force of mortality or failure rate. A hazard rate measures instantaneously the risk of death at a specific time. When $S(t)$ represents the probability of survival from time $= 0$ to time $= t$, then the hazard rate is

$$\text{hazard rate} = \lambda(t) = -\frac{dS(t)/dt}{S(t)}. \tag{1.17}$$

A hazard rate does not differ in principle from the general definition of a rate [expression (1.2)] and measures instantaneous mortality or disease risk relative to a survival probability. A hazard rate is sometimes called an "instantaneous death rate." The survival probability and hazard rate are important elements in the description of epidemiologic data and will be reintroduced in the context of life tables and survival analysis in Chapters 10, 11, and 12.

The relationships among an average mortality rate, a survival probability, and a hazard rate are illustrated by a simple model. The probability of surviving up to time t (the survival probability) is given by the theoretical relationship (made-up to be purely illustrative)

$$S(t) = 1 - \frac{t}{100} \tag{1.18}$$

where $0 \leq t \leq 100$ weeks. The survival curve $S(t)$ describes the probability of surviving at least t weeks. For example, the probability a person survives beyond 40 weeks is $S(40) = 1 - 40/100 = 0.6$. Note that $S(0) = 1$, $S(100) = 0$ and that the probability of survival is linearly related to time (intercept $= 1$ and slope $= -1/100$; Figure 1–3, top). In terms of numbers of individuals N, the number of persons expected to survive beyond time t is $N \times S(t)$. The number of deaths occurring between two times (t_0 and t_1 with $t_0 < t_1$) is then

$$\text{number of deaths} = N[S(t_0) - S(t_1)] = \frac{N(t_1 - t_0)}{100}. \tag{1.19}$$

The number of person-weeks accumulated by N individuals between times t_0 and t_1 is

$$\text{time at risk} = N(t_1 - t_0)\{S(t_1) + 0.5[S(t_0) - S(t_1)]\}$$

$$= N(t_1 - t_0)\left(1 - \frac{0.5(t_0 + t_1)}{100}\right). \tag{1.20}$$

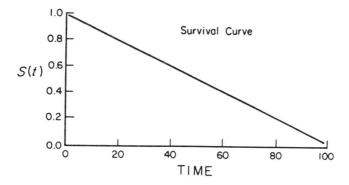

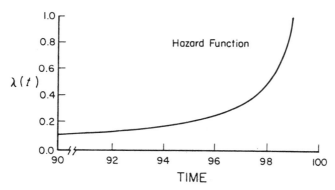

Figure 1–3. Survival curve and hazard function associated with the survival function $S(t) = 1 - t/100$

Therefore, the average mortality rate between times t_0 and t_1 is

$$\text{average rate} = \frac{\text{number of deaths}}{\text{time at risk}} = \frac{\mathcal{N}(t_1 - t_0)/100}{\mathcal{N}(t_1 - t_0)\left(1 - \frac{0.5(t_0 + t_1)}{100}\right)}$$

$$= \frac{1}{100 - 0.5(t_0 + t_1)}. \tag{1.21}$$

A hazard rate $\lambda(t)$ is an instantaneous rate at specific time t. An average mortality rate becomes a more precise approximation of the hazard rate as the length of the time interval considered decreases. The linear survival rate [expression (1.18)] example shows the relationship between the average rate and the hazard rate. Consider an average rate calculated for the period starting at $t_0 = 60$ weeks for a series of selected time intervals where:

$$t_0 = 60 \text{ weeks} \quad t_1 = 70 \text{ weeks} \quad \text{average rate}/1{,}000 = 28.6$$
$$t_0 = 60 \text{ weeks} \quad t_1 = 68 \text{ weeks} \quad \text{average rate}/1{,}000 = 27.8$$
$$t_0 = 60 \text{ weeks} \quad t_1 = 66 \text{ weeks} \quad \text{average rate}/1{,}000 = 27.0$$
$$t_0 = 60 \text{ weeks} \quad t_1 = 64 \text{ weeks} \quad \text{average rate}/1{,}000 = 26.3$$
$$t_0 = 60 \text{ weeks} \quad t_1 = 62 \text{ weeks} \quad \text{average rate}/1{,}000 = 25.6$$
$$t_0 = 60 \text{ weeks} \quad t_1 = 60 \text{ weeks} \quad \text{average rate}/1{,}000 = 25.0.$$

The last line $(t_0 = t_1 = 60)$ is the hazard rate (instantaneous). Ultimately, when $t_1 = t_0 = t$, the average rate becomes exactly the hazard rate associated with the survival curve $S(t)$ and for the illustrative case [using expression (1.21)] is

$$\text{average rate} \approx \frac{1}{100 - t} = \text{hazard rate} = \lambda(t). \tag{1.22}$$

Of course, directly applying the definition of the hazard rate as the derivative with respect to t of the survival function divided by $S(t)$ (multiplied by -1) yields the same expression. This hazard rate is displayed in Figure 1–3 (bottom) for the weeks 90 to 99, because the curve is almost flat for the first 90 weeks.

Statistical Properties of Probabilities Calculated from Mortality or Disease Data

Statistical properties of an estimated value arise from an underlying statistical model. A common model that is the source of many statistical properties of a probability calculated from mortality or disease data involves two assumptions. First, the probability of death or disease is assumed to be the same for each individual in a defined group. Second, the occurrences of death or disease are assumed to occur in a statistically independent manner. If these two assumptions are tenable, the observed number of deaths (D) in a sample of individuals is accurately described by a binomial probability distribution (see Appendix B for more detail). In such a population, the expected number of deaths in a sample of n individuals is nq, and the variance associated with the observed number of deaths is variance $(D) = nq\,(1 - q)$, where q represents the probability of death. The variance of an estimated value is the key to the assessment of statistical precision, an essential part of any conclusions drawn from data.

A number of statistical properties follow from the binomial model. The probability of death is estimated by

$$\hat{q} = \frac{D}{n} \quad \text{with variance } (\hat{q}) = \frac{q\,(1 - q)}{n} \approx \frac{\hat{q}}{n} = \frac{D}{n^2}, \tag{1.23}$$

because for most mortality or disease data the probability q is small (i.e., $1 - q \approx 1$). Other approximate measures of variability also follow such as:

$$\text{standard error } (\hat{q}) \approx \frac{\hat{q}}{\sqrt{n}} \tag{1.24}$$

and

$$\text{variance } (D) \approx n\hat{q} = D \quad \text{or standard error } (D) \approx \sqrt{D}. \tag{1.25}$$

These variances, generated from a binomial model, are used to evaluate estimates made from mortality or disease data. The approximate standard error of an observed number of deaths is estimated by the square root of the number of deaths and is an often-used "rule of thumb" for assessing isolated mortality counts. If $D = 5$ deaths occur in a specific county, for example, an estimate of the standard error associated with this observation is $\sqrt{5} = 2.236$. The binomial model is also the key element in expressions of the variances of more complicated measures of mortality such as the standardized mortality ratio and the direct adjusted standardized mortality rate ([3] or [4]).

The utility of the binomial model must be tempered by two issues. Variance is most easily interpreted when the situation addressed is related to a normal, or at least an approximately normal, distribution. When the probability q is small, the distribution of the estimate $\hat{q}$ becomes skewed so that the normal distribution does not represent accurately the distribution of $\hat{q}$. The phrase "plus or minus two standard deviations," suggesting likely ranges of a statistic, has little meaning when q is small, particularly when the sample size is also small. William Cochran, who is responsible for many modern statistical techniques, produced a table to be used as a "working rule" for application of the normal approximation to estimated binomial probabilities [5]. Table 1–4 is constructed so that approximate 95% confidence intervals limits have less than a 5.5% error.

If the sample size n is large enough, then confidence limits based on a normal distribution approximation are an accurate assessment of the impact of random variation on the estimated probability $\hat{q}$ (e.g., an approximate 95% confidence interval is $\hat{q} \pm 1.96\sqrt{\hat{q}(1 - \hat{q})/n}$. When the sample size for a given value of q is smaller than the value in

Table 1–4. Sample sizes for accurate use of the normal approximation

q	0.50	0.40	0.30	0.20	0.10	0.05
Sample size (n)	30	50	80	200	600	1,400

Cochran's table, the distribution associated with $\hat{q}$ is sufficiently skewed that alternatives to procedures based on the normal distribution should be used. Tables of exact confidence limits exist [6] and more accurate approximations are possible [3]. Since the probability of death or disease q is small for most studies involving human data, exact methods are often required or, at the very least, care is necessary in the application of approximate methods.

The second issue involves the assumption that the population of interest is homogeneous with respect to the probability q. Most disease data are divided into roughly homogeneous groups. It is common to form categories according to sex, age, and race to reduce the heterogeneity of q by forming homogeneous groups. The reduction in heterogeneity aids in the statistical analysis but, more important, aids in the interpretation. The statement that "the probability of breast cancer is 102 cases per 100,000 women" is meaningful only if the women sampled to estimate this probability have similar risks. When most women in the data set have a risk of 1 case per 100,000 while a few have a risk of 10 cases per 1,000 (1,000 cases per 100,000), a summary value of 102 cases per 100,000 is not very meaningful (it applies to practically no one because of the heterogeneity of the sampled population).

A consequence of the assumption of homogeneity of risk (constant q) is that it makes analyses based on estimates of q conservative. By "conservative," it is meant that the variability is overestimated when heterogeneity of q is ignored. Overstating the actual variability makes it less likely that systematic patterns in disease frequencies will be detected when they exist. That is, treating a population that is heterogeneous for q as if it were homogeneous exaggerates variability, and the evaluations of measures of association tend to be biased toward the conclusion of no association. A simple but artificial model illustrates.

Two populations are considered, each with four subgroups; one population is perfectly homogeneous and the other heterogeneous with respect to q, shown in Table 1–5.

First consider the homogeneous case. If four individuals are sampled, then the number of "deaths" can equal 0, 1, 2, 3, or 4 with the

Table 1–5. Four hypothetical levels of risk

Population	q_1	q_2	q_3	q_4	$\bar{q}$
Homogeneous	0.09	0.09	0.09	0.09	0.09
Heterogeneous	0.20	0.10	0.05	0.01	0.09

Table 1–6. Distribution of possible outcomes

"Deaths"	$D = 0$	$D = 1$	$D = 2$	$D = 3$	$D = 4$
Probability	0.68575	0.27128	0.04025	0.00265	0.00007

binomial probabilities for the five possible outcomes that are shown in Table 1–6. Then the variance $(D) = 4(0.09) = 0.328$, where D is the observed number of "deaths" among a sample of four.

For the heterogeneous case the calculation is not as simple. To account for the four levels of heterogeneity of q, a sample of one observation is taken from each of the four strata. Table 1–7 lists all possible outcomes of a sample of four and their associated probabilities. These probabilities are calculated under the assumption that the four sampled observations are independent so that the probability of any one outcome is the product of the associated probabilities [e.g., number 10, $P(0101) = P(D = 2) = (0.80)(0.10)(0.95)(0.01) = 0.00076$]. The distribution of 0, 1, 2, 3, and 4 "deaths" is produced by summing the probabilities associated with each of these outcomes and is shown in Table 1–8. The variance associated with the observed number of "deaths" accounting for the heterogeneity is variance $(D) = 0.307$.

The number of "deaths" (D) sampled from the heterogeneous population is less variable (0.307) than the variability (0.328)

Table 1–7. All possible samples from the hypothetical heterogeneous population

i	1	2	3	4	D	Probability
1	1	1	1	1	4	0.00001
2	1	1	1	0	3	0.00099
3	1	1	0	1	3	0.00019
4	1	0	1	1	3	0.00009
5	0	1	1	1	3	0.00004
6	1	1	0	0	2	0.01881
7	1	0	0	1	2	0.00171
8	0	0	1	1	2	0.00036
9	1	0	1	0	2	0.00891
10	0	1	0	1	2	0.00076
11	0	1	1	0	2	0.00396
12	0	0	0	1	1	0.00684
13	0	0	1	0	1	0.03564
14	0	1	0	0	1	0.07524
15	1	0	0	0	1	0.16929
16	0	0	0	0	0	0.67716

Table 1–8. Distribution of possible outcomes

"Deaths"	$D = 0$	$D = 1$	$D = 2$	$D = 3$	$D = 4$
Probability	0.67716	0.28701	0.03451	0.00131	0.00001

associated with the number of "deaths" sampled from a homogeneous population. The relationship between these two variances in general is

$$\text{variance } (D \mid q = \text{homogeneous}) \geq \text{variance } (D \mid q = \text{heterogeneous}) \quad (1.26)$$

since

$$n\bar{q}(1 - \bar{q}) = \sum_{i=1}^{k} n_i q_i (1 - q_i) + (k - 1)\sigma_q^2, \quad (1.27)$$

where $\sigma_q^2 = [1/(k-1)] \sum n_i(q_i - \bar{q})^2$ measures the amount of variability among the subgroups (heterogeneity of q), n_i is the number of individuals sampled from each subgroup ($n = \sum n_i$), and k is the number of subgroups. The value $\bar{q}$ is the mean probability of death, where $\bar{q} = (1/k) \sum n_i q_i$. The variance based on this value, variance $(D) = n\bar{q}(1 - \bar{q})$, will always be greater than the variance $(D) = \sum n_i q_i (1 - q_i)$, when heterogeneity ($\sigma_q^2 \neq 0$) with respect to the probability of death exists within the population sampled. Only when the population is exactly homogeneous ($\sigma_q^2 = 0$) is the variance estimate based on the binomial model and $\bar{q}$ strictly correct; otherwise the estimated variance is biased (slightly biased in many cases) toward overstating the true variability.

Returning to the simple example with four subgroups, where $k = 4$, $\bar{q} = 0.09$ and $q_1 = 0.20$, $q_2 = 0.10$, $q_3 = 0.05$, and $q_1 = 0.01$ with $n_1 = n_2 = n_3 = n_4 = 1$, then

$$\text{variance } (D \mid q = \text{heterogeneous}) = \sum n_i q_i (1 - q_i) = 0.3074$$
$$(k - 1)\sigma_q^2 = \sum n_i (q_i - \bar{q})^2 = 0.0202 \quad \text{and}$$
$$\text{variance } (D \mid q = \text{homogeneous}) = n\bar{q}(1 - \bar{q}) = 4(0.09)(0.91) = 0.3276$$
$$= 0.3074 + 0.0202.$$

Suppose that $D = 676$ deaths occur during a specific year in a county among $n = 14,700$ residents at risk. An estimate of the probability of death is $\hat{q} = 676/14,700 = 0.046$ and, as mentioned, the estimated standard error of this estimate is $\sqrt{\hat{q}(1 - \hat{q})/n} = 0.00173$ based on the assumption that all persons at risk have the same probability of death. However, it is likely that the 676 deaths result from combining heterogeneous subgroups such as the city residents, suburban residents, and rural residents, who undoubtedly have differing probabilities of death (i.e., the q_i values are in reality heterogeneous). Because $\hat{q}$ and its standard error are based on the assumption of homogeneous q (the only choice when information is lacking on any heterogeneous subgroups), the estimated standard error is too large, giving an upper limit to the value that would be calculated if the heterogeneity of the q-values was known and taken into account.

Special Case: Probability Equals Zero

The statistical properties of an estimated probability when the observed value is small require special attention, as mentioned. The most extreme case occurs when a value of zero is observed. Confusion sometimes arises between an impossible event and a rare event. If the event is impossible, then an observed value of zero is exactly what is expected (no variance); but when a zero value is observed for an event that is rare, a statistical evaluation of the estimate $\hat{q} = 0$ is called for. In the first case, the size of the sample is not relevant, but in the second case, it is the sample size, as always, that primarily determines the precision of the estimate.

Colon cancer incidence data for the city of Oakland, California, recorded as part of a community action project aimed at decreasing the stage-specific cancer incidence among black females, are given in Table 1–9. The "background" rate of localized colon cancer among black females was 15.5 per 100,000 for the San Francisco area over the decade 1970–80. Is there anything special about absence of cases of local colon cancer in Oakland (1977), or is this lack of cases an expected occurrence for a rare disease? It is difficult to answer this question without evaluation. One method to evaluate the influence of chance fluctuations on a statistical estimate is a confidence interval. However, a confidence interval is typically developed in terms of a normal approximation (e.g., estimated parameter $\pm 2 \times$ standard error). If an estimated probability is zero, then a confidence interval based on the normal distribution is logically impossible, because the confidence interval lower bound will be less than zero. As indicated earlier, the distribution of an estimated proportion near zero also becomes skewed, further reducing the utility of the normal distribution as an

Table 1–9. Rate of localized incidence of colon cancer (Oakland, California, 1977)

Site	Number of Cases	Population	Rate per 100,000
Colon	0	20,183	0.0

approximation. However, it is entirely possible to develop an exact confidence interval based on an observed value of zero. The process begins with the fundamental concept underlying the construction of confidence intervals in general.

The 95% confidence interval limits are created from estimated values to have a probability of 0.95 of containing the true parameter. The interval is subject to random variation, but the parameter is not. To construct a confidence interval, the sample data are considered as fixed, and the likelihood associated with different parameters is considered. For the colon cancer example, if the probability of colon cancer is 5 per 100,000, then the probability of observing zero cases among 20,183 women is $(1 - 0.00005)^{20,183} = 0.365$. A value of zero is not unlikely when data on 20,183 black women are collected. If the probability is 10 per 100,000, then the probability of observing zero cases decreases to $(1 - 0.0001)^{20,183} = 0.133$. Table 1–10 shows the probability of observing zero cases in a population of 20,183 individuals for a number of selected cancer probabilities (same data set but different parameters). Clearly, as the probability of colon cancer increases, the probability of observing zero cases of disease decreases.

Confidence limits are bounds for possible values of the true probability q for which the observed data are likely. When zero observations occur among n individuals, these bounds are zero and q_{upper}. For an exact 95% confidence interval the value of q_{upper} is the cancer probability such that the probability of observing zero cases among n individuals is 0.05 and is given by

$$(1 - q_{upper})^n = 0.05, \quad \text{then} \quad q_{upper} = 1 - (0.05)^{1/n}. \quad (1.28)$$

Values of q greater than q_{upper} are considered inconsistent with the data, because the observed result (zero cases) becomes "unlikely"

Table 1–10. Probability of zero cases for different probabilities of localized colon cancer

Probability of Cancer	Probability of Zero Cases
1/100,000	0.817
3/100,000	0.546
5/100,000	0.365
10/100,000	0.133
15/100,000	0.048
20/100,000	0.018
25/100,000	0.006
30/100,000	0.002

(i.e., less than 0.05). For the colon cancer example, $q_{upper} = 1 - 0.05^{1/20,183} = 0.000148$. That is, the probability of observing zero cases is 0.05 when the probability of colon cancer is 0.000148. The probability of zero cases is less than 0.05 for any rate above 14.842 per 100,000, and greater than 0.05 for rates less than 14.842 (see Table 1–10). Rates that exceed q_{upper} are, somewhat arbitrarily, considered unlikely explanations of the observed data because they are unlikely candidates for the parameter producing no observed cases of disease. A confidence interval can be viewed as a way of dividing all possible values of a parameter into two groups based on a specific set of data; those values that are likely (e.g., rate < 14.48 per 100,000 person-years) and those that are not (e.g., rate > 14.48 per 100,000 person-years).

Note that since

$$x^{1/n} = 1 + \frac{\log [x]}{n} + \frac{(\log [x])^2}{2!n^2} + \dots \quad \text{a result from algebra,} \quad (1.29)$$

then, approximately

$$q_{upper} = 1 - (0.05)^{1/n} \approx 1 - \left(1 + \frac{\log [0.05]}{n}\right) = \frac{3}{n}. \quad (1.30)$$

An approximate 95% confidence interval for a zero rate is therefore $(0.0, 3/n \times 100,000)$ per 100,000. Other approximate limits are $2.3/n$ for a 90% confidence interval, $4.6/n$ for a 99% confidence interval, and $5.3/n$ for a 99.5% confidence interval. For the localized colon cancer data, the approximate confidence interval $(0.0, 0.000148)$ is almost equal to the exact 95% confidence interval based on expression (1.28).

A confidence interval indicates a set of likely parameters giving some idea of the range of possible parameter values that could have produced the observed data. The "usual" rate of 15.5 cases of localized colon cancer per 100,000 black women is not a very plausible explanation of the Oakland data, because rates higher than 14.84 rarely produce zero cases (i.e., the 95% confidence interval does not contain the background rate). That is, the true and unknown rate for localized colon cancer in Oakland for the year 1977 likely differs from the rate 15.5 cases per 100,000 based on the observation of zero cases among a population of 20,183 black women.

ANALYSIS OF RATES: SMOOTHING, TRANSFORMING, AND ADJUSTMENT

Three techniques—smoothing, transforming, and adjusting—are ways to describe and evaluate a set of rates. Smoothing is a simple and useful descriptive tool. A transformation is effectively used to test specific hypotheses. Adjustment procedures yield a summary "rate" that accounts for the influence of other variables, usually age. These methods apply not only to rates but also to a vareity of data, and they are only three possibilities among a large number of statistical strategies for analyzing rates.

Smoothing

A sequence of rates can be viewed as a series of numbers with two components: an underlying pattern disrupted by nonsystematic fluctuations. These fluctuations are due to such influences as random variation, bias, or outlier observations. Regardless of their nature, the fluctuations frequently obscure underlying patterns in a sequence. Smoothing techniques dampen the roughness in a sequence so that any underlying pattern is more clearly seen. Most smoothing techniques operate on a simple and general principle. Each observation in the sequence is replaced by a more "typical value." A "typical value" is established by combining adjacent values to produce a new value influenced to some extent by neighboring observations. The extent of this influence depends on which particular smoothing technique is applied.

One "typical-value" calculation is called a running median. For a sequence of n observations $\{y_1, y_2, y_3, \ldots, y_n\}$, each value y_i is replaced by the median of the three consecutive values y_{i-1}, y_i, y_{i+1}. Consider the sequence of 20 observations in Table 1–11 (also see Figure 1–4).

The smoothed values (Smooth 1 in Table 1–11) represent a running-median smoothing of the data. For example, y_2 is replaced with the median of $y_1 = 1.71$, $y_2 = -14.47$ and $y_3 = 10.20$, namely 1.71. This process is repeated for all observations except the first and the last. For this illustration the first and last observations are left unchanged, but other possibilities exist for smoothing these two end values ([7] or [8]). The resulting smoothed sequence is displayed in Figure 1–4 (middle). An immediate consequence of this process is the elimination of extreme values. For example, $y_{17} = 93.43$ no longer disproportionately influences the data pattern because it is replaced by the locally more consistent value of 224.71.

An important feature of most smoothing techniques is that they are model free. The smoothed sequence of estimates in Table 1–11 comes from applying the running median, and no assumptions are made about the underlying form of the data. For contrast, a second-degree polynomial $(y = b_0 + b_1 x + b_2 x^2)$ is estimated and fitted to the data (displayed in the second column of Figure 1–4). The clear advantage

Table 1–11. Data, median-smoothed, moving-average smoothed, and residual values

Data	1.71	−14.47	10.20	4.68	18.56	26.22	10.09	73.57	42.69	59.19
	37.35	168.01	152.86	127.23	227.44	224.71	93.43	331.17	415.17	471.02
Smooth 1	1.71	1.71	4.68	4.68	18.56	18.56	18.56	42.69	42.69	42.69
	42.69	152.86	152.86	152.86	224.71	224.71	224.71	331.17	415.17	471.02
Smooth 2	1.71	2.45	4.12	8.01	15.92	17.90	24.43	38.12	41.55	42.40
	70.16	132.18	147.69	169.53	210.92	221.26	250.48	331.99	408.34	471.02
Residual	—	−16.92	6.08	−3.33	2.64	8.32	−14.34	35.45	1.14	16.79
	−32.81	35.83	5.17	−42.30	16.52	3.45	−157.05	−0.82	6.83	—

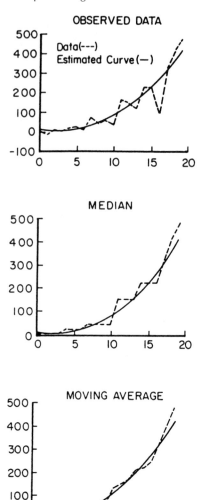

Figure 1–4. Illustration of median/average smoothing process and a fitted curve for data given in Table 1–11

of the median-smoothing approach is that it does not require the specification and estimation of a possibly complex mathematical function. Figure 1–4, however, indicates two features of median smoothing that are not particularly desirable. A tendency towards level spots appears in the smoothed "data." Also, median smoothing has no influence on a sequence of numbers that strictly increases. For example, the sequence 5, 10, 15, 30, 60, 100 is unaffected by applying the median-smoothing process.

A second smoothing improves the running-median approach. This iteration involves applying a moving average to the sequence of median-smoothed values. One version of a moving average is defined by $y_i = 0.25y_{i-1} + 0.50y_i + 0.25y_{i+1}$ (called hanning after Julius von Hanning, an early scientist). Other versions of a moving average use different weights or different numbers of adjacent observations, but all work essentially in the same manner. Like the median-smoothing process, a moving average makes each observation more consistent with its neighboring observations. Applying the hanning moving average to the illustrative data (Smooth 1) yields another set of smoother values (the median-smoothed "data" is again smoothed). For example, the once-smoothed second value $y_2 = 1.71$ is replaced by $0.25(1.71) + 0.50(1.71) + 0.25(4.68) = 2.45$. This process is also applied to all but the first and last observations producing a second set of smoothed "data" (Smooth 2 in Table 1–11), which is shown in Figure 1–4. The estimated polynomial is included for comparison.

The median smoothing removes extreme observations. The moving average is effective in removing the level patterns that arise from the median smoothing and smoothing increasing sequences. The combination produces a relatively smooth, model-free representation of the data and, as seen from the example, the sequence of smoothed values can be similar to estimating a mathematical function.

Median smoothing followed by moving-average smoothing can be applied to the already smoothed "data," producing yet a smoother curve. The median/averaging process can be applied a number of times (iteratively) until little or no difference is observed in the resulting smoothed "data." To illustrate, a series of multiply smoothed distributions of cancer incidence rates are displayed in Figure 1–5. These age-specific rates are from incidence cases collected routinely by nine U.S. cancer registries (Surveillance Epidemiology End Results, SEER [9]) for the years 1974 through 1983. Incidence rates of cancer are given by age, sex, race, and site for both the observed data and the multiply smoothed "data." Clear age-specific patterns emerge from the smoothed race/sex groups. The smoothing process has the most pronounced effect on the cancer sites with the fewest cases (e.g., thyroid cancer and leukemia), because the relatively large fluctuations associated with small numbers of observations are reduced. Sites with more stable rates (e.g., brain cancer) are less dramatically affected by the smoothing process.

Smoothing sacrifices detail for a clearer picture of the underlying pattern. This property does not imply that detail is unimportant. In many cases the detailed characteristics of a sequence of rates are its

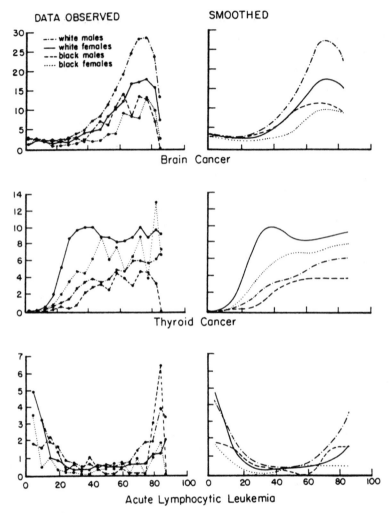

Figure 1–5. Incidence rates by age, by sex, and by race for selected sites of cancer from the SEER data (1974–83)

most important feature. Almost paradoxically, a smoothed curve allows the easy identification of the values that do not "fit" the observed pattern. Once a smoothed pattern is established, it is possible to go back and investigate the detail that was eroded away by the smoothing process. One approach is to subtract the smoothed "data" points from the original values. An exploration of these differences, called residuals, is a productive way to understand specific characteristics of a sequence of rates. For example, large residual values may identify unnoticed atypical values. Residual values for the illustrative data are given in Table 1–11. The analysis of residual values is an important statistical technique further explored in Chapter 4.

Logistic Transformation

Rates can be transformed giving them valuable statistical properties that produce easy and accurate assessments of specific hypotheses. In general, transformations are an important tool in statistical analysis. A short list of reasons for considering a transformation follows:

1. Transformations can be used to make a distribution of observations or a distribution of estimated values more symmetric. Symmetric distributions are then more accurately approximated by a normal distribution, leading to easier statistical assessment. Many approaches to evaluating statistical measures depend on using a normal distribution as an approximation to a more complicated distribution. Perhaps a more important property of a symmetric distribution is that the mean and the variance take on concrete meaning. The mean is the center of a symmetric distribution (the most "typical" value), and the variance provides a way to judge the likelihood that observations deviate from the mean.

2. Transformations can reduce the impact of extreme observations that could disproportionately influence an analysis if left in the data set. Extreme observations usually present a problem. Removing them from the data set potentially introduces bias, and leaving them in the analysis can distort the conclusions. One solution is to use a transformation that reduces the impact of outlier observations but does not eliminate them entirely, making the analysis "resistant" to the effects of extreme observations.

3. Transformations can promote additivity (minimize interactions). Additivity is a desirable property involving several technical issues and is discussed in later chapters.

4. Transformations can equalize or stabilize the variance among a set of groups. It is generally difficult to compare groups with unequal variances. Statistical procedures are more complicated and the interpretation of results is more difficult if comparisons involve data with unequal variability. Even comparisons based on visual inspection of the data are difficult when groups differ widely in variability.

5. To facilitate the analysis of collected data, transformations sometimes produce simple relationships among the variables being studied. For example, either of two values x and y might be transformed to obtain a linear relationship, making interpretation and analysis simpler. A logistic transformation can produce a relatively simple relationship between a binary measure of disease outcome and associated risk factors (Chapters 7, 8, and 9). In general, transformations can produce "data" that are better represented by an analytic model.

To illustrate a specific transformation, consider the 1980 colon cancer incidence data presented in Tables 1–12, 1–13, and 1–14. Average rates are calculated from data collected in three communities (Oakland, the rest of the East Bay, and San Francisco), for two races (white and black) and both sexes (male and female).

Analysis of rates is enhanced by applying a logistic transformation, suggested and discussed by Cox [10]. The data are transformed using the relationship

$$y_j = \log\left(\frac{x_j + 0.5}{l_j - x_j + 0.5}\right),\tag{1.31}$$

where x_j represents the number of observed cases and l_j represents the number at risk for the jth category. The value 0.5 is added to both the number of cases and noncases making the y_j less biased (again,

Table 1–12. Cases of colon cancer (during 1980): location by race by sex

Place	White		Black	
	Male	Female	Male	Female
Oakland	23	18	15	14
Other East Bay	112	98	6	13
San Francisco	58	60	5	12

Table 1–13. Population (at the beginning of 1980): location by race by sex

Place	White		Black	
	Male	Female	Male	Female
Oakland	19,789	21,783	18,701	21,395
Other East Bay	172,074	182,596	11,933	13,271
San Francisco	63,356	63,681	12,214	13,423

Table 1–14. Rates of colon cancer per 100,000: location by race by sex

Place	White		Black	
	Male	Female	Male	Female
Oakland	116.3	82.7	80.2	65.5
Other East Bay	65.1	53.7	50.3	98.0
San Francisco	91.6	94.3	40.9	89.4

see Cox [10]). This transformation is actually applied to the probability of disease (x_j/l_j) and not strictly to the rates [e.g., for the Oakland white males $y_1 = \log(23.5/19{,}789.5) = -6.736 \approx \log(\text{rate}) = \log(116.3/100{,}000) = -6.757$]. The estimated variance of the transformed value y_j is

$$\text{variance } (y_j) = v_j = \frac{(l_j + 1)(l_j + 2)}{l_j(x_j + 1)(l_j - x_j + 1)}. \qquad (1.32)$$

For mortality and disease data, x_j is almost always much less then $l_j(x_j \ll l_j)$; this variance is then simply estimated by

$$\text{variance } (y_j) = v_j \approx \frac{1}{x_j + 1}. \qquad (1.33)$$

Although it is mathematically complex, it can be demonstrated that this logistic transformation creates "data" that are simply and accurately analyzed with basic statistical techniques.

Applying the logistic transformation to the colon cancer data gives the values shown in Table 1–15, along with the variance estimates given in Table 1–16. These 12 transformed values are easily contrasted in terms of summaries (represented by $\hat{c}$) that have approximate normal distributions. That is, a contrast is

$$\hat{c} = \sum_{j=1}^{k} a_j y_j, \qquad (1.34)$$

Table 1–15. Logit transformed (y_j): location by race by sex

	White		Black	
Place	Male	Female	Male	Female
Oakland	$y_1 = -6.73$	$y_2 = -7.07$	$y_3 = -7.09$	$y_4 = -7.30$
Other East Bay	$y_5 = -7.33$	$y_6 = -7.52$	$y_7 = -7.51$	$y_8 = -6.89$
San Francisco	$y_9 = -6.99$	$y_{10} = -6.96$	$y_{11} = -7.71$	$y_{12} = -6.98$

Table 1–16. Logit transformation variance (v_j): location by race by sex

	White		Black	
Place	Male	Female	Male	Female
Oakland	$v_1 = 0.042$	$v_2 = 0.053$	$v_3 = 0.063$	$v_4 = 0.067$
Other East Bay	$v_5 = 0.009$	$v_6 = 0.010$	$v_7 = 0.143$	$v_8 = 0.072$
San Francisco	$v_9 = 0.017$	$v_{10} = 0.016$	$v_{11} = 0.167$	$v_{12} = 0.077$

where the a_j values are chosen to identify specific issues, and k represents the number of contrasted cells from the table. The variance of $\hat{c}$ is estimated by

$$\text{variance } (\hat{c}) = \text{variance} \left(\sum_{j=1}^{k} a_j y_j \right) = \sum_{j=1}^{k} a_j^2 \text{ variance } (y_j) \approx \sum_{j=1}^{k} \frac{a_j^2}{x_j + 1} \quad (1.35)$$

when the values y_j are independent, which is the case for the colon cancer data and usually the case when rates are calculated from individuals classified into a series of categories. The test statistic $z = \hat{c}/\sqrt{\text{variance } (\hat{c})}$ has an approximate standard normal distribution (mean $= 0$ and variance $= 1$) if the expected value of $\hat{c}$ is zero.

The construction of a contrast arises naturally from specific questions asked about the subject matter generating the table of rates. Differences in the y_j values are weighted so they have expected value of zero when the rates (or logit transformed values) do not systematically differ. For example, male and female transformed rates, contrasted for each community and each race in Table 1–15, yield six contrasts (i.e., $y_{\text{male}} - y_{\text{female}}$). These differences can then be summed from the relevant parts of the table to form a contrast $\hat{c}$ which is used to evaluate observed differences between male and female rates from the entire table.

Specifically, the question of whether the colon cancer incidence rates differ by sex is addressed by calculating $\hat{c}$ from the 12 transformed values y_j, forming six contrasts $y_i - y_{i+1}$, where the contrast using all rates in the table is

$$\hat{c}_{\text{sex}} = y_1 - y_2 + y_3 - y_4 + y_5 - y_6 + y_7 - y_8 + y_9 - y_{10} + y_{11} - y_{12} \quad (1.36)$$

with

$$\text{variance } (\hat{c}_{\text{sex}}) = v_1 + v_2 + v_3 + v_4 + v_5 + v_6 + v_7 + v_8 + v_9 + v_{10} + v_{11} + v_{12}, \quad (1.37)$$

and $z = \hat{c}_{\text{sex}}/\sqrt{\text{variance } (\hat{c}_{\text{sex}})}$ has an approximately standard normal distribution when no systematic difference exists between male and female colon cancer rates (i.e., when the expected value of $\hat{c}_{\text{sex}}$ is 0). The estimated contrast $\hat{c}_{\text{sex}} = -0.651$ with variance $(\hat{c}_{\text{sex}}) = 0.734$ calculated from Tables 1–15 and 1–16 produces $z = -0.760$ with a p-value $= 0.447$, showing no evidence of a difference between male and female colon cancer rates.

Similarly, the difference between races can be investigated where

$$\hat{c}_{\text{race}} = y_1 + y_2 - y_3 - y_4 + y_5 + y_6 - y_7 - y_8 + y_9 + y_{10} - y_{11} - y_{12} \quad (1.38)$$

and the estimated variance has the same value as the contrast for sex [expression (1.37)]. Again, if no systematic differences exist between white and black rates, the expected value of $\hat{c}_{race}$ is zero. Here, $\hat{c}_{race} = 0.872$, giving $z = 1.018$ with p-value $= 0.309$, also showing little evidence of an important difference.

A slightly more complicated contrast is illustrated by investigating the differences among the three communities where the 12 transformed rates give

$$\hat{c}_{places} = y_1 + y_2 + y_3 + y_4 - 2(y_5 + y_6 + y_7 + y_8) + y_9 + y_{10} + y_{11} + y_{12} \quad (1.39)$$

with

$$\begin{aligned}\text{variance } (\hat{c}_{places}) &= v_1 + v_2 + v_3 + v_4 \\ &+ 4(v_5 + v_6 + v_7 + v_8) + v_9 + v_{10} + v_{11} + v_{12}.\end{aligned} \quad (1.40)$$

The contrast $\hat{c}_{places} = 1.698$ with $z = 1.418$ produces a p-value $= 0.156$, again showing no strong evidence of a difference among the three communities. This contrast is basically a sum of contrasts between two differences or

$$\begin{aligned}c_i &= (y_i - y_{i+4}) - (y_{i+4} - y_{i+8}) = y_i - 2y_{i+4} + y_{i+8} \quad \text{and} \\ \hat{c}_{places} &= \hat{c}_1 + \hat{c}_2 + \hat{c}_3 + \hat{c}_4,\end{aligned} \quad (1.41)$$

which has expected value zero when only random differences exist among the rates from the three communities. This contrast could also be constructed as the comparison of the mean of two areas with a third area [i.e., $\frac{1}{2}(y_1 + y_9) - y_5$]. Other useful contrasts (with estimated variances) can be similarly formed from the logistic transformed data to explore more complex issues and do not differ in principle from the contrasts illustrated by the colon cancer analysis.

The example data illustrate the ease with which specific issues are assessed, from just about any table containing a set of rates, by contrasting a series of logit-transformed values. The logistic transformation, more formally referred to as the fully saturated logistic model (discussed in Chapters 7, 8, and 9), provides an introduction to a general and important approach to the analysis of binary outcome data (data with two outcomes: cancer case and not a cancer case).

Age Adjustment of Rates

The process of age adjustment is an integral part of the evaluation of mortality and disease rates, because age almost always strongly influences disease risk and potentially interferes with the assessment of the role of other variables. An adjustment process produces a

Table 1-17. Hypothetical deaths and populations at risk

	Population I			Population II		
Age	Deaths	Person-years	Rates	Deaths	Person-years	Rates
40–50	1	1,000	0.001	1	1,000	0.001
50–60	3	1,500	0.002	10	5,000	0.002
60–70	8	2,000	0.004	40	10,000	0.004
70–80	20	2,500	0.008	160	20,000	0.008
Total	32	7,000	0.00457	211	36,000	0.00586

single summary value unaffected by differences in age distributions. Observed differences in adjusted rates are then attributable to the influence of factors other than age. The two most common approaches, called the direct and indirect methods, are discussed extensively elsewhere; see [3] and [4], for example.

The problem of relying on only a crude rate (total deaths divided by total person-years of risk) for the comparison of mortality or disease risk among groups is seen from a simple hypothetical example. "Data" from populations I and II are given in Table 1-17.

These two populations are constructed with identical age-specific rates but with differing age structures. The larger proportion of older individuals in population II leads to a higher crude mortality rate (457.1 versus 586.1 deaths per 100,000 person-years at risk), where the risk of death is clearly the same for populations I and II, because the age-specific rates are the same for both groups.

Crude rates furnish simple, direct summaries of a set of age-specific disease data but fail to reflect risk exclusively. A mixture of the age-specific risk and the age structure confounds observed differences in crude rates. An ideal strategy is to compare directly the age-specific rates or to construct a model summarizing the relationship between age and rates of disease. Many times directly comparing the age-specific rates does not provide sufficient summarization, and a modeling approach is usually complex. Although detail and potentially important characteristics of the groups being compared can be lost, a single summary is nevertheless often useful.

Direct Method

Direct adjustment is achieved by using a standard population as a basis of comparison. Two populations that frequently serve as standards are the U.S. 1950 or 1970 populations (Table 1-18). An

Table 1–18. Standard million population of the United States for 1950 and 1970

Age	1950	1970
0–4	107,258	84,416
5–9	87,591	98,204
10–14	73,785	102,304
15–19	70,450	93,845
20–24	76,191	80,561
25–29	81,237	66,320
30–34	76,425	56,249
35–39	74,629	54,656
40–44	67,712	58,958
45–49	60,190	59,622
50–54	54,893	54,643
55–59	48,011	49,077
60–64	40,210	42,403
65–69	33,199	34,406
70–74	22,641	26,789
75–79	14,725	18,871
80–84	7,025	11,241
85+	3,828	7,435

alternative to choosing a U.S. population or some other external standard is to use the total observed population, or even a specific group within a data set, as a standard. For example, the total population could serve as a standard for comparing populations I and II in Table 1–17 (i.e., age group totals: 2,000, 6,500, 12,000, and 22,500).

The direct method produces a single summary value for each of a series of groups "free" from the confounding influences of the age distribution based on the age-specific population counts of the standard. An age-specific number of deaths in each group is calculated as if all groups had the same population distribution, namely the standard. The numbers of "deaths" are computed by applying age-specific rates to the corresponding age groups of the standard population. The total number of these "deaths" divided by the total population of the standard is the direct age-adjusted rate.

In symbols, if the ith age category from the standard contains P_i individuals, and the age-specific rate for the ith age category in the jth comparison group is r_{ij}, then the direct adjusted rate for group j is

$$\text{direct adjusted rate for group } j = \frac{\text{"deaths"}}{P} \times \text{base} = \frac{\sum_{i=1}^{k} r_{ij} P_i}{P} \times \text{base}, \quad (1.42)$$

where k is the number of age categories and $P = \sum P_i$ is the total population of the standard.

Indirect Method

Indirect age adjustment is based on deriving an expected number of deaths using a standard population and contrasting this value to the number of deaths observed in a specific comparison group. The ratio of the total observed number of deaths to the number expected is called the standard mortality ratio (SMR). An indirect adjusted rate is found by multiplying the SMR by the crude rate from the standard population (denoted by R). In symbols, the indirect adjusted rate for group j is

$$\text{indirect adjusted rate for group } j = \text{SMR} \times R = \frac{d_j}{e_j} R = \frac{\sum\limits_{i=1}^{k} d_{ij}}{e_j} R. \quad (1.43)$$

The value $d_j = \sum d_{ij}$ is the total number of deaths observed in the jth comparison group, where d_{ij} represents the number of deaths occurring in the ith age category of the jth group. The expected number of "deaths" is

$$e_j = \sum_{i=1}^{k} R_i p_{ij}, \quad (1.44)$$

where R_i represents the rate from the ith age category of the standard, and p_{ij} represents the population of the ith age category in the jth comparison group. The product $R_i p_{ij}$ is the expected number of deaths in the ith age category of the jth comparison group. The value e_j is then the total expected number of deaths, based on the rates of the standard and the age-specific populations from the jth comparison group. The important element of an indirect age-adjusted rate is the SMR where, to repeat,

$$\text{SMR} = \frac{\text{total observed deaths}}{\text{expected number of deaths}} = \frac{d_j}{e_j}$$

for the group denoted by j.

To illustrate, breast cancer incidence counts among women residents of the San Francisco Bay Area (1977–83) are compared between whites and blacks for two stages of cancer in Table 1–19. The race-, age-, and stage-specific incidence rates from these data are shown in Table 1–20. The age-adjusted incidence rates are given in Table 1–21.

Table 1–19. Breast cancer by race, age, and stage (local and regional): cases and person-years (1977–83)

Age	White			Black		
	Local	Regional	Person-years	Local	Regional	Person-years
40–49	1,429	1,082	1,625,812	1,006	999	1,767,995
50–59	1,825	1,394	1,437,511	809	913	996,536
60–69	1,048	667	565,078	258	212	235,442
70–79	484	273	229,203	245	162	171,292
79+	176	87	84,698	44	38	31,789
Total	4,962	3,503	3,942,302	2,362	2,324	3,203,054

Table 1–20. Breast cancer by race, age, and stage (local and regional): age-specific incidence rates/100,000 (1977–83)

Age	White		Black	
	Local	Regional	Local	Regional
40–49	87.89	66.55	56.90	56.50
50–59	126.96	96.97	81.18	91.62
60–69	185.46	118.04	109.58	90.04
70–79	211.17	119.11	143.05	94.58
79+	207.80	102.72	138.41	119.54
Crude rate	125.87	88.86	73.74	72.56

Table 1–21. Breast cancer by race, age, and stage (local and regional): age-adjusted incidence rates/100,000 (1977–83)

	White		Black	
	Local	Regional	Local	Regional
Direct adjusted	121.00	86.22	77.23	75.38
Observed deaths	4,962	3,503	2,362	2,324
Expected deaths	3,770.4	3,770.4	2,805.7	2,805.7
SMR	1.316	0.929	0.842	0.828
Indirect adjusted	121.11	85.50	77.49	76.24

The adjusted rates are based on the internal standard created by summing the two populations at risk for all five age categories to form a single standard population. An overall crude rate from the standard is $R = 92.02$ deaths per 100,000. The direct and indirect age-adjusted rates are not appreciably different for the breast cancer data (Table 1–21). The highest mortality is found among the white, local-stage patients. The age-adjusted rate among whites for regional stage is somewhat lower. The age-adjusted rates within blacks show still lower values which are similar for the two stages. In all comparisons, differences in the age structure between whites and blacks is not an issue.

Another example of age-adjustment is provided by the question of whether cancer rates have increased since 1940. A relevant set of data and a series of summary values for U.S. cancer mortality among white males are given in Table 1–22 (extracted from *Vital Statistics of the United States 1940 and 1960*, published by the National Center for Health Statistics).

The crude rates (166.09 in 1960 and 119.53 in 1940) show an apparently important increase in cancer mortality (about 40%). However, the U.S. age distribution also has changed over the twenty-year period, 1940 to 1960. Specifically, higher proportions of individuals are found in the older age categories in 1960, where the cancer mortality is highest. To assess more clearly the observed increase in cancer mortality, this difference in age distributions must be taken into account.

A natural standard is the 1960 population. That is, the number of "deaths" is computed using the rates from the 1940 data and the age-specific population counts from 1960. These "1940 deaths" are given in the table ("deaths"—direct; column 8 of Table 1–22). The crude rate based on these theoretically derived "deaths" (the direct adjusted rate) is $109,127/78,367,144 = 139.25$ per 100,000. Once the 1940 "rate" is based on the age distribution of the 1960 population, the difference in cancer mortality is less striking but not attributable to differences in age distributions. A large part of the remaining difference is undoubtedly due to the smoking-related cancers, which dramatically increased over the twenty years between 1940 and 1960.

An indirect adjustment produces essentially the same result. When the 1960 rates are applied to the 1940 age-specific population counts, a set of expected "deaths" is produced ("deaths"—indirect; column 9 of Table 1–22). The standard mortality ratio based on these "deaths" and the deaths observed in 1940 is $71,058/85,557 = 0.831$, and an indirect adjusted rate becomes SMR × 1940 crude rate = $0.831(166.09) = 137.94$ deaths per 100,000. Incidentally, direct standardization viewed as a ratio of total expected "deaths" to observed deaths (i.e., $109,127/130,158 = 0.838$) multiplied by the 1960 crude rate also produces the direct adjusted rate of $0.838(166.09) = 139.25$, as before. Table 1–23 summarizes the rates from the two time periods.

Table 1–22. Comparison of United States cancer mortality for the years 1940 and 1960 (white males)

Age	1960			1940			"Deaths" Direct	"Deaths" Indirect
	Deaths	Population	Rate*	Deaths	Population	Rate*		
<1	141	1,784,033	7.9	45	906,897	5.0	89	72
1–4	926	7,065,148	13.1	201	3,794,573	5.3	374	497
5–14	1,253	15,658,730	8.0	320	10,003,544	3.2	501	800
15–24	1,080	10,482,916	10.3	670	10,629,526	6.3	661	1,095
25–34	1,869	9,939,972	18.8	1,126	9,465,330	11.9	1,182	1,780
35–44	4,891	10,563,872	46.3	3,160	8,249,558	38.3	4,047	3,819
45–54	14,956	9,114,202	164.1	9,723	7,294,330	133.3	12,149	11,970
55–64	30,888	6,850,263	450.9	17,935	5,022,499	357.1	24,462	22,647
65–74	41,725	4,702,482	887.3	22,179	2,920,220	759.5	35,715	25,911
75–84	26,501	1,874,619	1,413.7	13,461	1,019,504	1,320.3	24,751	14,412
85+	5,928	330,915	1,791.4	2,238	142,532	1,570.0	5,196	2,553
Total	130,158	78,367,144	166.09	71,058	59,448,516	119.53	109,127	85,557

*Rate per 100,000 person-years.

Table 1–23. Summary: 1940 and 1960 cancer rates per 100,000

	Crude	Direct	Indirect
1940	119.53	139.25	137.94
1960	166.09	166.09	166.09
Difference	46.56	26.84	28.15

When a comparison group contains a small number of deaths or only the total number of deaths is known (i.e., d_j) then indirect age-adjustment is typically used. It is worthwhile to note that under certain circumstances indirect standardization does not completely remove the influence of differences in population composition [3], making it possible to construct contradictory examples. Two populations (A and B) can be constructed so that the age-specific rates in A are all larger than those of B, but the indirect age-adjusted rates show the opposite relationship. In applied situations, however, both the direct and the indirect adjustment procedures usually provide an effective and similar measure of the average level of mortality, conveying much of the essential information contained in the age-specific rates. The choice of a standard is not critical but can make a difference [4]. The absolute values of both types of age-adjusted rates have little meaning; rather, the relative magnitude of an adjusted rate is a useful summary of a set of age-specific mortality data. A model-based age-adjustment procedure that does not depend on a standard population is discussed in Chapter 11.

2 Variation and Bias

A designed experiment begins with the random assignment of individuals to a series of groups. Each group then receives one of a series of treatments. Subsequent differences observed among these groups likely result from treatment effects, because it is probable that the randomization process produced groups essentially equivalent with respect to other factors. Or from another point of view, if the treatments under investigation have no influence, then comparisons among values calculated from groups of randomly assigned individuals will show only random differences. The balancing of variables producing comparable groups is the essence of randomized data.

The analysis of nonexperimental data, often called observational data, also involves the comparison of a series of groups, but, for one reason or another, individuals are assigned to these groups in nonrandom ways. Individuals can select group membership themselves (e.g., smokers versus nonsmokers) and this self-selection tends to make groups different regardless of "treatment" influences. Others may assign group membership. For example, physicians may place patients on one versus another therapy. As with self-selection, the reasons for the choice of a particular therapy tend to make groups different for a range of characteristics. In other situations, groups are selected in some sort of natural way (e.g., low-weight infants versus normal-weight infants) and undoubtedly differ by other characteristics. The fact that nonrandomized groups differ with respect to a number of variables makes isolation of a specific influence difficult and also makes direct comparisons of specific measures of association hard to interpret. The interpretation of measures arising from the analysis of observational data, therefore, is almost always complicated by potential biases arising from the lack of randomization.

Another important property of both experimental and observational data is the lack of uniformity in the study subjects. Variation tends to obscure systematic influences among groups, also making it difficult to isolate reasons for observed differences. In an experimental setting, individuals chosen to be as similar as possible are randomly assigned to comparison groups, diminishing the influence of extraneous variation. It is rare that observational data are controlled to the same extent. Observational studies rely on statistical techniques to deal with differences that result from lack of randomization and to minimize extraneous variation. Such techniques as matching, stratifying, and statistical modeling are typical analytic approaches to observational data.

This chapter reviews several basic analytic methods by postulating a statistical model to justify the data analysis; at the same time, these statistical structures are employed to define and illustrate the possible consequences of specific approaches associated with observational data.

Two types of mathematical structures are referred to as models. Both employ mathematical expressions to describe relationships within a set of data but with different goals. One attempts to reflect biological or physical reality, whereas the other is essentially a mathematical convenience used to make predictions or to represent a set of relationships in a parsimonius way. Galileo postulated a mathematical explanation for the behavior of the solar system. His model described the paths of planetary movements around the sun. If his model had been simply a mathematical convenience to make predictions, presumably the Catholic Church would not have objected to such an exercise. Mendel's genetic model is another example of a mathematical structure postulated to reflect reality and ranks among the most important scientific theories because of its correspondence to the biological mechanisms underlying inheritance. Models used in most statistical analysis are carefully constructed to reflect the observed data, providing a mathematically convenient way to study complex issues when detailed knowledge of underlying mechanisms is lacking. The relationships surrounding the occurrence of disease, for example, are not governed by mechanisms with simple mathematical expressions. However, simple mathematical expressions are often the statistical basis for summarizing, analyzing, and, in general, understanding these relationships in a convenient way.

A Simple Model

In research situations complete knowledge about the true relationships under study is generally not available. A statistical model provides a mathematical framework to make decisions, despite this lack of concrete knowledge about how data might be collected and analyzed. Such models suggest ways to choose among analytic strategies and allow estimation of relevant summary statistics. Although a statistical model describing the measurement of two pieces of string is not a critical element in epidemiologic analysis, it is a good place to start.

Suppose two lengths of string are to be measured with two measurements. Can one do better than making one measurement on each piece of string? A simple statistical model provides a justification for a specific approach. Assume that the lengths of these strings cannot be measured perfectly. That is, if a large number of independent measurements is made on the same piece of string, the mean value will approach the true length of the string (unbiased), but the individual measurements differ (error variability: some too large and some too small). Let μ_1 represent the true length of piece 1 and μ_2 represent the true length of piece 2. Assume also that the measurement errors are not related to the length of the string. A mathematical structure describing this situation is

$$\text{string } 1: y_1 = \mu_1 + e_1 \quad \text{and} \quad \text{string } 2: y_2 = \mu_2 + e_2, \tag{2.1}$$

where y_1 and y_2 are the measured lengths with e_1 and e_2 representing the contribution of random measurement error (mean $= 0$ and variance represented by σ^2). The variance of the observed length (σ^2) is the variability associated with the distribution of repeated independent measurements on a single length. This elementary model contains a systematic (μ_i) and a random component (e_i)—a property of statistical models in general.

Suppose the two lengths of string are measured first by laying them end to end and measuring the total length (denoted by L), then by laying strings side by side and measuring the difference in lengths (denoted by D). The average of these two measurements

$$\frac{L + D}{2} \quad \text{estimates} \quad \frac{(\mu_1 + \mu_2) + (\mu_1 - \mu_2)}{2} = \mu_1 \quad \text{or} \quad \hat{\mu}_1 = \frac{L + D}{2} \tag{2.2}$$

is an unbiased estimate of the true length of string 1 (μ_1) because the mean of the errors (e_i's) is zero. Similarly, $\hat{\mu}_2 = (L - D)/2$ estimates the length of string 2 (μ_2). The trick is to note that the variance of the estimated length $\hat{\mu}_1$ based on the combined measurements is

$$\text{variance } (\hat{\mu}_1) = \text{variance} \left(\frac{L + D}{2} \right) = \frac{\sigma^2 + \sigma^2}{4} = \frac{\sigma^2}{2}, \tag{2.3}$$

which is half the variance of measuring a single piece of string, denoted by σ^2. Similarly, the variance $\hat{\mu}_2 = (L - D)/2$ is also $\sigma^2/2$. Since the error in measurement is the same for any length, it is possible to reduce the variability associated with the estimated lengths by an averaging process. Therefore, the averages $\hat{\mu}_1 = (L + D)/2$, and $\hat{\mu}_2 = (L - D)/2$ produce less variation, resulting in more precise estimates of the lengths of two pieces of string by a factor of 2 over measuring each string separately. If the pieces of string are sampled from a distribution and the measurement process is perfect (another model), then combining the strings does not produce gains in precision. The question of how to measure two strings becomes clearer when a statistical model is postulated and investigated. Also, a focused discussion on the measuring process generated by a model can suggest important issues. Although this model is designed to be as simple as possible, the process has many of the characteristics of more complex situations.

A statistical model is a conceptual process. It is derived from knowledge or speculation about how the data might behave rather than directly from the data itself. It is not costly, involves no risk, requires no experimentation, and is easily modified, making it a basic tool in the struggle to understand the complexities of the "real" world reflected by collected data.

t-Test

The *t*-test, sometimes called Student's *t*-test and the accompanying *t*-distribution are fundamental to statistical analysis.

> Aside: The *t*-test procedure was pioneered by William Sealy Gosset (1876–1937) who used the pseudonym "Student." Around the turn of the century, Gosset developed several significant biometric solutions to problems in agriculture and genetics. His most important contribution, the *t*-test, was essentially contained in a 1908 paper entitled "On Probability Error of a Mean," which opened the door to the analysis of small samples of data. W. S. Gosset was not only a statistician but a master brewer. He worked for the famous Guinness brewing firm and ultimately became the chief brewer for the London Branch. Gosset was part of a select group of scientists who came together during the first part of the twentieth century to "invent" statistical analysis. Others in this group were Karl Pearson, Ronald A. Fisher, E. J. G. Pitman, J. B. S. Haldane, and later, Jerzy Neyman and E. S. Pearson.

The *t*-test procedure employed to compare two groups (two-sample *t*-test) is based on a specific statistical model. Random assignment of individuals to treatment and control groups gives two samples of data, and a statistical model representing this two-sample situation is

Control individual: $y_{1j} = \mu + e_{1j}$

Treatment individual: $y_{2j} = \mu + \delta + e_{2j}$,

where y_{ij} is the observed response for the jth individual belonging to either control group $(i = 1)$ or treatment group $(i = 2)$. The value represented by μ is the overall mean level of the variable being studied, and the term δ represents the influence of the treatment on the response variable. If there is no treatment effect, then δ is zero. Otherwise, the value δ can be either positive or negative. The term e_{ij} symbolizes one of a series of independent random error terms assumed to have normal distributions with mean zero and with the same variance (σ^2) for both treatment and control groups. The response variables (y-values) are also normally distributed, because the model requires that the contributions of μ and δ be constant (i.e., not affected by the probability distribution associated with the error contribution). A statistical analysis explores the magnitude of the treatment effect (δ) while accounting for the variation in response (e). This analytic structure is called the "shift" model, because the treatment shifts all participants in the treatment group δ units from the overall mean μ.

A natural comparison of treatment and control groups is the difference in mean values, or $\bar{y}_2 - \bar{y}_1$, where $\bar{y}_2$ is a mean value based on n_2 treatment responses, and $\bar{y}_1$ is a mean value based on n_1 control responses. Under the conditions postulated by the "shift" model, the difference in mean values is an unbiased estimate of the treatment effect or $\hat{\delta} = \bar{y}_2 - \bar{y}_1$. The estimate $\hat{\delta}$ is unbiased because the random errors (e_i's) have mean zero and balance each other (in the long run), producing no net effect. When the treatment does not influence the response variable, or, more formally, under the null hypothesis that no treatment effect exists $(H_0: \delta = 0)$, then

$$T = \frac{\hat{\delta} - 0}{S_{\hat{\delta}}} = \frac{\bar{y}_2 - \bar{y}_1}{\sqrt{\text{variance}(\bar{y}_2 - \bar{y}_1)}}, \qquad (2.4)$$

and the variable T has a t-distribution with $n_1 + n_2 - 2$ degrees of freedom.

> Aside: Like all but the most advanced texts on statistical analysis, the concept of "degrees of freedom" will not be developed. The degrees of freedom relate to rather complicated considerations which involve the number of constraints used to define a statistical structure. Rules, however, on how the degrees of freedom are calculated will be given (e.g., for the two sample t-test, the degrees of freedom = total sample size -2). Therefore, the degrees of freedom can be simply thought of as a given parameter of the statistical distribution under consideration.

Extreme (unlikely) values of T lead to the inference that the difference observed between two mean values is not due to random variation; evidence exists that δ is not equal to zero. The test-statistic T is judged extreme when it exceeds the points $t_{1-\alpha}$ or $-t_{1-\alpha}$ selected from a t-distribution so that the null hypothesis is mistakenly rejected with a specified probability α (more discussion follows in the next chapter).

> Aside: Note that the subscript on the t-value refers to the probability to the left of a specific point. For example, $t_{1-\alpha}$ is the point on the t-distribution such that $1 - \alpha$ of the distribution is to the left of that point. Specifically for $\alpha = 0.025$, $t_{0.975} = 2.024$ for 38 degrees of freedom means that 97.5% of the t-distribution is less than 2.024. In the case of a standard normal distribution, $z_{0.95} = z_{1-0.05} = 1.645$, for example, because 95% of all standard normal values are less than 1.645 (to the left).

The "shift" model explicitly states that the variance is unchanged by the treatment. This assumption, necessary for small sample sizes, is less important as the sample sizes in both groups increase. Properties of the variance produce three forms of the two-sample test-statistic:

1. If the variance for the treatment and control groups are equal $(\sigma_1^2 = \sigma_2^2 = \sigma^2)$, then for any sample size the estimated variance is

$$\text{variance} \ (\bar{y}_2 - \bar{y}_1) = S_p^2 \left(\frac{1}{n_1} + \frac{1}{n_2} \right), \qquad (2.5)$$

where S_p^2 is a pooled estimate of the variance (σ^2) given by

$$S_p^2 = \frac{\displaystyle\sum_{j=1}^{n_1} (y_{1j} - \bar{y}_1)^2 + \sum_{j=1}^{n_2} (y_{2j} - \bar{y}_2)^2}{n_1 + n_2 - 2}. \qquad (2.6)$$

2. If the variances are not equal but the sample sizes are large (both n_1 and $n_2 > 30$ or so), then an estimate of the variance is

$$\text{variance} \ (\bar{y}_2 - \bar{y}_1) = \left(\frac{S_2^2}{n_2} + \frac{S_1^2}{n_1} \right), \qquad (2.7)$$

where S_1^2 and S_2^2 are the variances estimated separately from each group by

$$S_i^2 = \frac{\displaystyle\sum_{j=1}^{n_i} (y_{ij} - \bar{y}_i)^2}{n_i - 1}. \qquad (2.8)$$

The test-statistic T no longer has a t-distribution but an approximate normal distribution; a standard normal distribution (mean $= 0$ and variance $= 1$) under the hypothesis that the treatment has no influence $(\delta = 0)$.

3. If either n_1 or n_2 is small and the variances unequal, then T has a complicated distribution requiring special approximations (see [1]).

Data from the Western Collaborative Group Study (WCGS) yield a concrete application of a two-sample t-test (see Appendix A for a complete description of this data set which is repeatedly used in the following). Cholesterol determinations for the 40 heaviest men in the data set (all 225 pounds or more) are recoded along with an indicator of their behavior type (type-A and type-B; see Appendix A) in Table 2–1.

To assess the association between cholesterol and behavior type, the "shift" model is assumed appropriate and a null hypothesis is postulated that no difference exists in cholesterol levels between the two behavior-type groups (i.e., $\delta = 0$). Without prior knowledge of whether the type-A individuals have higher cholesterol than the type-B individuals or vice versa, large positive or large negative values of $\hat{\delta}$ lead to the inference that cholesterol and behavior type are associated. The mean values are: $\bar{y}_A = 245.050$ for the $n_1 = 20$ type-A individuals and $\bar{y}_B = 210.300$ for the $n_2 = 20$ type-B individuals, making $\hat{\delta} = \bar{y}_A - \bar{y}_B = 34.750$. Assuming that the variability in cholesterol levels is the same for both type-A and type-B individuals leads to a pooled estimate of variance, $S_p^2 = 1839.557$. Since $n_1 = n_2 = 20$, then $t_{0.975} = 2.024$ (degrees of freedom $= 38$) and the t-statistic is

$$T = \frac{34.750}{\sqrt{1839.557\left(\frac{2}{20}\right)}} = 2.562. \tag{2.9}$$

A value of $T = 2.562 > 2.024$ indicates that type-A individuals are likely to have higher cholesterol levels than type-B individuals—behavior type is associated with cholesterol level among heavy men. The probability of observing a value of T more extreme when no

Table 2–1. WCGS data: cholesterol (mg/100 ml) and behavior type

	Chol	A/B		Chol	A/B		Chol	A/B		Chol	A/B		Chol	A/B
1	344	B	9	246	B	17	224	A	25	242	B	33	252	A
2	233	A	10	224	B	18	239	A	26	252	B	34	202	A
3	291	A	11	212	B	19	239	A	27	153	B	35	218	A
4	312	A	12	188	B	20	254	A	28	183	B	36	202	B
5	185	B	13	250	B	21	169	B	29	234	A	37	212	A
6	250	A	14	197	A	22	226	B	30	137	B	38	325	A
7	263	B	15	148	B	23	175	B	31	181	A	39	194	B
8	246	A	16	268	A	24	276	A	32	248	A	40	213	B

difference exists in levels of cholesterol is 0.014 (again from a *t*-distribution with 38 degrees of freedom). A significance probability of 0.014 (*p*-value) indicates it is unlikely that a difference more extreme ($\hat{\delta}$ less than -34.750 or greater than 34.750) would have occurred by chance alone.

However, this inference results from the analysis of a set of observational data. Individuals were not assigned to groups A and B at random, raising the possibility that influences (biases) from variables other than behavior type (variables which differ between these two groups), might account for all or part of the differences seen in cholesterol. For example, type-A and type-B individuals likely differ with respect to dietary habits, possibly causing part of the observed differences in cholesterol levels.

Another measure of the association between behavior type and cholesterol level is a correlation coefficient; that is, the correlation behavior (A = 1 and B = 0) and level of cholesterol is $r = 0.384$.

Aside: The term correlation coefficient almost always refers to the measure of association originated by Karl Pearson in 1897 and more formally called the Pearson product-moment correlation coefficient. This important measure of linear associated is defined by

$$r_{xy} = \frac{S_{xy}}{\sqrt{S_{xx}S_{yy}}} \quad \text{with} \quad S_{xy} = \sum_{i=1}^{n} (x_i - \bar{x})(y_i - \bar{y}),$$

$$S_{xx} = \sum_{i=1}^{n} (x_i - \bar{x})^2 \quad \text{and} \quad S_{yy} = \sum_{i=1}^{n} (y_i - \bar{y})^2, \tag{2.10}$$

where n pairs of (x_i, y_i) values are observed. The value r is most often calculated for continuous variables x and y where these pairs are thought to have a bivariate normal distribution. This case produces a rigorous and rich interpretation of the correlation coefficient r. However, the variables x and y can represent any sort of numeric values, and the value of r remains a summary value between -1 and $+1$ that measures association within observed pairs. Specialized product-moment correlation coefficients are typically given specific names (e.g., when x and y are binary variables, r is called a "ϕ-correlation"; when x and y are sets of ranks, r is called a rank correlation coefficient; when x and y are linearly adjusted values, r is called a partial correlation coefficient). The correlation coefficient is only one of the numerous contributions to statistics made by Karl Pearson, who many believe was the founder of modern statistical thought. Perhaps Karl Pearson's most significant contribution is the chi-square goodness-of-fit test used to compare a series of expected to observed values.

A correlation coefficient of 0.384 reflects the degree of association between the binary variable "A/B" and the continuous variable cholesterol in heavy men (r in this case is called a point biserial correlation coefficient—one variable dichotomous and one variable continuous).

The value r produces a measure of association between -1 and 1, while the t-test allows interpretation of the results in terms of a probability. A t-test and a point biserial correlation are different ways an association between two variables can be expressed, but produce identical statistical significance tests (p-values) because they are related. Specifically,

$$T^2 = \frac{r^2}{1 - r^2} (n_1 + n_2 - 2) \tag{2.11}$$

so that any probability associated with T is also associated with r (e.g., if the observed value of T is determined to be a rare event, then the corresponding value of r will be equally unlikely).

Another issue worth noting concerns the allocation of individuals to the two comparison groups. In experimental settings a total of $n = n_1 + n_2$ observations are assigned to either the treatment or control groups; but how are the sample sizes n_1 and n_2 best determined? If the variances in both groups are equal ("shift" model), using $n_1 = n_2 = n/2$ is best. Allocating equal numbers to both groups minimizes the variance of $\bar{y}_2 - \bar{y}_1$ (i.e., the component of the variance $1/n_1 + 1/n_2$ is minimized). Reducing the denominator of the t-test statistic increases the chances of detecting a difference in response in the numerator $\bar{y}_2 - \bar{y}_1$ when one exists. In general,

$$n_1 = \frac{n\sigma_1}{\sigma_1 + \sigma_2} \quad \text{and} \quad n_2 = n - n_1 \tag{2.12}$$

best allocates the sample sizes for the comparison of two groups when the variances are known. Expression (2.12) shows the sensible result that the group with the most variability receives proportionally more observations. Observational studies, where control over allocation of data is rarely possible, often produce disproportionate values of n_1 and n_2, reducing the effectiveness of the t-test comparison of mean values.

Test-Direction Bias

The selection of which t-test—one-sided or two-sided—to use should be based only on prior knowledge about the influence of the treatment. If it is known that the treatment can not possibly decrease the mean response $(\delta \geq 0)$, then a one-sided test is usually chosen; the null hypothesis is rejected only if T is a large positive number, greater than $t_{1-\alpha}$. Likewise, if it is known that the treatment cannot possibly increase the mean response $(\delta \leq 0)$, then a one-sided test is also chosen; the null hypothesis of no treatment influence is rejected only if T is a large negative number, less than $-t_{1-\alpha}$. However, if no *a priori* knowledge is available about the direction of the treatment response, then a two-sided test is used; the null hypothesis is rejected if T is either greater than $t_{1-\alpha/2}$ or less than $-t_{1-\alpha/2}$. The decision to use a one- or two-sided test must be made in advance of the data analysis. Basing this decision on information from the collected data incurs test-direction bias.

To illustrate, consider the following procedure: If $\hat{\delta} = \bar{y}_2 - \bar{y}_1 > 0$, then conduct a one-sided test, but if $\hat{\delta} = \bar{y}_2 - \bar{y}_1 < 0$, then conduct a two-sided test. The probability of rejecting the null hypotheses is a combination of two probabilities derived from a t-distribution or normal distribution. It is

$$\alpha^* = P \text{ (reject } H_0 \text{ when } H_0 \text{ is true)} = P \text{ (one-sided}|\hat{\delta} > 0)P(\hat{\delta} > 0)$$
$$+ P \text{ (two-sided}|\hat{\delta} < 0)P(\hat{\delta} < 0).$$

If an "α level $= 0.05$" test is based on the normal distribution, then the actual error rate is

$$\alpha^* = P(Z > 1.645|\delta > 0)(1/2) + P(Z < -1.960|\delta < 0)(1/2)$$
$$= 0.10(1/2) + 0.05(1/2) = 0.075.$$

However, reporting this "options-open" test as an "$\alpha = 0.05$ level" procedure clearly ignores the test-direction bias.

Selection Bias

Implicit in the "shift" model is the assumption that all individuals sampled come from the same population. Consequently, all individuals have a common underlying mean level of the variable being studied (μ). If individuals are not randomly assigned to treatment and control groups, a selection bias occurs when individuals in the two comparison groups do not have the same underlying mean value. The "shift" model becomes

"Control" individual: $y_{1j} = \mu_1 + e_{1j}$

"Treatment" individual: $y_{2j} = \mu_2 + \delta + e_{2j}$.

A t-statistic based on this model is

$$T = \frac{(\bar{y}_2 - \bar{y}_1) - (\mu_2 - \mu_1) - \delta}{\sqrt{\text{variance } (\bar{y}_2 - \bar{y}_1)}}, \qquad (2.13)$$

and when there is no treatment effect, $\delta = 0$, then

$$T = \frac{(\bar{y}_2 - \bar{y}_1) - (\mu_2 - \mu_1)}{\sqrt{\text{variance } (\bar{y}_2 - \bar{y}_1)}}. \qquad (2.14)$$

The probability of rejecting the null hypothesis $(H_0: \delta = 0)$ in the presence of this specific selection bias depends on the values of μ_1 and μ_2 and is approximately [based on expression (2.14)]

$$\alpha' = 1 - P(-z_{1-\alpha/2} + b < Z < z_{1-\alpha/2} + b), \qquad (2.15)$$

where Z has a standard normal distribution with percentiles represented by $z_{1-\alpha/2}$. The bias b is

$$\text{bias} = b = \sqrt{n/4}\left(\frac{\mu_2 - \mu_1}{\sigma}\right), \qquad (2.16)$$

when $n_1 = n_2 = n/2$ is the number of observations in each group. Some selected values of α' are shown in Table 2–2.

Figure 2–1 shows the impact of this bias on a t-test. The actual probability α' is always greater than or equal to the nominal level of α (0.05 in this illustration). Selection bias inflates the probability of falsely declaring a difference. Furthermore, this bias increases as the sample size increases, a not uncommon property of bias. The assumption that no selection bias exists $(\mu_1 = \mu_2 = \mu)$ is clearly critical for a valid two-sample t-test (middle column of Table 2–2).

Misclassification Bias: Specificity and Sensitivity

In measuring or classifying a disease there is always the possibility of an error. A disease can be declared present when it is absent or declared absent when it is present. More formally, consider the following table

Table 2–2. Selection-biased values α'

$(\mu_1 - \mu_2)/\sigma$	-1.0	-0.5	0.0	0.5	1.0
$n = 10$	0.352	0.124	0.05	0.124	0.352
$n = 20$	0.609	0.201	0.05	0.201	0.609
$n = 30$	0.782	0.278	0.05	0.278	0.782
$n = 40$	0.885	0.352	0.05	0.352	0.885

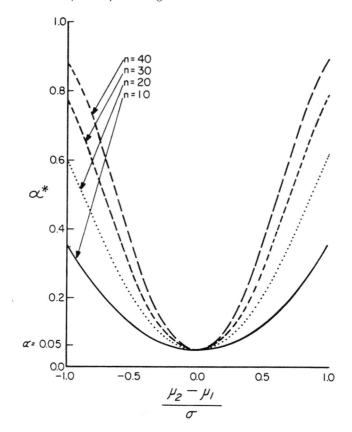

Figure 2–1. Selection bias α^* for $n = 10, 20, 30,$ and 40 observations for an α-level test of 0.05

where a diagnostic test is used to determine disease status. There are four possibilities, noted in Table 2–3. The values a, b, c, and d represent the counts of four possible outcomes of diagnosing n individuals. The counts b and c represent errors; that is, individuals are diagnosed as positive when they are disease-free (b), and individuals are diagnosed as negative when they in fact have the disease (c). The

Table 2–3. Diagnostic test—the test is positive or negative, and the disease is either present of absent among n individuals

	Disease Present (D)	Disease Absent ($\bar{D}$)	Total
Test positive (" $+$ ")	a	b	$a + b$
Test negative (" $-$ ")	c	d	$c + d$
Total	$a + c$	$b + d$	n

two possibilities where no error occurs (a and d) get special names. The probability of a positive test when the disease is present is called *sensitivity*. Clearly, a good diagnostic test should have a high degree of sensitivity. In addition, when a person is free of the disease, a good diagnostic test should give a negative result. The probability of a negative test among those individuals who are disease-free is called *specificity*. In symbolic terms,

$$\text{sensitivity} = P(\text{``}+\text{''}|D) = \frac{a}{a+c} \quad \text{and}$$

$$\text{specificity} = P(\text{``}-\text{''}|\bar{D}) = \frac{d}{b+d}, \tag{2.17}$$

where notation "$+$" means the individual is declared positive for the disease, and similarly the symbol "$-$" means an individual is declared as disease-free. It is necessary to know the "true" disease status of a set of individuals to assess the accuracy of a diagnostic test in terms of specificity and sensitivity.

To be concrete, data are presented in Table 2–4 showing medical records that were carefully searched and compared for the diagnosis of a specific malformation reported on the birth certificates among newborns. It is assumed that the medical records are complete and correct (perhaps, not the best assumption in all cases); therefore, 27 individuals are known to have a birth defect and 387 are known to be free of the birth defect out of the 414 records searched. Giving,

$$\text{sensitivity} = P(\text{''}+\text{''}|D) = \frac{8}{27} = 0.296 \quad \text{and}$$

$$\text{specificity} = P(\text{``} - \text{''}|\bar{D}) = \frac{374}{387} = 0.966.$$

The specificity and sensitivity associated with the determination of disease status is obviously a key issue in the analysis of any disease data. Furthermore, the issues of sensitivity and specificity are not

Table 2–4. Diagnostic test—malformation found on birth certificates compared to whether or not the malformation appears in the medical records

	Medical Records Malformation Present	Medical Records Malformation Absent	Total
Birth certificates—present	8	13	21
Birth certificates—absent	19	374	393
Total	27	387	414

restricted to only the determination of the presence and absence of a disease. The same questions arise in determining the classification based on any variable. For example, it is entirely possible that the determination of the presence or absence of a risk factor is subject to error which will certainly affect the results of any subsequent analysis.

False positive is another term associated with errors in classification when determining an individual's disease status. The probability of a false positive observation is sometimes defined as the lack of sensitivity. A false positive, however, occurs when the disease is in fact absent among the test results that are positive. A similar quantity is a false negative which occurs when a disease is present among the test results that are negative. In symbolic terms,

$$\text{probability of a false positive} = P(\bar{D}|\text{``}+\text{''}) \quad \text{and}$$

$$\text{probability of a false negative} = P(D|\text{``}-\text{''}).$$

These probabilities can be calculated from Table 2–4 if both the probability of the disease (i.e., $P(D)$) and the probability of a diagnostic test give a positive result (i.e., $P(\text{``}+\text{''})$) are known.

In the situation where disease status, risk factor status, or the status of any relevant variable cannot be determined perfectly, the validity of any calculated statistical summary is affected. Two types of misclassification occur—differential misclassification and nondifferential misclassification. For the sake of simplicity it is assumed that only the disease is subject to misclassification, but other more complex situations certainly arise and are described elsewhere (e.g., [2] and [3]).

The notation for a 2 × 2 table where no misclassification occurs in categorizing two binary variables is given in Table 2–5 (which is not very different from Table 2–3), and is a common representation of the four possible outcomes associated with two binary variables.

Let p_1 represent specificity and p_2 represent sensitivity when the risk factor is present (F), and let P_1 represent specificity and P_2 represent sensitivity when the risk factor is absent $(\bar{F})$. If $p_1 \neq P_1$ or if $p_2 \neq P_2$, the misclassification is called differential. The probability of

Table 2–5. Notation for a 2 × 2 table—risk factor **F** and disease **D**

	Disease Present (D)	Disease Absent $(\bar{D})$	Total
Risk factor present (F)	a	b	$a + b$
Risk factor absent $(\bar{F})$	c	d	$c + d$
Total	$a + c$	$b + d$	n

misclassification depends on the level of the risk factor. If $p_1 = P_1$ and $p_2 = P_2$, the misclassification is called nondifferential, because the probability of misclassification is the same for both levels of the risk factor. Misclassification is unrelated to the risk factor.

When the misclassification is differential, the magnitude and the direction of the misclassification bias can lead to overestimation or underestimation of the strength of an association. For example, the odds ratio (a complete description is given in Appendix C) is either biased upwards or downwards leading to spurious conclusions, depending on the relative values of sensitivity and specificity. For example, consider a sample of women recruited for a clinical trial who were either assigned a special diet (treátment) or assigned to a control group (nondiet) and classified as improved or not improved for benign breast disease. The possibility of differential misclassification occurs when the person doing the classification knows whether the participant was assigned to the diet or nondiet group. The investigator might exaggerate the improvement in the patients on the diet which would introduce differential misclassification—classification depends on the risk factor.

The simpler but, perhaps, less realistic case involves nondifferential misclassification and is represented in Table 2–6. Nondifferential classification occurs when the probability of misclassification does not depend on the risk factor (p_1 and p_2 apply regardless of the level of the risk factor). In the previous example, if the investigator did not know the diet status of the person diagnosed, then misclassification of benign breast disease would be the same for those on the diet as well as those not on the diet—nondifferential. In the case of nondifferential misclassification, the disease and the nondisease groups will appear more alike, producing an underestimate of the association between risk factor and disease. For example, the odds ratio will always be biased towards 1.0. That is, the odds ratio calculated from Table 2–6 will always be closer to 1.0 than an odds ratio calculated from Table 2–5,

Table 2–6. Expected counts for risk factor F and disease D for nondifferential misclassification of the disease

	Disease Present (D)	Disease Absent $(\bar{D})$	Total
Risk factor present (F)	$ap_1 + b(1 - p_2)$	$a(1 - p_1) + bp_2$	$a + b$
Risk factor absent $(\bar{F})$	$cp_1 + d(1 - p_2)$	$c(1 - p_1) + dp_2$	$c + d$
Total	$(a + c)p_1 + (b + d)(1 - p_2)$	$(a + c)(1 - p_1) + (b + d)p_2$	n

Table 2–7. Selected examples of the effect of nondifferential misclassification on the odds ratio

		Cells	Example 1	Example 2	Example 3
		a	40	60	80
		b	60	40	20
		c	15	20	30
		d	45	40	30
Sensitivity	Specificity				
1.0	1.0	or	2.0	3.0	4.0
0.95	0.95	or_{bias}	1.83	2.67	3.35
0.95	0.80	or_{bias}	1.58	2.27	2.96
0.80	0.95	or_{bias}	1.73	2.33	2.51
0.80	0.80	or_{bias}	1.46	1.91	2.13

where no misclassification occurs ($p_1 = 1$ and $p_2 = 1$). Table 2-7 illustrates this property. The simple illustration (Table 2–7) indicates that substantial bias can result from misclassification, and the best that can be said is that an understatement of the association occurs when the misclassification is nondifferential. Of course, if other variables such as confounding variables or other risk factors are misclassified, the results of an analysis will also be biased. Continuous variable measurement error also biases the study of a risk factor and a disease and is a subject of extensive investigation (e.g., [4]). Suggestions exist for correcting misclassification bias [5], but application of these techniques can give misleading results [6]. Of course, the best way to deal with misclassification bias is to avoid it in the first place by soundly designed studies with correctly measured variables.

Comparison of k Groups

A natural extension of the two-sample t-test is the comparison of more than two groups. Envision k groups, where one or more of the groups, for example, does not receive a treatment, thereby producing a control group. A basic model describing the k-sample situation is

$$\text{Observed individual:} \quad y_{ij} = \mu + \delta_i + e_{ij},$$

where i indicates the group and j indicates the observation within the group. The parameters of this statistical structure are analogous to those of the two-sample "shift" model (where $\delta_1 = 0$ and $\delta_2 = \delta$). Again y_{ij} represents a measured response variable. Comparison among

k groups using a t-test can detect which, if any, of the treatments have important influences on the response variable (e.g., $\delta_1 \neq \delta_2$?). Like the two-sample "shift" model ($k = 2$), the values y_{ij} are required to be normally distributed with the same variance in all k groups.

Each group produces a sample mean ($\bar{y}_i$) based on n_i observations, where the total number of observations is $n = \sum n_i$. Parallel to the two-sample t-test, hypotheses are generated concerning the values of the δ_i's. These hypotheses can take the form of contrasts. A contrast, as before, is a weighted sum of values (e.g., $\sum a_i \bar{y}_i$ or $\sum a_i \delta_i$), where the sum of the coefficients is zero ($\sum a_i = 0$). For example, if group 1 is a treatment group and groups 2, 3, ..., k are various kinds of control groups, then

$$\bar{y}_1 - \frac{1}{k-1}(\bar{y}_2 + \bar{y}_3 + \cdots + \bar{y}_k) \qquad (2.18)$$

is a contrast comparing of the estimated mean of the treatment group with the estimated mean level from $k - 1$ control groups.

If interest is focused on a constrast of m mean values ($\sum a_i \bar{y}_i$), then

$$T = \frac{\sum\limits_{i=1}^{m} a_i \bar{y}_i - \sum\limits_{i=1}^{m} a_i \delta_i}{\sqrt{\text{variance}\left(\sum\limits_{i=1}^{m} a_i \bar{y}_i\right)}} \qquad (2.19)$$

has a t-distribution with $n - k$ degrees of freedom. When the groups contrasted have the same level of treatment effect, then $\delta_i = \delta$, making $\delta \sum a_i = 0$.

The variance of a contrast is estimated by

$$\text{variance}\left(\sum\limits_{i=1}^{m} a_i \bar{y}_i\right) = S_p^2 \sum\limits_{i=1}^{m} \frac{a_i^2}{n_i} \qquad (2.20)$$

when all k groups have the same associated variance. When the variability in response (y_{ij}) is the same for all k groups (not influenced by the treatments), an estimate of the common variance (σ^2) is derived by pooling the k-sample variances [expression (2.8)] using a weighted average (weights $= n_i - 1$) or

$$S_p^2 = \frac{\sum\limits_{i=1}^{k} (n_i - 1)S_i^2}{n - k} \qquad (2.21)$$

Table 2–8. Mean disease-severity scores

	Diet	Nondiet
Assigned to treatment	$\bar{y}_1$	$\bar{y}_2$
Assigned to control	$\bar{y}_3$	$\bar{y}_4$

which is alternatively expressed as

$$S_p^2 = \frac{\sum\limits_{i=1}^{k} \sum\limits_{j=1}^{n_i} (y_{ij} - \bar{y}_i)^2}{\sum\limits_{i=1}^{k} (n_i - 1)}. \tag{2.22}$$

Illustrative data come from a clinical trial concerning the efficacy of a caffeine-free diet in reducing the severity of the benign breast disease (adapted from [7]). Participating women with the disease were assigned randomly to a control group (usual diet) or a treatment group (caffeine-free diet). These women were measured at the beginning and at the end of the trial to produce a response score reflecting changes in severity of the disease. Compliance with the diet was accurately determined by biochemical analysis, producing the four groups of participants in Table 2–8.

The symbol $\bar{y}_i$ represents the mean response score or the mean difference between scores measured at the beginning and the end of the trial for each group. Negative scores indicate a decrease in severity of disease. Summary data from the trial are shown in Table 2–9. Two contrasts are of interest:

1. The difference in mean scores between those who followed the diet and those who did not, based on biochemical determinations.

Table 2–9. Benign breast disease summary data

Group	Status	Biochemical	$\bar{y}_i$	n_i	S_i^2
$i = 1$	Treatment	Diet	-5.0	62	12.44
$i = 2$	Treatment	Nondiet	0.6	7	13.65
$i = 3$	Control	Diet	-2.0	15	16.34
$i = 4$	Control	Nondiet	1.0	48	17.41
$i = 1 + 3$	—	Diet	-4.416	77	—
$i = 2 + 4$	—	Nondiet	0.949	55	—
$i = 1 + 2$	Treatment	—	-4.432	69	—
$i = 3 + 4$	Control	—	0.286	63	—

2. The difference in mean scores between those assigned to the treatment versus those assigned to the control group.

An important issue with regard to bias arises in the interpretation of these clinical trial data. The nurse examiner knew whether a patient had been assigned to the diet or to the control group. The "nonblind" aspect of this study leads to the possibility of observer bias (a type of misclassification bias), since the disease-severity score could be influenced (consciously or unconsciously) by the examining nurse.

> Aside: A study is usually called blind when the person measuring the outcome is unaware of the treatment/control status of the individual being measured. A trial is called double blind if, in addition, the patient is unaware of his or her own treatment/control status. The purpose of a blinded study is so far as possible to reduce bias introduced by the tendency of the patient or the investigator to report results based on preconceived notions. This type of bias is referred to as observer bias. A placebo effect is the tendency to report favorable results from a treatment regardless of its efficacy and is an example of observer bias. The ability to conduct a double-blind study depends on the treatment and the control being similar. In many cases, it is not possible to carry out a double-blind study, because the treatment is clearly distinguishable from the control. For example, a caffeine-free diet cannot be concealed from the participants. In this situation the strength of evidence from a clinical trial is diminished, and observer bias is an issue. However, the diet/nondiet status could have been concealed from the person evaluating the degree of improvement in disease status, which would decrease the possible influence of spurious effects on the trial results.

Also present in the breast disease data is misclassification bias. That is, individuals assigned to the treatment group did not conform to the diet (7 individuals), potentially diluting any impact of the diet on the differences in mean response. Also, some members of the control group voluntarily conformed to the diet, causing the nondiet group to contain some participants on the diet (15 individuals), also diluting differences between mean response. The observer bias affects the classification of the disease, and the misclassification of the treatment/control status affects the classification based on diet status.

It is tempting to argue that patients who complied with the diet should be compared with those who did not comply (based on the biochemical analysis), ignoring the original assigned treatment/control categories. This comparison restricts analysis to those actually receiving and not receiving the treatment, eliminating misclassification bias. The average difference in mean scores between those who followed the diet and those who did not is -4.3 (groups 1 and 3 versus groups 2 and 4—Table 2–9). A t-test to assess this difference is

$$T = \frac{(\bar{y}_1 + \bar{y}_3)/2 - (\bar{y}_2 + \bar{y}_4)/2}{\sqrt{\frac{S_p^2}{4}\left(\frac{1}{n_1} + \frac{1}{n_2} + \frac{1}{n_3} + \frac{1}{n_4}\right)}} = \frac{-4.3}{\sqrt{0.909}} = -4.511. \tag{2.23}$$

The estimate of the variance in scores (σ^2) is based on the assumption that all four groups are subject to the same variability, and the pooled estimate of the common variance is

$$S_p^2 = \frac{\sum\limits_{i=1}^{k} (n_i - 1)S_i^2}{n - k} = \frac{1887.739}{128} = 14.748. \tag{2.24}$$

The t-test provides sufficient evidence (p-value < 0.001) that the observed difference is not likely a result of random variation and is likely due to systematic influences differing between diet and nondiet groups. This result, however, is potentially biased. Compliance or noncompliance with the diet is voluntary, and comparing these two groups no longer maintains the original randomization. Analyzing the difference between those who complied to the diet and those who did not avoids the misclassification bias at the cost of introducing a possible selection bias. The experimental data (randomized) becomes observational data (nonrandomized).

The comparison between the treatment and the control groups can be evaluated with a t-test despite the misclassification bias. The average difference in mean scores between treatment and controls is -1.7 (groups 1 and 2 versus groups 3 and 4—Table 2–9; ignoring the possible influence of misclassification). The t-test to assess this difference produces

$$T = \frac{(\bar{y}_1 + \bar{y}_2)/2 - (\bar{y}_3 + \bar{y}_4)/2}{\sqrt{\frac{S_p^2}{4}\left(\frac{1}{n_1} + \frac{1}{n_2} + \frac{1}{n_3} + \frac{1}{n_4}\right)}} = \frac{-1.7}{\sqrt{0.909}} = -1.783. \tag{2.25}$$

This difference between mean responses (-1.7) is also likely due to systematic differences between the treatment and control groups (p-value $= 0.074$). Even though misclassification exists, a comparison that maintains the original randomization is still useful as long as the misclassification of data is not large (less than 20% or 30%). The presence of two misclassified subgroups generally dampens observed effects, but any remaining difference is not caused by selection bias because there is none. Maintaining randomization by contrasting the original treatment and control groups likely produces a reduced measure of the treatment effect but maintains the balance of other variables between groups that could bias the comparison. It is usually preferable to incur a reduction in sensitivity to avoid a biased comparison.

The contrast, however, of the original treatment and control mean values does not discriminate between observer bias and an effect from the diet. The observed decrease in scores could be due to a combination of bias introduced by the examiner and the influence of a caffeine-free diet.

One last note: The statistical analysis indicates that the diet may be associated with a reduction in the severity of the disease (not likely a random reduction). The reduction observed, however, is not clinically important. A reduction in the severity score of 5.0 or so was judged by both physician and patient to have no important consequence. Statistical significance does not always lead to biologically important results. Statistical inferences are limited to questions of whether an observed phenomenon is or is not likely a result of chance variation.

Interaction Contrast

Combining data is governed by a simple and rather obvious principle: *Data that systematically differ with respect to the quantity being studied should not be combined.* Forming larger groups by combining smaller sets of data improves precision of an estimated quantity that is free of bias only when the groups combined provide estimates of the same quantity. Data collected on levels of hypertension in the white and black populations of part of Alameda county, California illustrate this principle (adapted from [8]). Each individual is classified by race (white or black) and whether the census tract of residence is predominantly white or black in racial comparison ("white" or "black" neighborhood). The average diastolic blood pressures for a sample of females, ages 35–49 are shown in Table 2–10.

Table 2–10. Hypertension: summary data

Group	Race	Neighborhood	$\bar{y}_i$	n_i	S_i^2
$i = 1$	White	"White"	77.2	167	62.4
$i = 2$	White	"Black"	78.9	47	74.6
$i = 3$	Black	"White"	83.3	45	86.4
$i = 4$	Black	"Black"	98.4	245	87.8

When interest is focused on a comparison of the white versus black levels of blood pressure, a natural contrast is achieved by comparing the mean from combining groups 1 and 2 to the mean from combining groups 3 and 4, or $(\bar{y}_1 + \bar{y}_2)/2 - (\bar{y}_3 + \bar{y}_4)/2$. This contrast produces an unbiased measure of racial differences in blood pressure only if $(\bar{y}_1 - \bar{y}_3) - (\bar{y}_2 - \bar{y}_4)$ is zero or at least small. That is, $\bar{y}_1 - \bar{y}_3$ (the difference between races in "white" neighborhoods) and $\bar{y}_2 - \bar{y}_4$ (the difference between races in "black" neighborhoods) must reflect the same quantity. If these two quantities substantially differ, then summary values are not easily interpreted. Failure to reflect the same relationship at different levels of another variable is called an interaction. Interactions limit the ability to summarize relationships within a data set.

A contrast measuring the magnitude of an interaction is the difference between the race-specific differences $(\bar{y}_1 - \bar{y}_3) - (\bar{y}_2 - \bar{y}_4)$ and yields a value of $(77.2 - 83.3) - (78.9 - 98.4) = 13.4$ mm from the blood pressure data. The size of this difference indicates a likely interaction between neighborhood and race. This difference can be statistically tested and analyzed formally in a number of ways.

Comparing the white/black levels of blood pressure without regard to neighborhood type obscures the fact that important racial differences appear to exist between neighborhoods. In the "white" neighborhoods the difference between black and whites (6.1 mm) is substantially smaller than the same difference (19.5 mm) occurring in the "black" neighborhoods. The differences in mean blood pressure levels differ depending on the neighborhood considered. The mean difference, averaged over "neighborhoods," is 12.8 mm but does not accurately reflect the black/white differences in either neighborhood. In the presence of an interaction, summary measures from combined data are biased and in some cases produce entirely spurious results (another example appears in Chapter 6, Table 6–28). The issue of interaction is central to a number of statistical methods and will appear in differing forms in the remainder of the text, particularly Chapters 7, 8, and 9.

Figure 2–2 shows the mean diastolic blood pressures plotted for both races within each type of neighborhood (one line for "white" and one line for "black" neighborhoods). The differences between mean blood pressure values for white and black women in the survey are clear (6.1 mm in "white" and 19.5 mm in "black" neighborhoods). If no interaction were present, then these differences would be the same or nearly the same in each neighborhood type, making the lines reflecting the influence of race within neighborhoods approximately parallel.

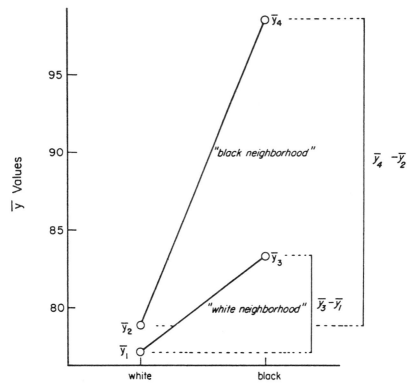

Figure 2–2. Mean diastolic blood pressure levels by neighborhoods and by race

Rates and Interaction

The data in Table 2–11 are age-adjusted mortality rates per 100,000 person-years showing the relationship of smoking and asbestos exposure to lung cancer deaths. The answer to the question of whether these two risk factors show any evidence of an interaction or whether they act independently depends on how the question is asked. One view postulates that risk factors affecting rates act independently

Table 2–11. Lung cancer mortality rates per 100,000 person-years by smoking status and asbestos exposure for Canadian insulation workers [9]

	Smoker	Nonsmoker	Ratio
Exposed	601.6	58.4	10.3
Unexposed	127.3	11.3	11.3
Ratio	4.7	5.2	—

if the consequence of possessing both risk factors is to produce a multiplicative increase in the measure of a risk, such as death rates. For example, if exposure to one risk variable increases the risk of death by a factor of 2 and exposure to a second risk variable increases the risk by a factor of 3, then the combined risk from possessing both risk factors is a 6-fold increase when these two variables act independently. A more than or less than 6-fold increase constitutes an interaction between the two variables.

Independent multiplicative effects become additive effects when mortality rates are expressed as the logarithm of the rates. To explore the independence of smoking and asbestos exposure as part of the risk of lung cancer mortality, the logarithm of the age-adjusted mortality rates are given in Table 2–12. The logarithms of the rates show that smoking and asbestos exposure have close to additive influences on the risk of lung cancer (multiplicatively in terms of the rates themselves). The difference in increased risk due to smoking is almost identical for both workers exposed and unexposed to asbestos (roughly 2.4 or $e^{2.4} = 11$-fold difference in rates). Similarly, the increase in risk due to asbestos exposure is also almost identical for smokers and nonsmokers (roughly 1.6 or $e^{1.6} = 5$-fold difference in rates). To repeat, additivity of effects (no interaction) of logarithms translates to independent multiplicative effects.

A measure of an interaction in a 2×2 table of logarithms of rates can be expressed as the difference between differences. The effect from asbestos exposure among smokers is $6.400 - 4.846 = 1.553$, and the effect among nonsmokers is $4.067 - 2.425 = 1.643$, showing almost the same effect (i.e., $1.553 - 1.643 = -0.089$). The same quantity emerges when the effect of smoking is compared between asbestos-exposed and unexposed workers (i.e., $6.400 - 4.067) - (4.846 - 2.425) = -0.089$). The small difference in effects of one variable at both levels of the other variable implies no important interaction between asbestos and smoking is present, and leads to the conclusion that the effects of smoking and asbestos have independent

Table 2–12. The logarithms of lung cancer mortality rates by smoking status and asbestos exposure for Canadian insulation workers

	Smoker	Nonsmoker	Difference
Exposed	6.400	4.067	2.33
Unexposed	4.846	2.425	2.42
Difference	1.55	1.64	—

multiplicative influences on the risk of a lung cancer death as measured by age-adjusted mortality rates.

Two-Way Analysis

To reduce variation and control bias, a simple approach is to classify data into a series of more or less homogeneous groups (also discussed in Chapter 9). For example, individuals could be classified by exposure to air pollution (e.g., high, medium, low, and no exposure), while at the same time classified by the number of years they have lived at a specific location (e.g., less than a year, 1–5 years, and more than 5 years). Data of this sort form a two-way or a two-dimensional table. The cells of such a table could contain counts of a discrete variable or measured values of a continuous variable. Continuing the air pollution example, the categories formed by a two-way classification could contain the numbers of individuals with respiratory problems, or the cells of the table could contain specific measurements such as exposure levels to household nitrous oxide. The analysis of discrete tabular data is a topic in itself (partially covered in Chapters 6 and 7). A brief look at the analysis of continuous data classified into a two-way table continues to illustrate the way statistical models guide the analytic approach to specific types of data.

The notation for data classified into a two-way table is displayed in Table 2–13. Each cell contains a continuous outcome measure represented by y_{ij} (i^{th} row and j^{th} column of the table where r represents the number of rows and c represents the number of columns). The row means are denoted by $\bar{y}_{i.}$ and equal $\dfrac{1}{c}\left(\displaystyle\sum_{j=1}^{c} y_{ij}\right)$; similarly the column means are denoted by $\bar{y}_{.j}$ and equal $\dfrac{1}{r}\left(\displaystyle\sum_{i=1}^{r} y_{ij}\right)$, and the overall

Table 2–13. Notation for a two-way classification of a continuous variable

	1	2	c	$\bar{y}_{i.}$
1	y_{11}	y_{12}	y_{1c}	$\bar{y}_{1.}$
2	y_{21}	y_{22}	y_{2c}	$\bar{y}_{2.}$
3	y_{31}	y_{32}	y_{3c}	$\bar{y}_{3.}$
⋮	⋮	⋮	⋮	⋮
r	y_{r1}	y_{r2}	y_{rc}	$\bar{y}_{r.}$
$\bar{y}_{.j}$	$\bar{y}_{.1}$	$\bar{y}_{.2}$	$\bar{y}_{.c}$	$\bar{y}$

mean is denoted by $\bar{y}$ and equals $\dfrac{1}{rc}\left(\displaystyle\sum_{i=1}^{r}\sum_{j=1}^{c} y_{ij}\right)$.

To examine the properties of data classified into a $r \times c$ two-way table, a useful statistical model is

$$y_{ij} = \mu + \gamma_i + \delta_j + e_{ij} \tag{2.26}$$

and, as before, μ represents a constant underlying mean value. The term γ_i represents the contribution of the row variable, and δ_j represents the contribution of the column variable. The random terms e_{ij}, as in the previous models, represent independent influences that have normal distributions with the same variance (σ^2) for all levels of the categorical variables (for all cells in the table). This model is referred to as an additive model, because the observed values result from only the addition of an overall, a row, and a column influence plus a random component.

A specific example of an additive model, with the column variable at three levels $(c = 3)$ and a row variable at two levels $(r = 2)$, produces the model values for a 2×3 table given in Table 2–14.

The mean values from the rows, columns, and total of a two-way table reflect the parameters of the additive model or, in symbols,

Columns means: $\bar{y}_{.j}$ estimates $\mu + \bar{\gamma} + \delta_j,$ (2.27)

Row means: $\bar{y}_{i.}$ estimates $\mu + \gamma_i + \bar{\delta}$ and   (2.28)

Total mean: $\bar{y}$ estimates $\mu + \bar{\gamma} + \bar{\delta}.$ (2.29)

The additive nature of the postulated model allows the influence of the column variable to be estimated free from the influence of the row variable. Specifically, note that the column mean minus the overall mean value is unaffected by row influences or

$$\bar{y}_{.j} - \bar{y} \quad \text{estimates} \quad \delta_j - (\delta_1 + \delta_2 + \delta_3)/3,$$

$$\text{or, in general,} \quad \bar{y}_{.j} - \bar{y} \quad \text{estimates} \quad \delta_j - \bar{\delta} \tag{2.30}$$

reflecting only the influence of the jth column variable. Also, the row mean minus the overall mean is unaffected by column variable influences or

$$\bar{y}_{i.} - \bar{y} \quad \text{estimates} \quad \gamma_i - (\gamma_1 + \gamma_2)/2,$$

$$\text{or, in general,} \quad \bar{y}_{i.} - \bar{y} \quad \text{estimates} \quad \gamma_i - \bar{\gamma} \tag{2.31}$$

reflecting only the influence of the ith row variable.

Expression (2.30) shows that the influences from the column variable

Table 2–14. Model values

	1	2	3	$\bar{y}_{i.}$
1	$y_{11}: \mu + \gamma_1 + \delta_1$	$y_{12}: \mu + \gamma_1 + \delta_2$	$y_{13}: \mu + \gamma_1 + \delta_3$	$\bar{y}_{1.}: \mu + \gamma_1 + (\delta_1 + \delta_2 + \delta_3)/3$
2	$y_{21}: \mu + \gamma_2 + \delta_1$	$y_{22}: \mu + \gamma_2 + \delta_2$	$y_{23}: \mu + \gamma_2 + \delta_3$	$\bar{y}_{2.}: \mu + \gamma_2 + (\delta_1 + \delta_2 + \delta_3)/3$
$\bar{y}_{.j}$	$\bar{y}_{.1}: \mu + (\gamma_1 + \gamma_2)/2 + \delta_1$	$\bar{y}_{.2}: \mu + (\gamma_1 + \gamma_2)/2 + \delta_2$	$\bar{y}_{.3}: \mu + (\gamma_1 + \gamma_2)/2 + \delta_3$	$\bar{y}: \mu + (\gamma_1 + \gamma_2)/2 + (\delta_1 + \delta_2 + \delta_3)/3$

are estimated without interference from the row variable when an additive model [expression (2.28)] accurately represents the structure of the collected data. For example, contrasting the means of columns j and k, produces an estimate of column variable effects, and the row variable plays no role in this estimate since

$$\bar{y}_{.j} - \bar{y}_{.k} \quad \text{estimates} \quad \delta_j - \delta_k. \tag{2.32}$$

For an additive model, contrasts of the row means are also not influenced by the variable used to construct the columns of the table.

When two factors fail to have additive effects, the factors interact and the direct comparison of column mean values, for example, does not measure the effect of the column variable free from the influence of the row variable. Again, the presence of an interaction limits the ability to summarize the data. Specifically, the column effect, averaged over the row variable, $\bar{y}_{.j} - \bar{y}_{.k}$, is no longer an unbiased estimate of $\delta_j - \delta_k$.

An example using a set of numerical values illustrates the properties of an additive model in a two-way table. "Data" are given in Table 2–15 illustrating an additive model.

The tabled values are accurately represented (in this case perfectly) by the additive model [expression (2.28)] where $\mu = 30$, $\delta_1 = -10$, $\delta_2 = 10$, $\gamma_1 = -10$, $\gamma_2 = 0$, and $\gamma_3 = 10$. The mean values of the columns of the table duplicate the relationships among the columns in each of the rows. The row variable has no influence on comparisons among the columns. In this example the difference between each column is 10, for each row and summarized by the column mean values. The fact that the column means reflect the influence of the column variable unaffected by the row variable is a direct result of additivity of the variables used to construct the table. It is also true that the row mean values are an unbiased summary of the relationship in each column.

Table 2–15. Numeric example of values that perfectly conform to an additive model

	$j = 1$	$j = 2$	$j = 3$	$\bar{y}_{i.}$
$i = 1$	$y_{11} = 10$	$y_{12} = 20$	$y_{13} = 30$	$\bar{y}_{1.} = 20$
$i = 2$	$y_{21} = 30$	$y_{22} = 40$	$y_{23} = 50$	$\bar{y}_{2.} = 40$
$\bar{y}_{.j}$	$\bar{y}_{.1} = 20$	$\bar{y}_{.2} = 30$	$\bar{y}_{.3} = 40$	$\bar{y} = 30$

Table 2–16. Numeric example of values that do not conform to an additive model

	$j = 1$	$j = 2$	$j = 3$	$\bar{y}_{i.}$
$i = 1$	$y_{11} = 10$	$y_{12} = 20$	$y_{13} = 30$	$\bar{y}_{1.} = 20$
$i = 2$	$y_{21} = 50$	$y_{22} = 40$	$y_{23} = 30$	$\bar{y}_{2.} = 40$
$\bar{y}_{.j}$	$\bar{y}_{.1} = 30$	$\bar{y}_{.2} = 30$	$\bar{y}_{.3} = 30$	$\bar{y} = 30$

For variables that are not additive, the row and column means do not reflect the influence of the row and column variables. Table 2–16 gives a set of numeric values that are not additive (interact).

Clearly, the column means do not reflect the influence of the column variable. The relationship among the column variable depends on the row variable (the relationship in row 1 is reversed in row 2). The dependency is illustrated by the fact that the column means are constant, which does not summarize the influence of column variable in a meaningful way. This simple example shows what is true in general. Mean values summarizing the rows or the columns of a 2-way table are useful descriptions of the data only when the effects of the variables used to create the table are at least approximately additive. If the influences of two variables are not additive (interact), the relationships among the columns depend on the rows and, visa versa. Therefore, the first question asked in exploring a two-way table should be: Do the variables have additive influences or not?

The variability associated with data classified into a two-way table involves two issues: the lack of fit of the additive model and the background variation. The difference between an observed data value and the corresponding value from the additive model [i.e., $e_{ij} = y_{ij} - (\mu + \gamma_i + \delta_j)$] measures this variability. Using the data to estimate the values of the parameters μ, γ_i, and δ_j gives

$$\hat{e}_{ij} = y_{ij} - [\hat{\mu} + \hat{\gamma}_i + \hat{\delta}_j] = y_{ij} - [\bar{y} + (\bar{y}_{i.} - \bar{y}) + (\bar{y}_{.j} - \bar{y})] = y_{ij} - \bar{y}_{i.} - \bar{y}_{.j} + \bar{y}.$$

(2.33)

Each cell produces a residual $\hat{e}_{ij}$ value. If these residual values are all zero, then the additive model fits the data perfectly (such as Table 2–15). The degree to which the residuals values are not zero measures the "lack of fit" of the additive model and/or the background variation intrinsic in the table. A summary estimate of these two sources of variability is

$$S^2 = \frac{\sum\limits_{i=1}^{r} \sum\limits_{j=1}^{c} \hat{e}_{ij}^2}{(r-1)(c-1)} = \frac{\sum\limits_{i=1}^{r} \sum\limits_{j=1}^{c} (y_{ij} - \bar{y}_{i.} - \bar{y}_{.j} + \bar{y})^2}{(r-1)(c-1)}.$$

(2.34)

The sum of the $\hat{e}_{ij}^2$ divided by $(r-1)(c-1)$ is an estimate of the background variability of outcome variable y_{ij} when the data conform to an additive model. The reason for dividing by $(r-1)(c-1)$ is beyond the scope of this presentation, except to note that by doing so S^2 becomes an unbiased estimate of the background variation of the tabled data under the additive model.

If the variables used to form the rows and the columns of the table do not behave in the additive way postulated by the model, the variance estimate S^2 is biased by influences not described by the model. When only one observation per cell is available, the random component and the "nonadditivity bias" cannot be separated. If more than one observation per cell is available, then a separate estimate of the variation σ^2 can be made and the impact of the "nonadditivity bias" assessed (see [1]).

In a clinical laboratory experiment three different methods to determine serum lead levels were examined. Data collected on six individuals, each tested by the three methods, are shown in Table 2–17. The estimate of the variance of serum lead levels assuming an additive model is $S^2 = 9.122$ [expression (2.34)]. To evaluate differences between the three methods a summary of three contrasts $\bar{y}_{.i} - \bar{y}_{.j}$ using a t-test is given in Table 2–18. Note that the estimated variance of the contrast $\bar{y}_{.j} - \bar{y}_{.k}$ is $variance (\bar{y}_{.j} - \bar{y}_{.k}) = 2S^2/r$ and gives a t-test of

$$T = \frac{\bar{y}_{.i} - \bar{y}_{.j}}{\sqrt{2S^2/r}}.$$

This t-test requires that an additive model describe the patient/method relationship to the serum lead levels, thus removing the influences from differences among patients from contrasts among the three laboratory methods and producing an unbiased estimate of variability.

Table 2–17. Three methods for determining serum lead: Data

	Method 1	Method 2	Method 3	$\bar{y}_{i.}$
Patient 1	20	26	28	24.67
Patient 2	34	32	38	34.67
Patient 3	54	61	68	61.00
Patient 4	38	40	46	41.33
Patient 5	19	25	31	25.00
Patient 6	40	38	54	44.00
$\bar{y}_{.j}$	34.17	37.00	44.17	38.44

Table 2–18. Three methods for determining serum lead: Contrasts

	$\bar{y}_{.2} - \bar{y}_{.1}$	$\bar{y}_{.3} - \bar{y}_{.1}$	$\bar{y}_{.3} - \bar{y}_{.2}$
Mean	2.833	10.000	7.167
Variance	3.041	3.041	3.041
t-test	1.625	5.735	4.110
p-value	0.135	<0.001	0.002

The variability of the difference between mean values (the denominator of the t-test statistic) is considerably reduced by taking into account the variation among the individual patients. If the data are treated as simple one-way classification (ignoring the distinctions among the six patients), then the estimated variability is $S_p^2 = 192.644$ rather than $S^2 = 9.122$. The reduction in variability increases the resolution power of the t-test applied to contrasts between means from a two-way table.

The two-way classification allows isolation of the effects of the three laboratory methods uninfluenced by differences in lead levels among patients. A two-way table in general allows the analysis of one variable "free" of influences associated with the another variable and usually produces a reduction in variability. However, these two properties of a two-way classification (separation of effects and reduction in variance), like many statistical approaches, depend on the adequacy of a model to represent the relationships in the data, specifically the assumption that the row and column effects are additive [no interaction—expression (2.26)].

A special case of a two-way classification is a matched pair design (described in detail in Chapter 9). Each column is a pair of matched observations and the two rows result from the presence or absence of an explanatory variable producing a $2 \times c$ table. An additive relationship between row and column variables is necessary so that the difference between column means $(\bar{y}_{.2} - \bar{y}_{.1})$ summarizes the within-pair differences associated with the explanatory variable.

Crossover Design

The way data are collected can lead to increased efficiency in detecting systematic influences when they exist. A crossover design, useful in comparative clinical studies, provides an example of manipulating the data collection process to produce elegant and powerful analyses. A crossover design involves a treatment given in one time period followed by a different treatment given in a second time period to the same individual. This pattern of collecting data is sometimes described as "using a person as his/her own control."

One version of this crossover design involves two time periods, two treatments, and a series of paired study participants. Suppose one "treatment" is a placebo (control) and the other treatment contains the agent under investigation. Two types of patients participate: patient type 1, who receives the placebo during the first period and then the treatment during the second period, and patient type 2, who receives the treatment during first period and the placebo during the second period. Both types of patients are subject to a time-period effect that can cause the first response to differ from the second regardless of whether the patient receives the treatment or placebo first. A statistical model describing the parameters of a crossover design for each pair of patients, where a placebo is evaluated against an experimental treatment, is given in Table 2–19. The term δ represents the treatment influence, the term τ the influence from time (period effect), and the term μ is again the common underlying mean value. Data from each of a series of pairs of patients collected in a crossover pattern would look like those represented in Table 2–20. Each patient is measured twice, producing n differences from a total $2n$ observations. Again, the response (y) is assumed to have a normal or near-normal distribution with the same variance for the four patient/time categories. A critical assumption implicit in the model (Table 2–19) is that no carryover effect exists (to be explored further). In other words, the order of the treatment has no importance. In terms of the model parameters, the value δ is the same for type 1 and type 2 patients. Furthermore, only the time period effect (τ) influences the mean response in time period 2 for those who received the treatment in time period 1. This property means that the individual fully "recovers" and the subsequent observation is uninfluenced by the treatment in time period 1. The "recovery" time between treatment and placebo is an important element for a successful (unbiased) estimate of the treatment effect and must be considered carefully when employing a crossover design.

Table 2–19. Crossover design: model

	Time 1	Time 2
Patient 1	μ	$\mu + \tau + \delta$
Patient 2	$\mu + \delta$	$\mu + \tau$

Table 2-20. Crossover design: Observed data

	Time 1	Time 2	Difference
Patient 1	y_0	$y_{\tau\delta}$	$y_{\tau\delta} - y_0$
Patient 2	y_δ	y_τ	$y_\delta - y_\tau$

The efficiency of a crossover design comes from the property that all subjects are used to evaluate the treatment. If individuals were simply assigned to treatment and control groups, typically more subjects would be necessary to achieve the same precision associated with detecting a treatment effect. The increased efficiency is purchased at the cost of the no carryover assumption.

The key to the analysis of the crossover design is the differences in observed values between time periods within each patient. These differences form a basis to estimate and evaluate the treatment and time parameters of the model. To evaluate the treatment note that

$D_1 = y_{\tau\delta} - y_0$ estimates $\tau + \delta$,   and $D_2 = y_\delta - y_\tau$ estimates $\delta - \tau$.

The mean values of the differences $(\bar{D}_i)$, each based on n individuals (type i), produce an estimate of δ where

$$(\bar{D}_1 + \bar{D}_2)/2 \quad \text{estimates} \quad \delta \quad \text{or} \quad \hat{\delta} = (\bar{D}_1 + \bar{D}_2)/2,$$

which is the estimated average change within subjects. A null hypothesis that the treatment has no effect is postulated $(H_0: \delta = 0)$ and assessed with the t-test statistic

$$T_\delta = \frac{\hat{\delta} - \delta}{S_\delta} = \frac{(\bar{D}_1 + \bar{D}_2)/2 - 0}{S_{(\bar{D}_1 + \bar{D}_2)/2}} = \frac{\bar{D}_1 + \bar{D}_2}{\sqrt{(S_{D_1}^2 + S_{D_2}^2)/n}}, \qquad (2.35)$$

which has a t-distribution with $2(n - 1)$ degrees of freedom when the null hypothesis is true. The estimated variance $S_{D_i}^2$ is calculated in the usual way using the n differences observed within each patient type [expression (2.8)].

It may be also of interest to investigate the influence of time periods. Again, the mean differences provide the key since

$$(\bar{D}_1 - \bar{D}_2)/2 \quad \text{estimates} \quad \tau \quad \text{or} \quad \hat{\tau} = (\bar{D}_1 - \bar{D}_2)/2.$$

The null hypothesis that there is no difference in response between time periods is postulated $(H_0: \tau = 0)$ and assessing the estimate $\hat{\tau}$ with a t-statistic gives

$$T_\tau = \frac{\hat{\tau} - \tau}{S_{\hat{\tau}}} = \frac{(\bar{D}_1 + \bar{D}_2)/2 - 0}{S_{(\bar{D}_1 + \bar{D}_2)/2}} = \frac{\bar{D}_1 + \bar{D}_2}{\sqrt{(S_{D_1}^2 + S_{D_2}^2)/n}}, \qquad (2.36)$$

which also has a t-distribution with $2(n-1)$ degrees of freedom when the null hypothesis is true.

Data adapted from Rivard [10] illustrate the analysis of a crossover design. An experiment was conducted to assess the influence of noise (treatment) on a person performing a stressful task. The task was a computer video game, and the treatment was an elevated level of noise (treatment $= 94$ dBA) versus background noise (control). The outcome was a performance score on the computer game. The observed scores for 20 participants are shown in Table 2–21.

To evaluate the influence of elevated noise level, the null hypothesis is postulated that $H_0: \delta = 0$ and the t-test statistic is

$$T_\delta = \frac{0.140 - 0.220}{\sqrt{(1.163 + 1.024)/10}} = -0.171.$$

The t-statistic indicates that noise is not a significant factor in the performance of the task (null hypothesis not rejected—p-value $= 0.866$). To assess the period effect, the t-test statistic is

$$T_\tau = \frac{0.140 - (-0.220)}{\sqrt{(1.163 + 1.024)/10}} = 0.770,$$

again indicating that no evidence exists that the participant's performance score on the computer game changed during the two time periods (p-value $= 0.452$). In both cases the degrees of freedom equal 18.

Table 2–21. Data from a crossover experiment on the effects of noise

Obs	Participant 1		Participant 2		Differences		Sums	
	y_0	$y_{\delta\tau}$	y_δ	y_τ	D_1	D_2	C_1	C_2
1	2.3	3.0	2.3	3.0	0.7	−0.7	5.3	5.3
2	3.0	2.0	1.3	1.3	−1.0	0.0	5.0	2.6
3	3.3	3.0	3.3	3.0	−0.3	0.3	6.3	6.3
4	2.0	2.7	3.3	5.7	0.7	−2.4	4.7	9.0
5	3.0	3.0	4.5	3.0	0.0	1.5	6.0	7.5
6	2.3	3.0	4.6	4.3	0.7	0.3	5.3	8.9
7	1.3	1.3	0.3	1.0	0.0	−0.7	2.6	1.3
8	3.3	3.0	2.0	2.7	−0.3	−0.7	6.3	4.7
9	3.3	5.7	2.7	2.7	2.4	0.0	9.0	5.4
10	4.5	3.0	3.7	3.5	−1.5	0.2	7.5	7.2
Means	2.83	2.97	2.80	3.02	0.140	−0.220	5.80	5.82
S^2	0.789	1.251	1.871	1.811	1.163	1.024	2.918	6.340

Crossover Design: Carryover Effect

As mentioned, the unbiased analysis of a crossover design depends on the absence of a carryover effect. If the treatment leaves carryover effects that influence the patient receiving the placebo in time period 2, a biased estimate of the treatment influence results. A term to represent this bias can be incorporated into the statistical model and assessed. Such a model is given in Table 2–22. The additional parameter π represents carryover effects from the treatment given in time period 1. The collected data for each pair of individuals has the same form as before. A series of the sums are calculated to estimate and test the magnitude of the carryover effect (π) prior to an investigation of the treatment influences. The data and the corresponding sums·are represented in Table 2–23.

The sums of the observations for time periods 1 and 2 for each patient produce an estimate of the carryover effect. Note that

$$C_1 = y_{\tau\delta} + y_0 \text{ estimates } 2\mu + \tau + \delta, \quad \text{and} \quad C_2 = y_\delta + y_{\tau\pi} \text{ estimates } 2\mu + \tau + \delta + \pi.$$

The difference of means of the C-values ($\bar{C}_i$ based on n within patient sums) estimates the amount of carryover effect since

$$\bar{C}_2 - \bar{C}_1 \quad \text{estimates } \pi \quad \text{or} \quad \hat{\pi} = \bar{C}_2 - \bar{C}_1,$$

which is the estimated difference in total mean response of type 1 and type 2 patients. The magnitude of this estimate is again evaluated with a t-test, and when $H_0: \pi = 0$ the test statistic

$$T_\pi = \frac{\hat{\pi} - \pi}{S_{\hat{\pi}}} = \frac{(\bar{C}_2 - \bar{C}_1) - 0}{S_{\bar{C}_2 - \bar{C}_1}} = \frac{\bar{C}_2 - \bar{C}_1}{\sqrt{(S_{\bar{C}_2}^2 + S_{\bar{C}_1}^2)/n}} \tag{2.37}$$

has a t-distribution with $2(n-1)$ degrees of freedom. Using the crossover design data from the noise experiment (Table 2–21) gives

$$T_\pi = \frac{5.820 - 5.800}{\sqrt{(2.918 + 6.340)/10}} = 0.020.$$

Clearly, the value of T_π indicates no evidence (p-value $= 0.982$) of a carryover effect from the 20 sampled individuals.

Table 2–22. Crossover design: carryover model

	Time 1	Time 2
Patient 1	μ	$\mu + \tau + \delta$
Patient 2	$\mu + \delta$	$\mu + \tau + \pi$

Table 2–23. Crossover design: observed data

	Time 1	Time 2	Sum
Patient 1	y_0	$y_{\tau\delta}$	$y_{\tau\delta} + y_0$
Patient 2	y_δ	$y_{\tau\pi}$	$y_\delta + y_{\tau\pi}$

If the null hypothesis is accepted $(\pi = 0)$, then it is common to behave as if no carryover effect exists and use the no-carryover model to analyze the data (Table 2–19). If the null hypothesis is rejected $(\pi \neq 0)$, it is recommended that only time period 1 be used in the analysis [11]. This strategy is not ideal, because the sample size is cut in half and no advantage is gained by the design. On the other hand, the time period 1 data does yield an unbiased estimate of the treatment effect.

An issue that occurs in a number of statistical analyses arises in connection with a crossover design. A bias results from using a preliminary statistical test to make decisions about further analyses. The test for a carryover effect determines how the analysis of the treatment will be conducted. Formal statistical tests (with some exceptions) require that decisions regarding the conduct of the test be made without knowledge derived from the collected data. Without employing special techniques, decisions based on the data at hand introduce bias into subsequent test procedures. That is, a test with a nominal significance level of α is no longer an α-level test. This test-direction bias was discussed earlier in a simpler context. However, if analyses are used without investigating the underlying assumptions, then potentially greater errors can occur. One solution, in the case of a crossover design, is to conduct both test (for carryover and treatment effects) at an $\alpha/2$ level and then the overall error rate for both tests will not exceed α. The complicated question of conducting multiple tests on a single set of data is an extensive topic (see [12]), and, other than pointing out the possibility of a bias, the topic will not be pursued further.

The crossover design illustrates a common approach to measuring and removing bias from a relationship under investigation. A model is formulated that describes the relationship of the bias to the outcome variable. Based on the postulated statistical structure the magnitude of the bias is estimated. If the bias has substantial impact, the analysis is adjusted to be "free" of the interfering influence. Frequently, this process is called statistical adjustment, and resulting estimates are referred to as adjusted estimates.

Confounder Bias: A Basic Description

The term confounder bias is widely used in epidemiologic analysis and will be described in several contexts, particularly Chapter 8. A simple model which provides a concrete illustration of this bias is

$$\text{Control individual:} \quad y_{1j} = \mu + bx_{1j} + e_{1j}$$
$$\text{Treatment individual:} \quad y_{2j} = \mu + \delta + bx_{2j} + e_{2j}.$$

(2.38)

The value y_{ij}, as before, represents the response of the variable of interest in the absence (y_{1j}) and presence (y_{2j}) of a treatment effect (δ). The symbol x_{ij} represents values of a variable related to y, which interferes with directly evaluating the treatment effect, sometimes called a confounder (i.e., producing confounder bias). This statistical model is an extension of the previous "shift" model where, again, the e_{ij} values represent a series of independent normally distributed influences (mean = 0, variance = σ^2).

If $\bar{x}_{1j}$ differs from $\bar{x}_{2j}$, then the difference $y_{2j} - y_{1j}$ does not exclusively reflect the influence of the treatment (δ), except when $b = 0$. The difference in mean response is a combination of influences from both the x-variable and the treatment. The inability to isolate and measure δ is an example of confounder bias. If the mean values of treatment and control groups are contrasted, then

$$\bar{y}_2 - \bar{y}_1 \quad \text{estimates} \quad \delta + b(\bar{x}_2 - \bar{x}_1)$$

for a two-sample model [expression (2.38)]. Clearly, if x_{ij} is unrelated to y ($b = 0$), the variable x does not play a role in measuring δ. There is no confounder bias. Also, if the x-variable is equally distributed between treatment and control groups, $\bar{x}_2 = \bar{x}_1$, then no confounder bias occurs. Otherwise, the x-variable distorts the difference between two means as an assessment of the influence represented by δ. The magnitude of the confounder bias is $b(\bar{x}_2 - \bar{x}_1)$. There are three fundamental methods to remove this confounder bias.

1. *Randomization to eliminate confounder bias.* The purpose of randomization is to balance between treatment and control groups variables associated with the response y so that the differences observed between groups are predominantly due to a treatment effect. Assigning observations randomly to the groups to be compared makes it likely that mean values of the x-variate in each group are similar. If $\bar{x}_1$ is approximately equal to $\bar{x}_2$, then the confounding influence of the x-variable is reduced. In terms of the model, when $\bar{x}_2 - \bar{x}_1$ has a difference of zero, $\bar{y}_2 - \bar{y}_1$ is an unbiased estimate of δ (no confounding from the value represented by x). Most epidemiologic data do not result from

randomized experiments, and the issue of confounder bias is dealt with using other approaches.

2. *Matching to eliminate confounder bias.* Another way to balance the x-values between treatment and control groups is to match each treatment individual with a control individual so that each pair has the same value of the x-variable. A difference in the mean values of y for a series of matched pairs then directly estimates δ free of confounder bias, because $\bar{x}_1$ must equal $\bar{x}_2$. For example, if x_{ij} represents a person's age and each pair of subjects is matched for age, then the mean ages for both treatment and control groups are identical. A difference in the mean responses measured by $\bar{y}_2 - \bar{y}_1$ directly estimates δ because it is not biased by the influence of age, even though age is related to y ($b \neq 0$ but $\bar{x}_1 - \bar{x}_2 = 0$).

A series of matched pairs can be statistically analyzed using a t-test applied to a sample of n within-pair differences such that

$$d_j = y_{2j} - y_{1j} \quad \text{and} \quad T = \frac{\bar{d}}{S_{\bar{d}}} = \sqrt{n}\,\frac{\bar{d}}{S_d}, \quad \text{where} \quad S_d^2 = \frac{1}{n-1} \sum_{j=1}^{n} (d_j - \bar{d})^2.$$

The resulting t-statistic has a t-distribution with $n - 1$ degrees of freedom when δ is 0.

A matched pair strategy is conceptually easy and leads to a simple analysis. However, there are some important disadvantages. Matches for individuals with unusual values for the confounder variable are sometimes hard to find, and imperfect matching removes only some of the confounder bias. A sample of matched pairs is not usually representative of any specific population which may reduce the general application of the analytic results. Also, in some situations statistical adjustment avoids the sometimes considerable logistical problems of collecting matched data. Chapter 9 describes in detail matching as a strategy to control for confounding bias.

3. *Statistical adjustment to eliminate confounder bias.* Adjustment is based strictly on a statistical model, and its success depends on whether the model accurately describes the underlying relationships in the data. For the present model, [expression (2.38)], two adjusted mean values remove the confounding bias of the x-variable. The adjusted mean values are

$$\bar{y}_1' = \bar{y}_1 - \hat{b}(\bar{x}_1 - \bar{x}) \quad \text{and} \quad \bar{y}_2' = \bar{y}_2 - \hat{b}(\bar{x}_2 - \bar{x}), \tag{2.39}$$

where $\bar{x}$ is the overall mean of the x-variable, then

$$\bar{y}_2' - \bar{y}_1' \quad \text{estimates} \quad \delta + (b - \hat{b})(\bar{x}_2 - \bar{x}_1). \tag{2.40}$$

Since it is likely, particularly for large samples of data, that $\hat{b}$ is essentially equal to b, then the difference between the adjusted mean values directly reflects the treatment effect or

$$\text{since} \quad b \approx \hat{b}, \quad \text{then} \quad \bar{y}_2 - \bar{y}_1 \quad \text{estimates} \quad \delta \quad \text{or} \quad \hat{\delta} = \bar{y}_2 - \bar{y}_1 \, (2.41)$$

regardless of the values of $\bar{x}_1$ and $\bar{x}_2$ ($\bar{x}_1 \neq \bar{x}_2$, but $b - \hat{b} \approx 0$).

When the confounding variable is linearly related to y [expression (2.38)], application of simple linear regression techniques produces an estimate of b. The coefficient b estimated from one group (b_1) is

$$\hat{b}_1 = \frac{S_{x_1 y_1}}{S_{x_1 x_1}} = \frac{\sum (x_{1j} - \bar{x}_1)(y_{1j} - \bar{y}_1)}{\sum (x_{1j} - \bar{x}_1)^2}, \tag{2.42}$$

and the coefficient b estimated from the other group (b_2) is similarly estimated by

$$\hat{b}_2 = \frac{S_{x_2 y_2}}{S_{x_2 x_2}} = \frac{\sum (x_{2j} - \bar{x}_2)(y_{2j} - \bar{y}_2)}{\sum (x_{2j} - \bar{x}_2)^2}. \tag{2.43}$$

Since the model postulates a single value for the parameter b, these two estimates are combined to give a single estimate ($\hat{b}$) as

$$\hat{b} = \frac{w_1 \hat{b}_1 + w_2 \hat{b}_2}{w_1 + w_2} = \frac{S_{x_1 y_1} + S_{x_2 y_2}}{S_{x_1 x_1} + S_{x_2 x_2}} \quad \text{with} \quad w_i = S_{x_i x_i}. \tag{2.44}$$

Therefore, $\bar{y}_1'$ and $\bar{y}_2'$ can be derived from the data, and the difference between these two adjusted mean values is an unbiased ("free" from confounding bias) estimate of the influence δ when the postulated model represents the relationships between groups, confounder, and outcome. Geometrically, the value $\bar{y}_2' - \bar{y}_1'$ is the distance between two straight lines with common slopes $\hat{b}$ and is a special case of a general approach to adjusting mean values called the analysis of covariance. Expressions for the variance and confidence interval for these adjusted mean values are found in [13] along with an extensive discussion of confidence intervals in general.

Ecologic Bias

The fact that the behavior of certain summary measures derived from a series of groups rarely reflects the behavior of the individuals who make up the groups was noted by Robinson [14] and subsequently called the ecologic fallacy or ecologic bias. In one form the ecologic fallacy appears as a bias in correlation and regression coefficients.

Correlation

Correlation coefficients are easily calculated from pairs of variables that summarize groups of observations. The correlation between the mean levels of air pollution and the mortality rates in a series of countries [15], or the correlation between the percentages of partici- pates in driver education courses and the rates of fatal automobile accidents among teenagers in a series of 27 states [3] are examples. Perhaps the most famous ecologic correlation is the association between the amount of fat consumption in the diet (percent of total calories) and the death rates from degenerative heart disease among a series of countries [16]. Japan had the lowest levels of both fat consumption and heart disease mortality with a more or less smooth increasing progression to the United States with the highest fat consumption and highest mortality rates. However, the interpretation of the resulting correlation coefficient is not simple.

A numeric example shows the difficulty of drawing conclusions from correlations between variables calculated from grouped data (e.g., means, percentages, or rates). Suppose that the following pairs of mean values were observed, one pair from each of four groups:

Group 1: $\bar{x}_1 = 3$ $\bar{y}_1 = 30$
Group 2: $\bar{x}_2 = 4$ $\bar{y}_2 = 40$
Group 3: $\bar{x}_3 = 5$ $\bar{y}_3 = 50$
Group 4: $\bar{x}_4 = 6$ $\bar{y}_4 = 60.$

The correlation between these four values is $\bar{r} = +1$. The quantity $\bar{r}$ represents the correlation among the four pairs of mean values of $\bar{x}$ and $\bar{y}$ and, as Robinson [24] pointed out, this correlation is unlikely to re- flect the relationships among the individuals that generated the grouped data. This property is clearly seen from the values in Table 2–24.

The mean values from each group in Table 2–24 are the above means $\bar{x}_i$ and $\bar{y}_i$ and, as before, the correlation coefficient is $\bar{r} = +1$. The correlation, however, among the individuals in each group is $r = -1$. In fact, the correlation r reflecting the association among individuals can take on any value between -1 and $+1$ regardless of the value of $\bar{r}$. Although the example is simple, it shows the essential problem of interpretation of a correlation based on grouped data. A correlation between fat intake and degenerative heart disease shows a relationship among countries but does not indicate the relationship between fat consumption and risk of degenerative heart disease in individuals. It is entirely possible that the individuals dying of degenerative heart disease are not the individuals consuming large quantities of fat. In any case, the correlation based on grouped data certainly does not indicate the relationship among individuals.

Observations from grouped data certainly have a role in epidemio- logy and play a part in many aspects of understanding the factors

Table 2–24. Artificial data illustrating differences between a correlation based on individual observations and a correlation based on grouped data

Group 1		Group 2		Group 3		Group 4	
x	y	x	y	x	y	x	y
1	50	2	60	3	70	4	80
2	40	3	50	4	60	5	70
3	30	4	40	5	50	6	60
4	20	5	30	6	40	7	50
5	10	6	20	7	30	8	40

underlying disease. Nevertheless, calculating a correlation coefficient directly from values derived from a grouped data $(\bar{r})$ is not a replacement for the correlation (r) within groups.

Regression

Ecologic bias also influences regression analysis. Consider the variables x_1 and x_2 entered as predictor variables into a linear bivariate regression equation or

$$y_i = a + b_1 x_{1i} + b_2 x_{2i} + e_i, \tag{2.45}$$

where e_i again represents a series of independent and normally distributed error terms with the same variance.

If k groups of size n are randomly formed from a set of N values (y_i, x_{1i}, x_{2i}), then estimates of the regression coefficients are not biased by the grouping process. In other words, the regression analysis based on mean values $(\bar{y}_i, \bar{x}_{1i}, \bar{x}_{2i})$ from randomly grouped data consistently reflects, with loss of precision, the underlying linear relationship. Even if the data are ordered into k groups based on x_1, the regression analysis employing means calculated from each group produces consistent estimates of the parameters of the linear model. Unlike the correlation coefficient estimated from group data, the estimated regression co-efficients are not biased and reflect the relationships among the dependent variable and the independent variables. However, if the variable used to form the groups is not included in the analysis, the resulting estimate of the remaining regression coefficient is biased. If x_1 is again used to order the data, for example, but not included in the regression analysis, then employing k pairs of mean values $(\bar{y}_j, \bar{x}_{2j})$ gives a biased estimate of the regression coefficient associated with x_2, where the bias is approximately $b_1 \bar{r}^2 / r$ or b_1 / r for large sample sizes where r is the correlation between x_1 and x_2, and $\bar{r}$ is the correlation between $\bar{x}_1$ and $\bar{x}_2$. This bias can be substantial.

A correlation coefficient calculated from grouped data is usually misleading when interpreted as the measure of the correlation that would have resulted if the nonaggregated data were employed (a good discussion is found in [17]). A similar bias in the regression coefficients occurs when the coefficients are estimated from grouped data and the analytic model fails to include measures that reflect the grouping process. The "ecologic fallacy" in terms of a regression coefficient can be considered as a special case of incomplete model bias [18]. From another point of view, the grouping process is a confounding influence on the relationships under investigation, and failure to account for this influence in the analysis produces confounder bias. Therefore, a fundamental question associated with applying linear regression analysis to summary measures derived from grouped data is whether the process underlying the formation of the groups is measured and included in the model. If the answer is yes, the estimated equation may be of value (no ecologic bias). If the answer is no (which is usually the case), the estimated regression equation has little value with respect to understanding the relationships among the individuals who make up the sampled groups (ecologic bias).

3 Statistical Power and Sample-Size Calculations

A primary goal of statistical analysis is to detect systematic influences in the presence of random variation. The likelihood that a statistical technique correctly detects nonrandom effects is called *power*. Statistical power is rigorously defined by two specific hypotheses, the null and the alternative. The null hypothesis asserts that all observed variation is due to the variability intrinsic in the material under investigation. The alternative hypothesis states that a systematic (nonrandom) influence explains at least some of the observed variation. Power is measured by the probability of rejecting the null hypothesis when the alternative is true. That is, power is the probability of identifying a systematic effect when it exists.

Technical Details

To explore the concept of power, a statistical structure is postulated consisting of a null and an alternative hypothesis. A statistical summary represented by X, with a normal or approximately normal distribution, will be used to choose between these two hypotheses. When the null hypothesis is true, this summary X has a normal distribution with mean $= \mu_0$ and variance $= \sigma_0^2$. When the alternative hypothesis is true, X also has a normal distribution but with mean $= \mu$ and variance $= \sigma^2$. In symbols,

Null hypothesis—H_0: mean of $X = \mu_0$ with   variance $(X) = \sigma_0^2$ and

Alternative hypothesis—H_1: mean of $X = \mu > \mu_0$ with   variance $(X) = \sigma^2$.

An observed value of X leads to a decision to accept or reject H_0 (reject or accept H_1). The first step in the process of deciding between these two hypotheses is to define a decision rule. A usual rule is: If the summary statistic X exceeds a specific point (called the α-level critical point, represented as $c_{1-\alpha}$), then the null hypothesis is rejected in favor of the alternative hypothesis and, conversely, if X is less than

$c_{1-\alpha}$, then the null hypothesis is accepted. In other words, if X is sufficiently large, then it is inferred that H_1 is a better description of the distribution that generated the data than H_0.

The critical point is determined so that the null hypothesis is mistakenly rejected with a predetermined probability, called a type I error rate or level of significance and symbolized as α. That is,

$$P(X > c_{1-\alpha}) = \alpha \tag{3.1}$$

is the probability of rejecting the null hypothesis when it is true. Since X is assumed to have a normal distribution (mean $= \mu_0$ and variance $= \sigma_0^2$ under H_0), then

$$P\left(Z > \frac{c_{1-\alpha} - \mu_0}{\sigma_0}\right) = \alpha, \tag{3.2}$$

where Z represents a variable with a standard normal distribution (mean $= 0$ and variance $= 1$). Therefore, the α-level critical point is

$$c_{1-\alpha} = z_{1-\alpha}\sigma_0 + \mu_0. \tag{3.3}$$

The symbol $z_{1-\alpha}$ represents the $(1 - \alpha)$-th percentile of the standard normal distribution. The value $c_{1-\alpha}$ is determined solely on the basis of H_0 and a selected value for probability α.

Since the power of the test statistic X is measured by the probability of rejecting the null hypothesis H_0 when the alternative hypothesis H_1 is true, then

$$\text{power} = 1 - \beta = P(X > c_{1-\alpha}) = P(X > z_{1-\alpha}\sigma_0 + \mu_0), \tag{3.4}$$

and, again, because X is assumed to have at least an approximate normal distribution,

$$\text{power} = P\left(Z > \frac{z_{1-\alpha}\sigma_0 + \mu_0 - \mu}{\sigma}\right) = P(Z > z_\beta), \tag{3.5}$$

where

$$z_\beta = \frac{z_{1-\alpha}\sigma_0 + \mu_0 - \mu}{\sigma}. \tag{3.6}$$

When the null hypothesis, the alternative hypothesis, and the type I error rate are known or postulated, the power of the test statistic X is the probability $P(Z > z_\beta) = 1 - \beta$. The symbol β represents the probability of rejecting the alternative hypothesis when it is true, called a type II error. A type II error occurs when sampling variation causes X to be less than $c_{1-\alpha}$ when the alternative hypothesis is true, leading to a mistaken acceptance of the null hypothesis. The expression (3.6) for z_β relates the null hypothesis, the alternative hypothesis, and the

α-level to the power of the test statistic X and is a key element in assessing the likelihood of identifying systematic influences in a data set. The expression for z_β also leads to sample-size calculations (following sections).

The power of a test statistic X does not depend in any way on the observed values from the sampled data. It is entirely determined by H_0, H_1, and α. Figure 3–1 illustrates a distribution of X under the null hypothesis $H_0: \mu_0 = 2$ with variance $= \sigma_0^2 = 2$ and under the alternative hypothesis $H_1: \mu = 5$ with variance $= \sigma^2 = 2$, where $\alpha = 0.05$. For this case, $c_{1-\alpha} = c_{0.95} = 4.326$. This hypothetical structure produces a type II error of $\beta = 0.317$, and the power to discriminate between random (H_0) and systematic (H_1) effects on the basis of an observed value of X is $1 - \beta = 0.683$. A summary of the hypothesis testing notation is shown in Table 3–1. Specifically, for the example (Figure 3–1), the four probabilities associated with a test of hypothesis are given in Table 3–2.

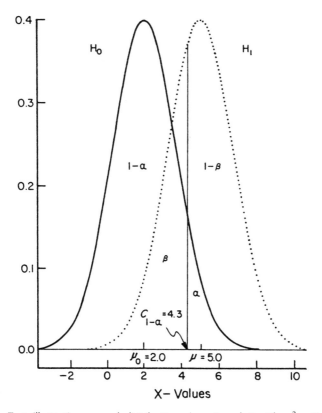

Figure 3–1. Two illustrative normal distributions ($\mu = 2$ and 5 with $\sigma^2 = 2$) generated under null and alternative hypotheses

Table 3–1. Notation

	H_0 is true	H_0 is false
	H_1 is false	H_1 is true
Accept H_0 (reject H_1)	$1 - \alpha$	Type II error = β
Reject H_0 (accept H_1)	Type I error = α	Power = $1 - \beta$

Table 3–2. Illustration

	H_0 is true	H_0 is false
	H_1 is false	H_1 is true
Accept H_0 (reject H_1)	0.95	0.317
Reject H_0 (accept H_1)	0.05	0.683

This section describes the power of a test statistic X where large values of X lead to rejecting the null hypothesis. The situation where small values of X lead to rejecting H_0 does not differ in principle and is similarly developed with only minor changes. The calculation of the power for a two-sided test (large values or small values lead to rejecting H_0) is a bit more complicated but does not differ in principle and is not presented.

Normal Distribution: Sample Mean

A potentially toxic material found in the workplace is benzene. The federal government has established a safety standard of 1.0 part benzene per million (ppm). The question arises: Is it likely that a company with a mean level of 1.5 ppm will be detected in violation of this standard using a sample of $n = 10$ measured exposures? The benzene exposure values have an approximate normal distribution; therefore the sample mean $\bar{x}$ also has an approximately normal distribution. The summary statistic $\bar{x}$ (i.e., $X = \bar{x}$) is used to discriminate between the null hypothesis that the workplace mean is at the standard versus the alternative hypothesis that the workplace mean exceeds the standard by 0.5 ppm or

Meets standard—H_0: expectation of $\bar{x} = \mu_0 = 1.0$ with $\sigma_0^2 = $ variance$(\bar{x}) = 1.4/10$

Exceeds standard—H_1: expectation of $\bar{x} = \mu = 1.5$ with $\sigma^2 = $ variance$(\bar{x}) = 1.4/10$, where the background variation $\sigma^2 = 1.4$ comes from a large previous data set. Using the values generated by H_0 and H_1 and choosing $\alpha = 0.05$ $(z_{1-\alpha} = z_{0.95} = 1.645)$ gives

$$z_\beta = \frac{1.645\sqrt{1.4/10} + 1.0 - 1.5}{\sqrt{1.4/10}} = 0.309 \tag{3.7}$$

and

$$P(Z > z_\beta) = P(Z > 0.309) = 0.379. \tag{3.8}$$

Companies with workplace means in violation of the standard by more than 0.5 ppm will be detected at least 38% of the time when a sample of 10 workers is used.

Perhaps the weakest link in the argument that produces a power calculation is the determination of the variance of the test statistic X. In most situations, it is difficult and sometimes impossible to get reliable estimates of the background variation under the null hypothesis and the alternative hypothesis. The variance of $\bar{x}$ for the benzene example is $\sigma_0^2 = \sigma^2 = 0.14$ based, as mentioned, on a large quantity of previously collected benzene data and assumed equal for both the null and alternative hypotheses. Occasionally, reasonable variance values are available from relevant literature or pilot studies but, by and large, it is rare that σ_0^2 and σ^2 are known with any degree of certainty.

Poisson Distribution: Relative Risk

A power calculation is often revealing in the investigation of an environmental exposure. Suppose a region is exposed to a toxic material suspected of causing a birth defect, such as an area in a county exposed to a water supply contaminant. Interest is focused on the probability that an infant born in the contaminated area will have a birth defect compared to the probability for unexposed newborns (e.g., the rest of the county). Such a comparison can be summarized by a relative risk; the ratio of the probability of the event in the exposed group divided by the same probability in the unexposed group.

When a rare event such as a birth defect is under consideration, a Poisson distribution (details in Appendix B) is often used to describe the distribution of the number of occurrences of these events.

> Aside: The Poisson distribution can be derived from basic considerations [1] or it can be viewed as an approximation for the binomial distribution where the probability of a specific event (p) is small and the number of possible events (n) is large (again see Appendix B). The expected value is np which in the context of a Poisson distribution is often symbolized

by λ (i.e., $np = \lambda$). The assumptions underlying these two distributions are the same, namely each of a series of n binary events occur independently with constant probability p. Both probability distributions describe the number of specific occurrences X among a series of events. For example, if $p = 0.03$ and $n = 100$, then the probability that $X = 2$ specific occurrences will occur among $n = 100$ possible events is

$$P(X = 2) = \binom{100}{2} p^2(1 - p)^{98} = 0.2252 \tag{3.9}$$

based on the binomial distribution or

$$P(X = 2) = \frac{e^{-\lambda}\lambda^2}{2!} = \frac{e^{-3}3^2}{2} = 0.2240 \tag{3.10}$$

based on the Poisson distribution. A feature of the Poisson distribution is that only the expected number of events λ needs to be specified to determine the probability distribution of X while values for both n and p are necessary to calculate binomial probabilities.

The mean and the variance of the Poisson distribution have the same value, namely the expected number of events in the population under consideration (see Appendix B). For pregnant women exposed to toxic material in the water supply, the expected number of newborns with malformations is represented by np, where n is the number of exposed mothers and p is the probability of a birth defect among those exposed mothers. If a toxic material has no adverse effects on pregnancy outcome, then the expected number of cases in the con-taminated area is np_0, where p_0 is the probability of a birth defect among unexposed mothers (the null hypothesis). The relative risk is defined as $\rho = p/p_0$. When p_0 (the "background" probability) is known or postulated, power calculations show the likelihood of detecting specific increases in relative risk for different numbers of exposed individuals for chosen error rates α and β.

The observed number of birth defects $(X = \hat{M})$ will be used to discriminate between the null hypothesis that no difference exists in frequency of birth defects in exposed and unexposed areas (i.e., $H_0: p = p_0$, then $\rho = 1$) and the alternative hypothesis that the exposed area has a greater frequency of birth defects (i.e., $H_1: p > p_0$, then $\rho > 1$). Applying the Poisson structure to describe the number of birth defects gives

No excess risk—H_0: expected number of defects $= np_0$ with variance$(\hat{M}) =$ np_0

Excess risk—H_1: expected number of defects $= np = n\rho p_0$ with variance$(\hat{M}) =$ $np = n\rho p_0$

and, as before, the approximate power is

$$P(\hat{Z} > z_\beta) = 1 - \beta \tag{3.11}$$

which is the probability of detecting an excess of birth defects based on $\hat{M}$ in the exposed area when the contaminant is associated with an increase (H_1 true: $p > p_0$). Applying expression (3.6) gives

$$z_\beta = \frac{z_{1-\alpha} + \sqrt{np_0(1 - \rho)}}{\sqrt{\rho}} \tag{3.12}$$

for this special Poisson case.

It is postulated that $\hat{M}$, the observed number of birth defects, has an approximately normal distribution which in many cases (np not too small) is a realistic assumption. That is, the normal distribution serves as an approximation to the Poisson distribution to facilitate the calculation of the power of the test. A direct calculation is also possible. When $\rho = 1$, then $z_\beta = z_{1-\alpha}$ so that the null hypothesis will be mistakenly rejected with probability α, P(type I error) $= \alpha$. Figure 3–2 shows four power curves associated with different relative risks and sample sizes (number of exposed pregnancies) when $p_0 = 0.01$ and $\alpha = 0.05$. These power curves are generated by using specific numeric values and expression (3.12). It can be seen, for example, that about an 86% chance exists of detecting a relative risk of 2.5 when 500

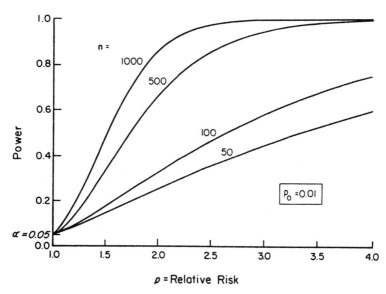

Figure 3–2. Power for detecting an excess relative risk ρ for sample sizes $n = 50, 100, 500,$ and 1000 for $p_0 = 0.01$

individuals are exposed but only a 46% chance when 100 individuals are exposed.

Sample Size: One-Sample Test of a Proportion

Power considerations can be used to calculate the sample size necessary to meet selected levels of type I (α) and type II (β) errors. The test of a single proportion illustrates a general pattern for a sample-size calculation. For a series of binary outcomes, the proportion of a specific result is commonly calculated (represented by $\hat{p}$). The statistic $\hat{p}$ could, for example, be the proportion of male infants recorded in a series of births, the proportion of times the white pieces win a chess match in a series of games, or the proportion of recessive genetic traits observed in a series of individuals. The test statistic $X = \hat{p}$ is used to discriminate between two hypotheses. The null hypothesis states that the observed proportion differs only because of chance variation from a specified proportion p_0. For example, playing the white or black chess pieces produces no difference in the probability of winning ($p = p_0 = 0.50$). The alternative hypothesis states that $\hat{p}$ differs only by chance from another population value, symbolized by p_1. That is, the observed difference between $\hat{p}$ and p_0 is due to a systematic effect—white pieces, for example, have an advantage ($p = p_1 > 0.50$, or say $p_1 = 0.60$). The test statistic $X = \hat{p}$ is used to choose between p_0 and p_1 as a description of the sampled population. In symbols,

Null hypothesis—H_0: proportion $= p_0$ with
$$\sigma_0^2 = \text{variance } (\hat{p}) = p_0(1 - p_0)/n$$

Alternative hypothesis—H_1: proportion $= p_1 > p_0$ with
$$\sigma^2 = \text{variance } (\hat{p}) = p_1(1 - p_1)/n,$$

where n represents the number of samples collected. Using these proportions and variances along with the expression for power [expression (3.6)] produces an approximate expression for the sample size n of

$$n = \frac{p(1 - p)(z_{1-\alpha} + z_{1-\beta})^2}{(p_1 - p_0)^2}, \qquad (3.13)$$

where $p = (p_0 + p_1)/2$. The value n is the approximate sample size necessary to attain the specified error probabilities α and β. It is assumed, for the sake of simplicity, that $p_0(1 - p_0) \approx p_1(1 - p_1) \approx p(1 - p)$, which is approximately true for proportions between 0.3 and 0.7. Specifically, the expression for sample size n is derived from the values $\mu_0 = p_0$, $\mu = p_1$, and $\sigma_0^2 \approx \sigma^2 \approx p(1-p)/n$ substituted into the expression (3.6), which is then solved for n. The resulting value for n is approximate because $\hat{p}$ has only an approximate normal distribution. Therefore, when p is small (<0.3) or large (>0.7) the approximation works less well (see Table 1–3). For p in the neighborhood of 0.0 or 1.0, alternative methods should be employed ([2] or [3]). Analogous to the Poisson case, the normal distribution is used to approximate a binomial distribution to easily calculate sample size.

The sample size n can be found for specified values p_0, p_1, α, and β. For example, if α is set at 0.05 ($z_{1-\alpha} = 1.645$), β at 0.10 ($z_{1-\beta} = 1.282$), $p_0 = 0.5$, and $p_1 = 0.6$, then from expression (3.13) the sample size is $n = 212$ using $p = 0.55$. A sample, therefore, of about 212 observations will correctly discriminate between population proportions 0.5 and 0.6 with a probability of 0.90 (power) and, at the same time, the probability of falsely declaring a difference exists is 0.05 (type I error—level of significance).

To get an idea of the relationship between the difference ($p_1 - p_0$) and sample size, consider the case where p_0 and p_1 are in the neighborhood of 0.5 with α and β set at 0.02. The sample size to attain these error rates is approximately

$$n \approx \frac{4}{(p_1 - p_0)^2}. \tag{3.14}$$

If $p_0 = 0.50$ and $p_1 = 0.51$, then $n \approx 4/0.01^2 = 40{,}000$ or if $p_0 = 0.50$ and $p_1 = 0.55$, then $n \approx 4/0.05^2 = 1{,}600$ or if $p_0 = 0.50$ and $p_1 = 0.60$, then $n \approx 4/0.1^2 = 400$. These normal-based sample-size calculations show the obvious underlying principle that as the distance between p_0 and p_1 decreases (for specific levels of α and β), then larger, sometimes considerably larger, sample sizes are required to detect reliably which value, p_0 or p_1, best represents the "true" proportion in the population sampled.

Sample Size: Two-Sample Test of Proportions

A two-sample situation occurs when two proportions, each from a different source, are estimated and compared. A difference between these observed proportions indicates one of two possibilities—the difference occurred by chance (null hypothesis) or a systematic difference exists between the two sources of data (alternative hypothesis). For example, $\hat{p}_1$ could be the proportion of *in situ* cervical cancer incidence cases in a specific community observed in 1980 and $\hat{p}_2$ the proportion observed in 1985. These two values undoubtedly differ, but is this observed difference due to the natural fluctuation of sampled values or due to a change in the cancer-staging distribution? The test statistic $X = \hat{p}_2 - \hat{p}_1$ is used to discriminate between H_0 and H_1 where $\hat{p}_1$ and $\hat{p}_2$ are the sample proportions from each of two sources of data. The formal hypotheses are:

No difference in proportions—H_0: $p_1 = p_2 = p$ with variance $(\hat{p}_1 - \hat{p}_2) = 2p (1 - p)/n$

Difference in proportions—H_1: $p_2 > p_1$ with variance $(\hat{p}_1 - \hat{p}_2) = p_1(1 - p_1)/n + p_2(1 - p_2)/n$.

Again using the expression (3.6), solving for n yields

$$n = \frac{(z_{1-\alpha}\sqrt{2p(1-p)} + z_{1-\beta}\sqrt{p_1(1-p_1) + p_2(1-p_2)})^2}{(p_2 - p_1)^2}, \quad (3.15)$$

where $p = (p_1 + p_2)/2$.

The value n is the approximate number of sample observations necessary from each source (assumed equal here but similar calculations can be made for the case of unequal sample sizes). If $p_1 = 0.10$ and $p_2 = 0.15$, then a sample of $n = 748$ observations from each population is necessary to achieve a type I error of $\alpha = 0.05$ and a type II error $= \beta$ of 0.10 (a total of $n = 1,496$ observations). Table 3–3 illustrates a series of sample sizes associated with $\alpha = 0.05$, $\beta = 0.10$, and $p_1 = 0.10$ for different values of p_2. Figure 3–3 shows plots of the sample-size curves (two versions of the same curve) associated with detecting a difference between two proportions.

If p_1 and p_2 are again about 0.5 with α and β set at 0.02, then

$$n \approx \frac{8}{(p_1 - p_2)^2}. \quad (3.16)$$

for each of the two samples. Comparing this result with the previous one-sample result [expression (3.14)] shows, not surprisingly, a fourfold increase in total sample size necessary to detect a difference between two sample proportions. As before, this sample-size calculation is approximate and only applies to restricted values of p; nevertheless, it indicates that the two-sample situation requires about four times as many observations to achieve the same error rates as the one-sample case.

Table 3–3. Sample size: two-sample situation

p_2	0.15	0.20	0.25	0.30	0.35	0.40	0.45	0.50	0.55	0.60	0.65	0.70	0.75	0.80	0.85	0.90
n	748	217	109	67	46	34	26	21	17	14	12	10	8	7	6	5

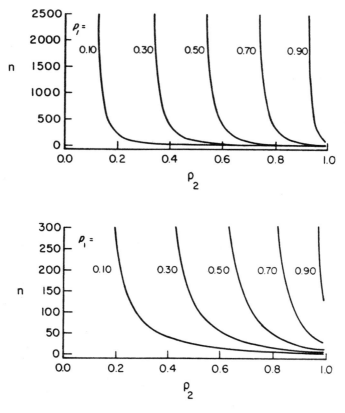

Figure 3–3. Sample sizes (n) for comparing p_1 (0.1, 0.3, 0.5, 0.7, and 0.9) to p_2 with type I error $= \alpha = 0.05$ and type II error $= \beta = 0.10$ (one set of curves plotted on different scales)

The odds are the ratio of the probability that an event occurs divided by the probability an event does not occur. The odds ratio is simply the ratio of two sets of odds (see Appendix C for a more complete description, additionally a number of texts completely describe the odds ratio measure of association, for example [4] and [5]). Occasionally it is desirable to calculate the sample size necessary to detect an elevated odds ratio (represented as *or*) given the probability of disease among those individuals unexposed to a risk factor (p_0). To estimate a sample size, the values *or* and p_0 are used to generate the probability of disease among those individuals with the risk factor (p_1). That is, for a given value of *or* and p_0

$$or = \frac{p_1/(1-p_1)}{p_0/(1-p_0)}, \quad \text{then} \quad p_1 = \frac{p_0(or)}{1 + p_0(or-1)}. \tag{3.17}$$

The values p_0 (given) and p_1 (calculates from the postulated odds ratio) can be used in expression (3.15) for computing the sample size (n) necessary to detect specific differences in two proportions for selected error rates $(\alpha$ and $\beta)$. Note that the value of n is the number of individuals in each group compared (a total of $2n$ observations is necessary, as before). For example, if the background frequency of a disease is $p_0 = 0.02$ and sufficient data must be collected to detect an odds ratio of 3.0, then

$$p_1 = \frac{0.02(3.0)}{1 + 0.02(3.0 - 1)} = 0.058, \tag{3.18}$$

implying that a sample size of approximately $n = 567$ must be collected from each sampled population for $\alpha = 0.05$ and $\beta = 0.05$; that is, 567 individuals with the risk factor and the same number without the risk factor. Once p_1 is calculated from or and p_0, the sample size n is calculated using the same normal approximation as the previous two-sample approach. Although this sample-size calculation gives some idea of the required number of observations, the estimate is not accurate in all situations. When the difference in proportions is in the neighborhood of -1 or $+1$, for example, the normal distribution fails to be a good approximation due to the asymmetry of the distribution of estimated values $\hat{p}_1 - \hat{p}_0$. A few illustrative values for $p_0 = 0.02$ are given in Table 3–4.

Two comments: The two earlier expressions for sample size [expressions (3.13) and (3.15)] are special cases of the general expression

$$n = \frac{(z_{1-\alpha}\sigma_0 + z_{1-\beta}\sigma)^2}{(\mu - \mu_0)^2}, \tag{3.19}$$

which is used in other situations where the null and the alternative hypotheses are defined in terms of normal distributions.

Table 3–4. Illustration of the odds ratio sample sizes $(\alpha = \beta = 0.05$ and $p_0 = 0.02)$

Odds Ratio	p_1	n
1.5	0.030	5,569
2.0	0.039	1,682
2.5	0.049	877
3.0	0.058	567
3.5	0.067	410
4.0	0.075	318
4.5	0.084	258
5.0	0.093	216

Applied power or sample-size calculations based on the assumption that the test statistic X is normally distributed are approximate (sometimes very approximate) and in certain cases can be "fine tuned" to be more accurate (e.g., [3]). However, it is not always possible to define the alternative hypothesis or the required variances with sufficient precision so that this "fine tuning" is worthwhile. These approximate calculations should be motivated by the desire to get a rough idea of the range of sample sizes (power) associated with a series of analytic strategies at the study design stage. The description of this range is an important part in planning an approach to data collection.

Additional Power

The question: How can the power to detect an association be increased? is easily answered. Increase the number of sampled observations. Power can also be increased, however, without collecting more data, by changing the α level of a statistical test. The tradition of setting α (type I error rate) at 0.05 is almost universal and rarely altered. A "5%" test is not usually required; in fact, the level of significance can certainly be set at any level. Increasing the level of significance increases the power of a test.

For example, if $\mu_0 = 2$ (H_0) and $\mu_1 = 5$ (H_1) are mean values from two normal distributions with equal variances ($\sigma_0^2 = \sigma^2 = 2$), then increases in significance level α produce increases in the power $1 - \beta$. Specifically, see the values in Table 3–5.

If the null hypothesis is rejected more often, then a direct consequence is that the alternative hypothesis will be accepted more often when it is true. While it is important to detect effects if they exist and not so important that effects are declared to exist when they do not, increasing the type I error is sometimes a useful strategy for increasing the power associated with a statistical procedure without collecting additional data.

Loss of Statistical Power and Bias from Grouping Continuous Data

For generally unclear reasons, investigators occasionally judge that, when a continuous variable is not measured precisely, grouping data

Table 3–5. Illustration of the relationship between α and $1 - \beta$

α	0.005	0.010	0.025	0.050	0.100	0.150	0.200	0.250	0.300
$1 - \beta$	0.325	0.419	0.564	0.683	0.799	0.861	0.900	0.926	0.945

into categories and using contingency table techniques is superior to analyses based directly on the continuous measures themselves. A statistical model gives some idea of the consequences of this decision in terms of loss of power and bias.

Assume that a continuous variable labeled Y, used to measure the disease process under investigation, has a normal distribution. For example, Y could represent the level of an individual's systolic blood pressure. Further, assume that a dichotomous risk factor E exists such as educational level—no college education ($E = 0$) versus college education ($E = 1$). The variables Y and E define a population model where Y is normally distributed with mean μ_0 when $E = 0$ and with mean μ_1 when $E = 1$ ($\mu_0 < \mu_1$). Both normal distributions are assumed to have the same variance, say $\sigma_Y^2 = 1.0$ for convenience. If a sample of k individuals is randomly selected from this population, the expected data would produce the 2×2 contingency table with the expected cell counts N_{ij} shown in Table 3–6. The prevalence of the risk factor E is represented as p [i.e., $p = P(E = 1)$].

The symbol $\bar{D}$ represents all observations when $Y \leq c$, and D represents observations when $Y > c$. A dichotomous variable (D and $\bar{D}$) results from grouping the continuous variable Y into "diseased" and "nondiseased" categories based on a cut-point c. For example, the point c could be the point midway between the two distribution [i.e., $c = \frac{1}{2}(\mu_0 + \mu_1)$]. A familiar example of such a practice is defining individuals as nonhypertensive (say, $Y \leq c = 140$) and hypertensive ($Y > c = 140$) based on systolic blood pressure. Then, if $c = \frac{1}{2}(\mu_0 + \mu_1)$,

$$\Phi = P(Y \leq \tfrac{1}{2}(\mu_0 + \mu_1) \,|\, E = 0) = P(Y > \tfrac{1}{2}(\mu_0 + \mu_1) \,|\, E = 1)$$

$$= \frac{1}{\sqrt{2\pi}} \int_{-\infty}^{(1/2)(\mu_1 - \mu_0)} e^{-(1/2)t^2} \, dt. \tag{3.20}$$

This statistical structure is represented in Table 3–6 and depicted in Figure 3–4.

Table 3–6. Expected frequencies

	$\bar{D}$ (no "disease")	D ("disease")
No college ($E = 0$)	$N_{00} = k(1 - p)\Phi$	$N_{10} = k(1 - p)(1 - \Phi)$
College ($E = 1$)	$N_{01} = kp(1 - \Phi)$	$N_{11} = kp\,\Phi$

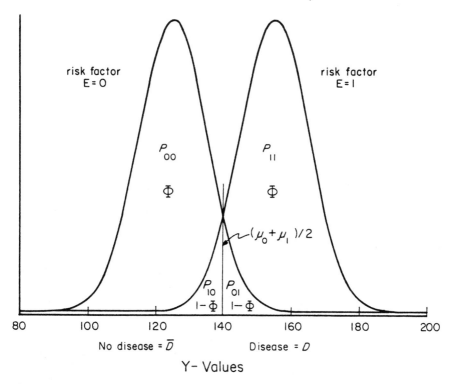

Figure 3–4. Model of a continuous variable grouped into four categories where two levels of a risk factor are investigated for a normally distributed outcome variable

To measure the association between the two binary variables E and D, the odds ratio is

$$\text{odds ratio} = \widehat{or} = \frac{\mathcal{N}_{00}/\mathcal{N}_{10}}{\mathcal{N}_{01}/\mathcal{N}_{11}} \tag{3.21}$$

and the value expected from the population model is $\widehat{or} = [\Phi/(1-\Phi)]^2$ or $\log(\widehat{or}) = 2\log[\Phi/(1-\Phi)]$. The variance of $\log[\widehat{or}]$ for the special case where $c = \frac{1}{2}(\mu_0 + \mu_1)$ is expressed as [applying expression (A.15) given in Appendix C]

$$\text{variance } (\log[\widehat{or}]) \approx [kp(1-p)\Phi(1-\Phi)]^{-1} \tag{3.22}$$

and, as before, k represents the total number of sampled individuals.

A typical α-level test of the hypothesis of no association between risk factor and disease generates

$$H_0: or = 1.0 \quad \text{versus} \quad H_1: or > 1.0,$$

and is used to assess the role of the risk factor E. If the power of this test is set at a level $1 - \beta$ or $P(\text{reject } H_0 | H_1 \text{ is true}) = 1 - \beta$, then the necessary sample size k to achieve a power of $1 - \beta$ with signficance level $= \alpha$ is approximately

$$k = \frac{\left[2z_{1-\alpha} + \dfrac{z_{1-\beta}}{\sqrt{\Phi(1 - \Phi)}} \right]^2}{p(1 - p)[\log{(or)}]^2} \tag{3.23}$$

from the expression (3.19).

For continuous rather than binary data, the comparison of two mean values (two-sample test) each based on samples from two normal distributions with equal variance is a classic problem in statistics. For example, to compare two mean values ($\bar{y}_1$ for the population defined by $E = 1$ and $\bar{y}_0$ for $E = 0$), the test statistic $\bar{y}_1 - \bar{y}_0$ is a common and statistically efficient choice. When sampling is conducted without knowledge of the risk factor (E) or disease status (Y), the variance of the difference between two mean values is

$$\text{variance} \, (\bar{y}_1 - \bar{y}_0) = [np(1 - p)]^{-1}, \tag{3.24}$$

where n represents the total sample size (note: $\sigma_Y^2 = 1$).

An α-level test of the hypothesis that no difference exists between the two sampled populations is based on

$$H_0: \mu_0 = \mu_1 \quad \text{versus} \quad H_1: \mu_0 < \mu_1,$$

which is used to assess the difference between $\bar{y}_1$ and $\bar{y}_0$; that is, to assess the role of the risk variable E. The sample size necessary for an α-level test with statistical power of $1 - \beta$ for this two-sample test is then

$$n = \frac{(z_{1-\alpha} + z_{1-\beta})^2}{p(1 - p)(\mu_1 - \mu_0)^2}, \tag{3.25}$$

again derived from expression (3.19).

An efficiency ratio (k/n), contrasting sample size for the dichotomous to the continuous approaches, is given by (for the special case of $\alpha = \beta$)

$$k/n = \frac{[2 + 1/\sqrt{\Phi(1 - \Phi)}]^2 / [\log{(or)}]^2}{4/(\mu_1 - \mu_0)^2} > \frac{\pi}{2}. \tag{3.26}$$

Furthermore, if the odds ratio is between 7.0 and 1/7, or $0 < \mu_1 - \mu_0 < 1.2$, then approximately, $k/n \approx \pi/2 = 1.571$ (i.e., <1.71). For this range, the efficiency ratio implies that if $n = 100$ observations are necessary to achieve a specific level of α and β, then at least 150 observations are required when a continuous variable is dichotomized and analyzed using an odds ratio as a measure of association. When

$(\mu_1 - \mu_0) > 1.2$, the efficiency ratio increases, and the odds ratio approach becomes more costly compared to the two-sample test in terms of additional data to maintain specified error rates or becomes less powerful for a fixed sample size.

The illustrative model is based on defining rather arbitrarily the "diseased" and "nondiseased" individuals by the midpoint between two normal distributions. It is certainly possible that other points are relevant and can be chosen to produce a binary variable reflecting "disease." However, the choice of this cut-point has a definite impact on the resulting odds ratio. For example, the odds ratio calculated for a few selected points c for exploring the relationship between the dichotomized variable Y and the binary variable E are shown in Table 3–7. To produce concrete odds ratios, two normal populations are assigned means $\mu_0 = 130$ and $\mu_1 = 150$ respectively, where $\sigma_Y^2 = 400$.

Clearly, the choice of the cut-point has a strong effect on the value of the odds ratio estimated from a binary variable and a dichotomized continuous variable. The same principle applies to some degree in almost all situations where a continuous variable is divided into a number of discrete categories. Although this illustration is certainly artificial, it shows that the influence introduced by the choice of the cut-point is an important consideration. Overshadowing the loss of power, the choice of a cut-point strongly affects the results and can introduce often unnecessary arbitrariness to an analysis.

Using an odds ratio to analyze a dichotomized continuous variable both reduces the probability of detecting the influence from a risk factor and introduces an arbitrary element to the resulting measure of association. On occasions, grouping continuous data into a table protects the analysis against unwanted effects of outliers. Outliers (out and out outliers) should be eliminated from a data set but should not

Table 3–7. Odds ratio calculated for the binary variable E and the variable Y dichotomized for selected values of the cut-point c

Cut-Point $= c$	Odds Ratio
110	8.1
120	6.2
130	5.3
140	5.0
150	5.3
160	6.2
170	8.1

dictate the analytic approach. Clarity of presentation and simplicity of measurement are other motivations for an odds ratio approach but again should not be the primary reason for choosing a specific analytic strategy. Certain groupings have medical or public health importance. For example, the definition of hypertension often involves a systolic blood pressure that exceeds 140 mm or a low birth-weight infant is almost always defined as a newborn who weighs less than 2,500 grams. It is important to note that the cost of using such traditional definitions is a less than fully efficient statistical analysis.

Lack of accuracy in outcome measures introduces additional variation to the analysis, but whether the effects are decreased by the analysis of continuous data with contingency table techniques is a question that has not been fully explored and, clearly, the presence of measurement error hurts any analytic approach. The best that can be said for creating a discrete measure of "disease" from a continuous outcome variable is that equivocal gains are paid for by a definite loss of statistical power. In addition, the results are influenced, sometimes substantially, by the definition of "disease." One last point: If a continuous variable is divided into more than two categories, the power lost decreases as the number of categories increases [6], and the choice of the cut-points has less impact.

Sample Size: Estimation

Sample sizes necessary to estimate a particular quantity with a specified precision can be derived from a confidence interval. The precision of an estimate is first described in terms of the length of an α-level confidence interval. The length is then used to calculate the number of observations necessary to obtain this desired degree of precision. No need exists to specify a null or an alternative hypothesis, but the results do not explicitly guarantee a specific level of power.

Generically, consider a parameter represented by θ. The estimate of θ is $\hat{\theta}$, based on a sample size of n observations. When the estimate is known or assumed to have at least an approximately normal distribution, a 95% confidence interval (95% is used here but any signficance level applies) is approximately

$$(\theta_{\text{lower}}, \theta_{\text{upper}}) = \left(\theta - 1.96\,\frac{\sigma}{\sqrt{n}},\ \theta + 1.96\,\frac{\sigma}{\sqrt{n}}\right), \qquad (3.27)$$

where σ represents the standard deviation associated with the sampled population. Such an interval has approximately a 0.95 probability of containing the population parameter θ. The length of this 95% confidence interval is

$$\text{length} = \theta_{\text{upper}} - \theta_{\text{lower}} = \left(\theta + 1.96\,\frac{\sigma}{\sqrt{n}}\right) - \left(\theta - 1.96\,\frac{\sigma}{\sqrt{n}}\right) = 3.92\,\frac{\sigma}{\sqrt{n}}$$

(3.28)

or

$$\text{width} = w = 1.96\,\frac{\sigma}{\sqrt{n}}.$$

(3.29)

Therefore, if a width (w) and a variance (σ^2) are specified, then the approximate sample size n to attain a confidence interval of width w follow as

$$n = \frac{3.84\sigma^2}{w^2}.$$

(3.30)

The translation of a width of a confidence interval into a sample size is used in a number of situations to achieve a specific level of precision associated with the estimate $\hat{\theta}$.

Example: Sample Mean

Many times a sample mean $\bar{x}$ (i.e., $\hat{\theta} = \bar{x}$) can be assumed to be calculated from a sample of observations with a normal distribution that has variance σ^2. For $w = 0.5$ units and $\sigma^2 = 10$, then

$$n = \frac{3.84(10)}{0.5^2} = 154.$$

(3.31)

A sample size of 154 observations is necessary to achieve an 95% confidence interval of width 0.5 units (length $= 2w = 1.0$). That is, there is an 0.95 probability that the interval centered at the sample mean ($\bar{x} \pm 0.5$ units), based on $n = 154$, contains the population mean.

Example: Sample Proportion

An estimated proportion $\hat{p}$ is a special type of mean made up of a sample of zeros and ones with variance $\sigma^2 = p(1 - p)$. The necessary sample size to achieve an approximate 95% confidence interval of width 0.1 for this estimate is

$$n = \frac{3.84(0.4)(0.6)}{0.1^2} = 93$$

(3.32)

when p is equal to 0.4.

Example: Difference between Two Sample Proportions

The estimated difference between two sample proportions $\hat{p}_2 - \hat{p}_1$ has associated variability $\sigma^2 = [p_1(1 - p_1) + p_2(1 - p_2)]/n$ when the same number of observations is sampled from the two populations. The sample size necessary to produce an approximate 95% confidence interval of length 0.5 ($w = 0.25$) is

$$n = \frac{3.84[(0.1)(0.9) + (0.4)(0.6)]}{0.25^2} = 21; \tag{3.33}$$

a total of 42 observations are needed when p_1 is 0.1 and p_2 is 0.4.

Some basic properties of this process are: (1) for a confidence interval with lower levels of α, increased numbers of observations are needed to achieve a given length, (2) increases in the variability associated with the sample estimate, cause increases in the sample size required to achieve a specified precision, and (3) if a smaller confidence interval length is chosen, then a larger sample size is necessary.

Using the length of a confidence interval as a measure of the level of precision for an estimate requires the knowledge or the assumption that the estimate has at least an approximately normal distribution. This is a reasonable assumption for many estimates or functions of estimates. More critically, the confidence interval approach to finding an approximate sample size requires two somewhat subjective decisions. First, a choice of an acceptable length (or precision) is required. This choice is usually made on nonstatistical grounds. Second, a choice must be made for a value of the variance σ^2. In the preliminary stages of an investigation it is not usual that an accurate assessment of variability is available. Therefore, sample-size calculations based on confidence intervals are usually only approximate and, like sample sizes based on power considerations, best serve as guidelines rather than hard and fast determinations.

4 Cohort Data: Description and Illustration

The term cohort describes a group collected to investigate a specific disease where the focus is on the frequency of disease after individuals have been classified as exposed or not exposed to a risk factor. For example, one type of cohort involves following a group of individuals over a period of time and observing the number of new cases of disease. Another type of cohort arises in the analysis of mortality data, also observed over a period of time, and is the topic of this chapter.

Two basic elements of cause-specific mortality data are age at death and year of death. Of course, other pieces of information are usually available, such as the place of residence and the sex of the person who died, but the focus here is on age at death and year of death as elements that provide a special perspective on the description of the cause of death. Using these two quantities, mortality rates can be classified into a two-way table where rows, for example, consist of different age categories and columns contain different calendar years of death. This simple table becomes more complex when it is realized that a third factor is present. Mortality data analyzed by specific calendar year do not directly account for the fact that individuals who died during a specific year were born at different times. This almost trivial fact has important implications in the study of certain diseases. Individuals born about the same time, a birth cohort, potentially have similar types and intensity of experiences during their lives. For example, individuals born around 1900 were in their late teens and early twenties during the influenza pandemic of 1919, while persons born after 1920 had no such "exposure." Men born in the 1920s show important cohort effects from serving in combat during World War II. Others born before 1920 and after 1930 were unlikely to have similar experiences. If an event occurring at a specific point in time puts certain individuals at increased risk of a disease throughout the rest of their lives, a related increase in mortality can occur which is often not apparent in data displayed in an age by calendar year tabulation. Increased risk associated with a group born during the same period is called a cohort effect. It was not until 1939 that tuberculosis mortality was noted (Frost [1]) to be influenced by a strong cohort effect. Other diseases, such as lung cancer (Levin [2]), Parkinson's disease (Poskanzer [3]), and prostatic cancer among nonwhites (Ernster [4]), have cohort influences that are now known to be part of their mortality pattern. It is the description and analysis of excess mortality associated with a specific birth cohort that is the topic of this chapter.

Cohort Effect: Model

To define and understand a cohort effect, consider the following hypothetical situation (model). Suppose the influence of calendar time produces the mortality rates per 100,000 person-years of risk shown in Table 4–1 (i.e., linear increase—10 deaths/year). If age does not influence the cause-specific mortality rates, then these rates are constant over age, and an age/year tabulation of the mortality data is given in Table 4–2. However, most causes of death are strongly influenced by age (older individuals die at higher rates). Suppose the influence of age produces the rates listed in Table 4–3 (i.e., again linear increase—15 deaths/year). If age is the only factor influencing mortality, then these rates are constant over time, and the age/year tabulation of the mortality data is given in Table 4–4.

Both age and time, for most diseases, simultaneously influence

Table 4–1. Mortality rates by time

Year	1935	1945	1955	1965	1975	1985
Rate	100	200	300	400	500	600

Table 4–2. Mortality rates by year and age: time effect only

Age	1935	1945	1955	1965	1975	1985
35–44	100	200	300	400	500	600
45–54	100	200	300	400	500	600
55–64	100	200	300	400	500	600
65–74	100	200	300	400	500	600
75–84	100	200	300	400	500	600
85+	100	200	300	400	500	600

Table 4–3. Mortality rates by age

Age	35–44	45–54	55–64	65–74	75–84	85+
Rate	50	200	350	500	650	800

Table 4–4. Mortality rates by year and age: age effect only

Age	1935	1945	1955	1965	1975	1985
35–44	50	50	50	50	50	50
45–54	200	200	200	200	200	200
55–64	350	350	350	350	350	350
65–74	500	500	500	500	500	500
75–84	650	650	650	650	650	650
85+	800	800	800	800	800	800

mortality. Age and time effects can be combined to illustrate a mortality pattern for a cause of death where both influences produce an additive increase on top of a background rate of 50 deaths per 100,000 person-years, producing the rates shown in Table 4–5. That is, the expected rate R_{ij} is represented as

$$R_{ij} = \mu + a_i + t_j, \tag{4.1}$$

where a_i represents the age effect (rows), and t_j represents the calendar time effects (columns). This is the same additive (no interaction) model described in Chapter 2 applied to mortality rates [expression (2.26)].

This age/year mortality table is strictly the sum of the three influences (background, age, and time). For example, the mortality rate for individuals ages 55–64 in 1965 is $R_{34} = 50 + 350 + 400 = 800$ deaths per 100,000. That is, the data are generated so that the age and time effects are additive; no interaction exists between age and

Table 4–5. Mortality rates by year and age: age and time influence

Age	1935	1945	1955	1965	1975	1985
35–44	200	300	400	500	600	700
45–54	350	450	550	650	750	850
55–64	500	600	700	800	900	1,100
65–74	650	750	850	950	1,050	1,150
75–84	800	900	1,000	1,100	1,200	1,300
85+	950	1,050	1,150	1,250	1,350	1,450

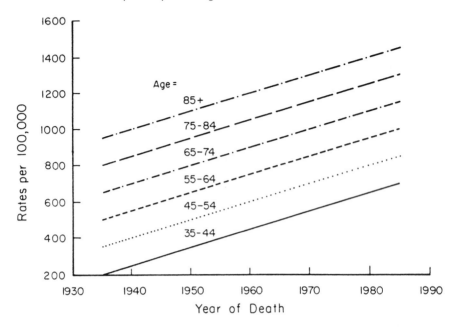

Figure 4–1. Age–specific curves for hypothetical data showing mortality rates per 100,000 population by year of death with no cohort effect

time for the fictional cause of death under investigation (Figure 4–1). The differences among age groups are the same for all calendar years and, conversely, the differences among rates for each calendar time are the same for all age groups. Additivity of age and time effects produces a pattern where plots of the row rates (or column rates) form parallel lines. In this artificial case, the lines are also straight lines, since both age and time have linearly increasing influences.

Suppose an exposure occurred around the year 1900 that subsequently increased the risk of death for individuals born about that time. Suppose further that the exposure around 1890 was moderate, by 1900 it was at its strongest, and by 1910 this exposure was again moderate. Assume also that the exposure did not exist prior to or following these twenty years. Such an exposure could produce the mortality pattern shown in Table 4–6 ignoring any other influences that are present.

Notice that this cohort effect is associated with the diagonal cells of an age/year tabulation of mortality data. Individuals on the diagonals of this age/year tabulation were born on or near the same year and thus form a birth cohort. Combining the age, time, and cohort effects, Table 4–7 emerges.

The cohort effect is seen in Figure 4–2 as an increase and then a

Table 4-6. Mortality rates by cohort influence only

Age	1935	1945	1955	1965	1975	1985
35–44	100	30	0	0	0	0
45–54	30	100	30	0	0	0
55–64	0	30	100	30	0	0
65–74	0	0	30	100	30	0
75–84	0	0	0	30	100	30
85+	0	0	0	0	30	100

Table 4-7. Mortality rates by age and time: age, time, and cohort influence

Age	1935	1945	1955	1965	1975	1985
35–44	300	330	400	500	600	700
45–54	380	550	580	650	750	850
55–64	500	630	800	830	900	1,000
65–74	650	750	880	1,050	1,080	1,150
75–84	800	900	1,000	1,130	1,300	1,330
85+	950	1,050	1,150	1,250	1,380	1,550

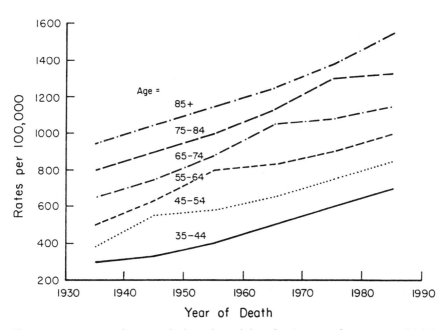

Figure 4-2. Age–specific curves for hypothetical data showing mortality rates per 100,000 population by year of death with a cohort effect present

decrease in the mortality rates at some point on each of the six age-specific mortality curves (in this case, straight lines). These regions of increased mortality occur at different points of calendar time for each age group. A cohort effect is a specific type of age/time interaction. In other words, the influence of age is not the same for all calendar years and, conversely, the calendar time influence is not the same for all ages. Geometrically, it is no longer possible to depict these rates as parallel lines. Figure 4–3 shows the same rates as Figure 4–2, but they are plotted by year of birth rather than year of death, which causes the cohort influence to appear directly above the birth years of those individuals who experience the excess mortality.

The view that a cohort influence is a specific type of age/time interaction suggests a statistical model to evaluate possible cohort influences on the pattern of mortality. A frequently postulated model states that a cause-specific mortality rate for a specific age and calendar time is proportional to the product of a background rate, an age influence, a time influence, and a cohort influence. In terms of the logarithm of the rate, the symbolic representation of the model is

$$\text{logarithm of the rate} = \log(R_{ij}) = \mu + a_i + t_j + c_{(k)}, \qquad (4.2)$$

where $\mu =$ the background rate, $a_i =$ the age effect (i^{th} row), t_j the

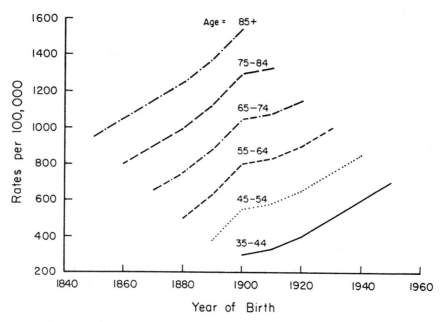

Figure 4–3. Age–specific curves for hypothetical data showing mortality rates per 100,000 population by year of birth with a cohort effect present

time effect (j^{th} column), and $c_{(k)}$ the effect associated with the kth cohort (the diagonal cells in the age/year table). For example, the birth cohort influence in the hypothetical data is $c_{(5)} = c_{(7)} = 30$, $c_{(6)} = 100$ and otherwise $c_{(k)} = 0$ (Table 4–6). Also note that when $c_{(k)} = 0$, no cohort influence exists, and the age and time effects are additive (no interaction).

Description of a Two-Way Table

Methods exist to estimate and to evaluate analytically the cohort parameters $c_{(k)}$ from mortality data based on cohort models such as expression (4.2) ([5], for example). Model-based approaches are not easily implemented and encounter computational difficulties. One method, however, designed to deal with two-way tables in general, is also useful in the analysis of mortality data with particular emphasis on describing a cohort effect. The method is called a median polish ([6] or [7] contain a complete development). This approach to an-alyzing a two-way contingency table makes no assumptions about the distribution or structure of the sampled data (distribution-free) and is effective when the tabled data are rates or logarithms of the rates.

The median polish involves computing a residual value for each cell in a table by removing from each observation the additive influence of the row variable and the additive influence of the column variable. In symbols, for each cell in the table, the residual is

$$\text{residual} = r_{ij} = (\text{tabled value}) - (\mu + a_i + t_j), \qquad (4.3)$$

where, as before, a_i represents the row influence and t_j represents the column influence. The residual values measure the failure of an additive model to reflect the values contained in each cell of the table. In a cohort analysis, this lack of additivity can come from the influence of a cohort effect that is typically assumed constant for each birth cohort. However, these residual values reflect nonadditivity in general and are meaningful indicators of any type of interaction associated with data classified into a two-way table.

The median polish calculation produces residual values by an iterative process. First, the row influences are estimated by the median value of each row. Each row median is then subtracted from each cell value in the same row of the table, producing a revised value for each cell. Then, column medians are found for each column of the revised table. The estimated column influences are subtracted from each corresponding cell value in the same column. The process is then repeated a number of times (usually less than five or so) until

Data:

	col 1	col 2	col 3	col 4
row 1	12	18	44	55
row 2	17	28	52	65
row 3	22	48	66	85
row 4	35	55	75	100

Step 1

	col 1	col 2	col 3	col 4
row 1	7.5	-2.0	2.0	-2.5
row 2	3.5	-1.0	1.0	-1.5
row 3	-8.5	2.0	-2.0	1.5
row 4	-3.5	1.0	-1.0	8.5

Step 3

	col 1	col 2	col 3	col 4
row 1	7.5	-2.0	2.0	-2.66
row 2	3.5	-1.0	1.0	-1.66
row 3	-8.18	2.31	-1.66	1.66
row 4	-3.5	1.0	-1.0	8.34

Step 2

	col 1	col 2	col 3	col 4
row 1	7.5	-2.0	2.0	-2.625
row 2	3.5	-1.0	1.0	-1.625
row 3	-8.25	2.25	-1.75	1.625
row 4	-3.5	1.0	-1.0	8.375

Step 4

	col 1	col 2	col 3	col 4
row 1	7.50	-2.00	2.00	-2.67
row 2	3.50	-1.00	1.00	-1.67
row 3	-8.17	2.33	-1.67	1.67
row 4	-3.50	1.00	-1.00	8.33

Figure 4–4. Illustrative data and iterative steps in the "median polish" process.

the residual values no longer appreciably change (i.e., until all medians ≈ 0). When the values remaining in the table become stable, they reflect the nonadditive component for each cell. The differences between these residual values and the original data produce a set of "data" that perfectly fits the additive model [expression (4.1)]. The process separates the data into an additive piece and a residual piece (data = additive "data" + residual). The cells with large residual values show the areas of the lack of fit of the additive structure and are potentially important in the understanding of the joint effects of the row and column variables.

Table 4–8. Data

	Column 1	Column 2	Column 3	Column 4
Row 1	12	18	44	55
Row 2	17	28	52	65
Row 3	22	48	66	85
Row 4	35	55	75	100

Table 4–9. Residuals

	Column 1	Column 2	Column 3	Column 4
Row 1	7.50	−2.00	2.00	−2.67
Row 2	3.50	−1.00	1.00	−1.67
Row 3	−8.17	2.33	−1.67	1.67
Row 4	−3.50	1.00	−1.00	8.33

A simple demonstration of the way a median polish works for a 4 × 4 table is given in Figure 4–4. The data used to demonstrate the mechanics of the median polish are shown in Table 4–8. The median polish produces the residual values given in Table 4–9 after four iterations (i.e., row medians = column medians = 0). Subtracting the stable residual values (Table 4–9) from each value in the original table (Table 4–8) produces a no-interaction table—strictly additive effects of the rows and the columns. The perfectly additive "data" are shown in Table 4–10.

Note that the difference between rows is constant for the columns of Table 4–10 and, similarly, the difference between columns is the constant for the rows. Necessarily, the row and column means perfectly reflect the relationships within the table. For example, the difference between columns 2 and 3 is 22 for all rows and for the row means. If the median polish technique were to be applied to this table, no changes would occur and the residual values would be exactly zero. Geometrically, a plot of the rows in Table 4–10 (or columns) produces four parallel lines. The median polish technique is one of several ways observations can be split into meaningful pieces. A median polish arbitrarily starts with determining the medians of the rows. If the residual estimation process starts with the median of each column, the final residual table can differ but, in most cases, not dramatically.

Table 4–10. "Additive data": no interaction

	Column 1	Column 2	Column 3	Column 4	Mean
Row 1	4.50	20.00	42.00	57.67	31.04
Row 2	13.50	29.00	51.00	66.67	40.04
Row 3	30.17	45.67	67.67	83.33	56.71
Row 4	38.50	54.00	76.00	91.67	65.04
Mean	21.67	37.17	59.17	74.83	48.21

Mean Polish

If mean values are used instead of median values in the process of dividing a two-way table into residual and additive components, stable residual values emerge after one iteration. The row means are subtracted from each cell value in the same row followed by calculating the column means and subtracting these values for each cell value in the same column, producing a residual value for each cell in a two-way table. Like the median polish, the difference between the residuals and the original observations produces perfectly additive "data" [expression (4.1)]. The estimated residuals have the same form as the e_{ij}-values estimated from the additive model used to analyse continuous data [i.e., $\hat{e}_{ij} = y_{ij} - [\bar{y}_{i.} + \bar{y}_{.j} - \bar{y}]$; Chapter 2, expression (2.33)].

The mean polish process is related to an analysis of variance applied to a two-way classification. The residual sum of squares for a two-way classification with one observation per cell is the sum of squared residual values that result when the additive influences of the row and the column variables are removed. If the data conforms to the analysis of variance assumptions (independence, normality, no interaction, and the null hypothesis is true), the residual sum of squares can be used to formally evaluate the influences from the row or column variables on a dependent variable. However, regardless of the structure underlying the data, the residual values provide an excellent descriptive tool to detect and interpret interactions (lack of additivity) between two categorical variables. The pattern of residuals is the focus of interest rather than the statistical testing of the effects, which is the main purpose of the analysis of variance approach.

Table 4–11 shows the additive values from the data given in Table 4–8 based on using the mean values to estimate the row and column influences rather than the medians. The resulting additive and residual values are similar to those using a median estimate but, as mentioned, require one iteration.

Examples from previous data sets (Table 2–10, Chapter 2—blood pressure data and mortality rates) show two simple applications of the mean polish (Tables 4–12 and 4–13). The moderate-size residual values (± 3.35) from the blood pressure data indicate the likely presence of an interaction which, as before, interferes with a general summary of either the "neighborhood" effect or the racial effect on blood pressure levels. On the other hand, the analysis of mortality rates from the Canadian insulation workers shows a remarkable lack of interaction (Table 4–13). The small residual values (± 0.02) lead to the inference that the effects of smoking and asbestos exposure are

Table 4-11. Applying the mean polish to the illustrative "data"—residual values are given in parentheses

	Column 1	Column 2	Column 3	Column 4	Mean
Row 1	5.188 (6.813)	20.938 (−2.938)	42.938 (1.603)	59.938 (−4.938)	32.25
Row 2	13.438 (3.563)	29.188 (−1.188)	51.188 (0.813)	68.188 (−3.188)	40.50
Row 3	28.188 (−6.188)	43.938 (4.063)	65.938 (0.063)	82.938 (2.063)	55.25
Row 4	39.188 (−4.188)	54.938 (0.063)	76.938 (−1.938)	93.938 (6.063)	66.25
Mean	21.500	37.250	59.250	76.250	48.563

Table 4–12. Mean polish showing evidence of an interaction between "neighborhood" and race for measurements of diastolic blood pressure (Chapter 2)

		White "Neighborhood"	Black "Neighborhood"
White			
	Observation	77.20	78.90
	Additive	73.85	82.25
	Residual	3.35	−3.35
Black			
	Observation	83.30	98.40
	Additive	86.65	95.05
	Residual	−3.35	3.35

Table 4–13. Mean polish showing essentially no interaction between smoking and asbestos exposure using the logarithms of the mortality rates (rates in parenthesis— Table 2–11, Chapter 2)

		Smoker	Nonsmoker
Exposed			
	Observation	6.400 (601.6)	4.067 (58.4)
	Additive	6.422	4.045
	Residual	−0.022	0.022
Unexposed			
	Observation	4.847 (127.3)	2.425 (11.3)
	Additive	4.824	2.447
	Residual	0.022	−0.022

essentially additive in terms of logarithms, which makes the effects multiplicative in terms of the mortality rates themselves.

The choice between using a median or a mean polish depends on the same issues that arise in choosing between the sample mean and the sample median as estimates of the population "location." If extreme values are to be deemphasized, the median polish gives little weight to these observations, while if extreme observations are to play a role in the calculations, the mean polish gives these values an important influence on the estimation process. Therefore, the choice becomes primarily one of deciding on the weight to be given to extreme values.

Illustration

Before returning to the topic of cohort analysis, consider a set of cell-type-specific leukemia data that provide an opportunity to use a

Table 4–14. Myeloid leukemia mortality rates by sex and type (U.S. whites, 1969–77): Rates per 100,000 and logarithms of the rates—logarithm of the rates in parentheses

| Age | Acute | | Chronic | |
	Male	Female	Male	Female
0–4	0.40 (−0.92)	0.41 (−0.89)	0.07 (−2.66)	0.06 (−2.81)
5–9	0.33 (−1.11)	0.27 (−1.31)	0.06 (−2.81)	0.04 (−3.22)
10–14	0.41 (−0.89)	0.36 (−1.02)	0.06 (−2.81)	0.04 (−3.22)
15–24	0.69 (−0.37)	0.55 (−0.60)	0.15 (−1.90)	0.04 (−3.22)
25–34	0.87 (−0.14)	0.77 (−0.26)	0.42 (−0.87)	0.10 (−2.30)
35–44	1.27 (0.24)	1.14 (0.13)	0.70 (−0.36)	0.26 (−1.35)
45–54	2.22 (0.80)	1.74 (0.55)	1.06 (0.06)	0.73 (−0.31)
55–64	4.66 (1.54)	2.98 (1.09)	1.89 (0.64)	1.24 (0.22)
65–74	9.98 (2.30)	5.59 (1.72)	4.00 (1.39)	2.26 (0.82)
75–84	16.47 (2.80)	9.98 (2.30)	8.00 (2.09)	4.46 (1.50)
85+	18.39 (2.91)	10.29 (2.33)	10.82 (2.38)	5.94 (1.78)

median polish to describe the mortality pattern associated with myeloid leukemia for both acute and chronic forms. The rates and the logarithms of the rates (in parentheses) for leukemia mortality in the United States during the years 1969–77 [8] are given in Table 4–14. A plot of the logarithms of the rates is shown later in Figure 4–6. Applying a median polish to the logarithms of the rates produces perfectly additive "data" which are shown in Table 4–15.

> Aside: The analysis of the logarithm of a rate, rather than dealing directly with the rate itself, is traditional and has some justification in the empiric behavior of risk. A wide range of studies of cancer and to a lesser extent other diseases show that influences on age-specific rates often act multiplicatively. For example, smoking appears to increase the risk of coronary heart disease in a multiplicative pattern (as will be seen in subsequent analyses) and, therefore, produces a linear relationship among the logarithms of the incidence rates. Certainly, no hard and fast reason exists requiring the analysis of disease data in terms of logarithms of the rate. The choice of scale (multiplicative, additive or others) is an issue in the description of all disease data.

Comparison of these "additive data" (displayed in Figure 4–5, bottom) with the observed data shows that the additive model produces a useful structure to examine the relationships of age, leukemia type, and sex to leukemia mortality. Although not shown, the residual values are generally small (i.e., Table 4–14 minus Table 4–15 = residual values using the logarithm of the rates).

The "additive data" indicate that death from acute myeloid

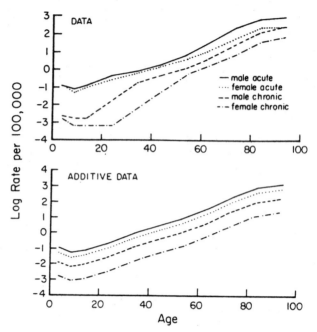

Figure 4–5. Age-specific curves for cell- and sex-specific myeloid leukemia mortality by age, logarithm of the rates per 100,000 population. Also shown are the same curves for strictly additive "data."

Table 4–15. Myeloid mortality leukemia by sex and type (U.S. whites, 1969–77) additive model "rates" per 100,000 and the logarithms of the "rates"

Age	Acute Male	Acute Female	Chronic Male	Chronic Female
0–4	0.38 (−0.97)	0.28 (−1.28)	0.15 (−1.87)	0.06 (−2.76)
5–9	0.28 (−1.27)	0.21 (−1.58)	0.11 (−2.17)	0.05 (−3.06)
10–14	0.31 (−1.16)	0.23 (−1.47)	0.13 (−2.06)	0.05 (−2.95)
15–24	0.51 (−0.68)	0.37 (−0.99)	0.20 (−1.59)	0.08 (−2.47)
25–34	0.95 (−0.05)	0.70 (−0.36)	0.38 (−0.96)	0.16 (−1.84)
35–44	1.55 (0.44)	1.14 (0.13)	0.63 (−0.46)	0.26 (−1.35)
45–54	2.49 (0.91)	1.83 (0.60)	1.01 (0.01)	0.42 (−0.88)
55–64	4.66 (1.54)	3.42 (1.23)	1.89 (0.64)	0.78 (−0.25)
65–74	9.92 (2.30)	7.28 (1.99)	4.02 (1.39)	1.66 (0.51)
75–84	18.03 (2.89)	13.22 (2.58)	7.31 (1.99)	3.02 (1.10)
85+	22.15 (3.10)	16.25 (2.79)	8.98 (2.19)	3.71 (1.31)

leukemia occurs about 2.5 times more frequently than the chronic form in males (difference in logarithms of 0.90 or $e^{0.90} = 2.5$) and about 4.4 times more frequently in females (difference in logarithms of 1.48 or $e^{1.48} = 4.4$). The influence of age is also easily summarized. For example, the rates of both forms of leukemia for both sexes increases about 11.6-fold between the ages 40 to 80 (difference in logarithms of 2.45 or $e^{1.86} = 11.6$).

The utility of an additive model is demonstrated by these median-polished leukemia "additive data" (Table 4–15). The effect of each variable is summarized without reference to the other. The difference in mortality associated with the acute and chronic forms is the same at all levels of age for both sexes. Similarly, age effects are described uninfluenced by leukemia type or sex. An additive model implies a type of independence among the variables under investigation, allowing a succinct description of the collected data based on separate assessments of each variable. Geometrically, the validity of assessing separately each influence results from the parallel relationships among the sex-, cell-type-specific curves (Figure 4–5, bottom). For example, the distance between log rates for acute and chronic types of leukemia among females is the same for all ages, since the logarithms of the rates for these two diseases form parallel lines when the "data" are additive. Therefore, it is not necessary to consider a specific age when summarizing differences in log rates between leukemia types. When the data are not adequately represented by an additive model (nonparallel lines), at least some of the residual values (r_{ij}) will be large, indicating more intricate relationships among the risk variables and disease rates. The major consequence is that it becomes difficult to isolate the impact of individual variables on a disease outcome.

Cohort Effect: Prostatic Cancer (Applied Example)

Ernster [4] demonstrated a cohort influence on the pattern of rates of prostatic cancer mortality among nonwhites in the United States. The data (rates/100,000) are given in Table 4–16 by age and year of death.

The logarithms of the rates are displayed in Figure 4–6 for the eight age categories by birth date. Median/average smoothed values are also displayed. Both plots indicate a cohort influence associated with the prostatic cancer mortality among nonwhites. This influence is most pronounced for individuals born around 1900 in the five younger age groups (<70 years old). Each age group has a maximum (or near maximum) mortality rate associated with individuals born near the beginning of the twentieth century. A quantitative description better

Table 4–16. Prostatic cancer mortality rates by age and time among U.S. nonwhites (1930–84)

Age/Year	1930–34	1935–39	1940–44	1945–49	1950–54	1955–59	1960–64	1965–69	1970–74	1975–79	1980–84
45–49	3.5	4.9	6.6	7.2	4.7	4.7	2.7	2.4	3.5	2.1	2.2
50–54	5.4	11.4	16.0	15.7	23.3	16.3	15.8	13.4	12.0	10.9	10.4
55–59	18.8	22.4	32.1	41.4	39.0	44.4	30.9	32.4	29.9	28.2	28.0
60–64	24.0	45.9	50.2	60.4	77.7	84.2	81.4	77.4	68.2	71.5	71.5
65–69	35.1	60.2	72.3	74.1	74.1	141.1	147.4	177.1	149.0	143.7	164.6
70–74	60.7	66.5	90.1	126.0	148.0	168.5	224.7	235.9	276.7	282.8	271.3
75–79	47.5	90.6	151.4	130.0	219.2	234.4	299.6	304.2	399.9	388.8	403.5
80+	56.7	124.5	152.1	155.6	299.1	328.6	371.6	359.1	471.3	557.9	673.6

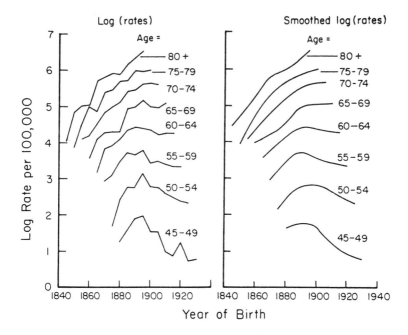

Figure 4–6. Age-specific curves for prostatic cancer mortality among nonwhites by year of birth, logarithm of the rates per 100,000 population. Also shown are the same curves median/average smoothed.

delineates this apparent cohort effect and provides an assessment of its magnitude.

A cohort effect, as previously stated, can be viewed as a specific type of nonadditivity in a table of mortality rates. This nonadditivity is likely to be reflected by the residual values. The median-polish technique applied to the prostatic cancer data produces an estimate of the magnitude of the observed cohort effect (nonadditivity). Residual values based on the logarithm of the rates for the prostatic cancer mortality are given in Table 4–17.

The residual values define the lack of additivity of age and time in determining the logarithm of the prostatic cancer rate. For example, the mortality rate for ages 45–49 for individuals who died between 1930 and 1934 is 3.5, and when the cohort effect is removed it becomes 1.5 deaths/100,000 [(i.e., estimate = rate $\times$ $e^{-\text{residual}}$ = $3.5e^{-0.880}$ = 1.5—expression (4.4)]. A value greater than zero indicates higher than additive influence and less than zero indicates lower than additive ·influence from age/time effects on the logarithm of the mortality rates. If no age/time interaction exists (no cohort influence), then the table of residual values will contain only small and essentially random

Table 4–17. Age, time, and cohort influences on prostatic cancer: residuals

Age/Year	1930–34	1935–39	1940–44	1945–49	1950–54	1955–59	1960–64	1965–69	1970–74	1975–79	1980–84
45–49	0.88	0.79	0.79	0.77	0.09	0.0	−0.60	−0.71	−0.26	−0.77	−0.79
50–54	0.70	0.39	0.43	0.31	0.44	0.0	−0.08	−0.24	−0.27	−0.37	−0.48
55–59	0.36	0.11	0.17	0.32	0.0	0.04	−0.36	−0.31	−0.31	−0.38	−0.45
60–64	0.0	0.22	0.01	0.09	0.08	0.08	0.0	−0.05	−0.09	−0.05	−0.12
65–69	−0.22	−0.11	−0.22	−0.30	−0.56	0.0	0.0	0.19	0.09	0.05	0.12
70–74	0.0	−0.34	−0.33	−0.09	−0.20	−0.15	0.09	0.14	0.38	0.40	0.29
75–79	−0.44	−0.22	−0.01	−0.26	0.0	−0.02	0.18	0.20	0.55	0.52	0.49
80+	−0.58	−0.23	−0.32	−0.40	−0.01	0.0	0.08	0.05	0.40	0.56	0.68

Table 4–18. Age, time and cohort influence on prostatic cancer: residuals ($+$, $-$)

Age/Year	1930–34	1935–39	1940–44	1945–49	1950–54	1955–59	1960–64	1965–69	1970–74	1975–79	1980–84
45–49	+	+	+	+	+	0	−	−	−	−	−
50–54	+	+	+	+	+	0	−	−	−	−	−
55–59	0	+	+	+	0	+	−	−	−	−	−
60–64	−	−	−	+	+	+	0	−	−	−	−
65–69	0	−	−	−	−	0	0	+	+	+	+
70–74	−	−	−	−	−	−	+	+	+	+	+
75–79	−	−	−	−	0	−	+	+	+	+	+
80+	−	−	−	−	−	0	+	0	+	+	+

121

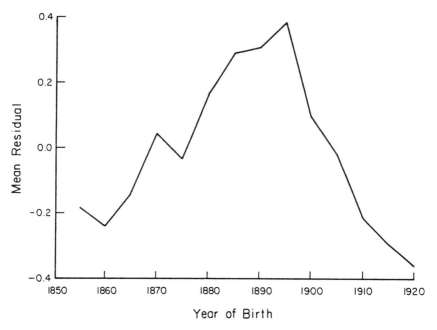

Figure 4–7. Average of the estimate residuals (the diagonal values in the age/time array) quantifying a specific nonadditive effect from the prostatic cancer data

(Table 4–18) using plus and minus signs clearly shows the systematic effect from the birth cohorts born around 1870 to 1900 on the pattern of prostatic cancer mortality.

Inspired by the cohort model [expression (4.2)], Figure 4–7 quantifies the influence of the observed cohort effect on the prostatic cancer rates using the average of the diagonal elements from the table of residual values (Table 4–17). These mean values estimate the nonadditive influence, which is assumed to be a constant component associated with each birth cohort (each diagonal of the age/time table). These average residual values consistently rise for the cohorts born before 1900, then rapidly and consistently fall for subsequent cohorts, describing the cohort effect influencing the prostatic cancer mortality rates among nonwhites.

Figure 4–8 shows the logarithm of the mortality rates by year of death and by year of birth where the estimated cohort influence has been statistically removed. That is, an "additive rate" is calculated by

$$\log(\text{additive rate}) = \log(\text{observed rate}) - \text{residual}$$

or

$$\text{additive rate} = (\text{observed rate}) \times e^{-\text{residual}}. \tag{4.4}$$

The estimated "additive rates" are given in Table 4–19.

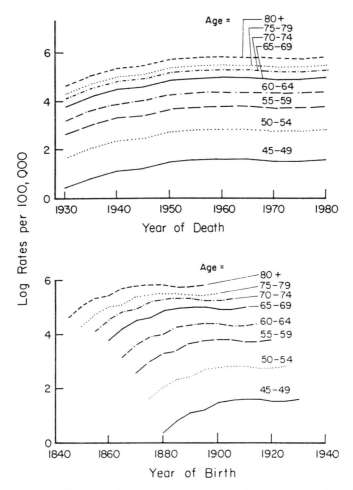

Figure 4–8. Age-specific curves for prostatic cancer mortality among nonwhites by year of death and by year of birth with the cohort effect removed (1969–77), logarithm of the rates per 100,000 population

The age/time interaction is no longer present, and the logarithms of these "rates" are a perfect additive function of age and calendar time; the curves representing the logarithm of the rates for each age group are parallel (rows). The "additive rates" produce a pattern of prostatic cancer mortality where no special "exposure" was experienced by any birth cohort ($c_{(k)} = 0$ for all k).

The nonwhite prostatic cancer data produce an essentially linear increase in the age-adjusted rates of mortality over the period 1930 to 1985. The direct age-adjusted prostatic cancer mortality rates per

Table 4-19. Prostatic cancer mortality "data" by age and time among U.S. nonwhites

Age/Year	1930–34	1935–39	1940–44	1945–49	1950–54	1955–59	1960–64	1965–69	1970–74	1975–79	1980–84
45–49	1.5	2.2	3.0	3.3	4.3	4.7	4.9	4.9	4.5	4.5	4.8
50–54	5.0	7.7	10.4	11.5	15.0	16.3	17.0	17.0	15.7	15.7	16.9
55–59	13.1	20.2	27.2	30.0	39.0	42.5	44.4	44.3	40.9	41.1	44.0
60–64	24.1	36.9	47.8	55.0	71.4	77.8	81.4	81.1	74.9	75.3	80.6
65–69	43.5	66.9	90.1	99.6	129.4	141.0	147.4	146.9	135.7	136.4	146.0
70–74	60.5	93.0	125.3	138.4	179.8	195.9	204.8	204.2	188.6	189.6	202.9
75–79	73.8	113.3	152.7	168.7	219.7	238.9	249.7	249.0	229.8	231.1	247.3
80+	101.5	155.9	210.1	232.1	301.6	328.6	343.6	342.5	316.2	317.9	340.3

Table 4-20. Age-adjusted prostatic cancer rates (with and without a cohort effect)

Age/Year	1930–34	1935–39	1940–44	1945–49	1950–54	1955–59	1960–64	1965–69	1970–74	1975–79	1980–84
Cohort	7.2	11.8	15.6	17.6	23.0	26.8	29.7	30.6	34.1	35.4	38.2
No cohort	8.5	13.0	17.4	19.3	25.1	27.3	28.5	28.5	26.3	26.4	28.3

100,000, using the U.S. 1970 standard population and based on the original data are given in Table 4–20 [expression (1.42)]. These age-adjusted rates are shown in Figure 4–9 (solid line, labeled "cohort" in Table 4–20). Also shown are the age-adjusted "rates" for of prostatic cancer among nonwhites with the observed cohort effect removed, based on the "additive data" from Table 4–19. The additive "rates" allow the calculation of age-adjusted "rates" without a cohort influence (plotted in Figure 4–9 as the dotted line, labeled "no cohort" in Table 4–20). The linearly increasing pattern of prostatic cancer mortality levels off around 1950 when the cohort effect is "removed." These "rates" then remain fairly constant after 1950, even decreasing slightly. Comparison of the patterns of these two sets of age-adjusted prostatic cancer mortality rates leads to the inference that the cohort effect in the nonwhite population is a principal reason for the increase in mortality after 1950.

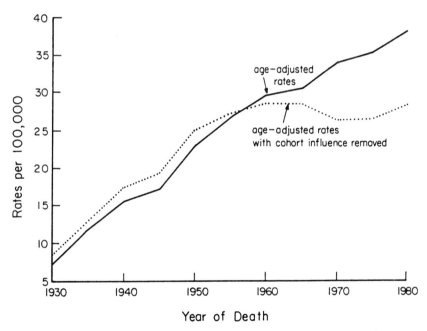

Figure 4–9. Age-adjusted curves for prostatic cancer mortality among nonwhites, rates by year of death with the cohort effect present and removed, rate per 100,000 population

5 Clustering:
Space and Time Data

The distribution of disease in a population is fundamental to epidemiology, as noted by Abraham Lilienfeld [1] who began his basic text:

> Epidemiology may be defined as the study of the distribution of disease or a pathological condition in human populations and the factors that influence this distribution.

Although Lilienfeld had in mind distribution in a broad sense, initial successes in epidemiology can be traced to the study of the spatial distribution of disease. John Snow identified the source of cholera in the nineteenth century primarily from the spatial distribution of cases in a specific area of London.

> Aside: British physician John Snow utilized what became the classic epidemiologic approach to study cholera in 1854. He postulated that cholera was caused by a contaminant in the water supply when bacterial disease was an unknown phenomenon. Dr. Snow then proceeded to collect data on customers of two water companies where one of these companies provided water that was relatively free of sewage. He also plotted the locations of deaths from cholera in central London on a map. By comparing the rates of death between groups served by the two companies and examining the spatial distribution of cases, he concluded that an "impurity" in the water was associated with an increase in cholera cases. The complete account of this remarkable analysis of a "natural experiment" is given in Snow's book *On the Mode of Communication of Cholera*.

Geographic distributions have played a central role in the epidemiology of a number of other diseases and are essential to evaluate data involving exposures to environmental pollutants. This chapter explores a few analytic techniques for identifying nonrandom spatial patterns of disease and, at the same time, introduces two important statistical techniques (permutation tests and jackknife estimation) that apply to a wide range of situations.

Poisson Model

The Poisson probability distribution (see Appendix B) is an effective description of objects distributed spatially at random. The spatial distribution of such things as stars, weeds, bacteria, and even flying-bomb strikes are described, sometimes quite accurately, by Poisson probabilities. The study of spatial patterns using a Poisson probability distribution begins by dividing the area of interest into a series of nonoverlapping subdivisions, so that the probability that a single random point falls within any one subdivision is small. In many cases this probability is easily made small by creating a large number of subdivisions. If the probability that a specific random point is found in a single subdivision is constant (denoted by p) and small (say, $p < 0.05$), then the number of subdivisions containing $0, 1, 2, 3, \ldots$ points follows an approximate Poisson probability distribution. Random means that each point has the same probability of falling into a specific subdivision. The size of each subdivision but not the location influences the probabilities associated with each point. More formally, if k represents the number of random points in a subdivision, then the number of subdivisions with k points is given by

$$\text{number of subdivisions with } k \text{ points} = m \times P(X = k) = m\,\frac{\lambda^k e^{-\lambda}}{k!}, \quad (5.1)$$

where m is the total number of subdivisions and $P(X = k)$ is a Poisson probability. The parameter λ represents the expected number of points in each subdivision.

The Poisson distribution as a description of random points on a plane is rigorously justified on theoretical grounds [2]. Without going into the mathematical details, two conditions must hold to justify the Poisson distribution: (1) the probability (p) that each point falls into one of a large number of a specific subdivisions must be constant and (2) the probability p must be small.

If spatial clustering exists, then p differs among the subdivisions; for some areas p will be large producing data that cluster, and for other areas p will be relatively small tending to make data sparse. The Poisson distribution is synonymous with the hypothesis that p is constant. Rejection of this hypothesis provides evidence that p is heterogeneous, implying that at least some points are not randomly distributed across the region of interest.

Figure 5–1 displays $n = 200$ computer-generated random points on a unit square. There are $m = 100$ subsquares with area $= 0.01$, so that every random point has a probability of $p = 1/m = 0.01$ of falling in a specific subsquare. The expected number of points per subsquare is

200 RANDOM POINTS

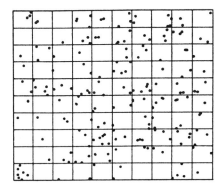

Figure 5–1. Two hundred random points distributed over a unit square divided into 100 equal subsquares

$\lambda = np = 200(0.01) = 2$. Or, more simply, since there are 200 points and 100 subsquares, the expected number of random points in any one square is $200/100 = 2$. The Poisson probabilities associated with an expected value of $\lambda = 2$ as well as the observed proportion of subareas with k points per subsquare (Figure 5–1) are shown in Table 5–1.

A classic study [2] of spatial distributions occurred during World War II, in which records of flying-bomb strikes in south London were analyzed. It was critical to know if the German bombs were falling at random $(p = \text{constant})$ or if these bombs possessed an accurate guidance system $(p \neq \text{constant—clustering})$. South London was divided into $m = 576$ small subdivisions of equal area, each 0.25 square kilometers. The World War II flying-bomb data is reproduced in Table 5–2. Again, the variable $X = count$ is the number of subareas with k strikes recorded.

The Poisson model cannot be applied without a value of the parameter λ or, at least, an estimate of this fundamental part of the Poisson distribution. An estimate of this parameter comes from using the observed mean number of hits per area $(\hat{\lambda})$ as an estimate of the

Table 5–1. Count of subareas with k points per square

k	0	1	2	3	4	5	6	7	Total
Counts	15	25	25	22	8	3	1	1	100
Probability	0.135	0.271	0.271	0.180	0.090	0.036	0.012	0.005	1.00
Proportion	0.150	0.250	0.250	0.220	0.080	0.030	0.010	0.010	1.00

Table 5–2. Flying-bomb hits in south London: data

k	0	1	2	3	4	≥ 5	Total
Count	229	211	93	35	7	1	576

unknown expected number of hits per area (λ). That is,

$$\hat{\lambda} = \frac{\text{total number of hits}}{\text{number of subdivisions}} = \frac{n}{m}$$

$$= \frac{0(229) + 1(211) + 2(93) + 3(35) + 4(7) + 5(1)}{576} = 0.929 \quad (5.2)$$

is the observed mean number of hits per subdivision among the 576 subdivisions (a bit less than one per subdivision). Note that ≥ 5 was set to 5 to estimate λ. An estimate of λ makes it possible to estimate the Poisson probabilities and expected number of random hits distributed among 576 areas, as shown in Table 5–3 for the data in Table 5–2.

A chi-square statistic or some other goodness-of-fit procedure to test the accuracy of the Poisson distribution as a model for the London data is hardly necessary. This example appears in a number of texts because of the extraordinary correspondence between the observed and the theoretically derived values. The conclusion some fifty years ago would have been that the data from south London indicated no evidence that these weapons were guided with any accuracy.

Situations certainly arise where it is not obvious whether a Poisson distribution serves as a description of a set of observations. Then, a summary statistic and a significance test are useful. Such a summary statistic is developed from the fact that the mean and the variance are identical for the Poisson distribution (again see Appendix B). Therefore, the sample mean and the sample variance from a Poisson distributed data should be about equal, give or take random variation. In other words, the sample mean value $\bar{x}$ and the sample variance S^2 should

Table 5–3. Flying-bomb hits in south London: probabilities and expected hits

k	0	1	2	3	4	≥ 5	Total
Probability	0.395	0.367	0.170	0.053	0.012	0.003	1.0
Expected counts	227.53	211.34	98.15	30.39	7.06	1.54	576
Observed counts	229	211	93	35	7	1	576

be approximately equal under the condition that the data are a random sample from a Poisson distribution or

$$\frac{S^2}{\bar{x}} \approx 1, \tag{5.3}$$

where $\bar{x}$ and S^2 are calculated in the usual way. The ratio $S^2/\bar{x}$ multiplied by $(m-1)$ has an approximate chi-square distribution when the population sampled has a Poisson distribution, where m is the total number of subdivisions each containing x_i-values. The degrees of freedom are the number of observed subdivisions minus one $(m-1)$.

The test statistic $X^2 = (m-1)S^2/\bar{x}$, sometimes called the test of variance for obvious reasons, can be justified from the common expression for the Pearson chi-square statistic,

$$X^2 = \sum \frac{(\text{observed} - \text{expected})^2}{\text{expected}}. \tag{5.4}$$

For the test of variance, the expected value represented by λ, is estimated by $\hat{\lambda} = \bar{x} = \sum x_i/m$. Substituting this estimate into the chi-square expression (5.4) gives

$$X^2 = \sum_{i=1}^{m} \frac{(x_i - \bar{x})^2}{\bar{x}} = (m-1)\frac{S^2}{\bar{x}}, \tag{5.5}$$

where $observed = x_i$ represents the count from one of the m subdivisions with estimated expected $= \bar{x}$.

To illustrate, the mean value of the data displayed in Figure 5–1 (also given in Table 5–1) is $\bar{x} = 2.010$, and the variance is $S^2 = 2.091$. Then, $X^2 = 99(2.091)/2.010 = 102.980$, which has a chi-square distribution with $m - 1 = 99$ degrees of freedom when the $n = 200$ points are distributed at random over the $m = 100$ subdivisions of the unit square. The associated p-value of 0.372 indicates that the magnitude of the deviations from the expected values are typical when no spatial pattern of points exists. The test of variance approach is effective even for fairly small samples of data $(n > 20$ or so) and is also useful in other contexts to evaluate the goodness-of-fit of a Poisson distribution.

Nearest Neighbor

Employing a Poisson distribution to detect clustering has a weakness. Distance is a continuous measure. As discussed earlier, employing discrete counts is not as effective as directly analyzing a continuous variable, particularly for small numbers of observations. One method to investigate the question of spatial randomness, which utilizes the actual distance between points, is a nearest-neighbor analysis.

A nearest-neighbor is basically what the name implies. For n points, distances to all other points under consideration are calculated. The nearest neighbor is the minimum distance among these $n - 1$ measurements. The collection of these n minimum distances constitutes a set of nearest-neighbor data. The expected mean and the variance of the distribution for a set of nearest-neighbor values can be derived under the conditions that the spatial distribution generating the data is random. A test of randomness results from the comparison of the mean from a set of observed nearest-neighbor distances to the mean expected when no spatial pattern exists.

Suppose, as before, that a sample of points is distributed at random over a specified area. For a specific point let the probability that no other points occur within a distance d units be symbolized by $P_0(d)$. The probability that no points are within an additional small distance δ can then be expressed as

$$P_0(d + \delta) \approx P_0(d)(1 - \lambda\delta), \tag{5.6}$$

where λ is the expected number of points per unit area. Then,

$$\frac{P_0(d + \delta) - P_0(d)}{\delta} \approx -\lambda P_0(d) \tag{5.7}$$

and a bit of mathematical manipulation, or noting that exponential growth (decay) occurs when the rate of change of a variable is proportional only to the level of that variable, gives

$$P_0(d) = e^{-\lambda d}. \tag{5.8}$$

Aside: This same expression, in an entirely different context, results from probably the most famous single differential equation. Thomas Malthus (1798) used this exponential relationship to support his view that populations tend to increase faster than the resources needed to sustain them. This theory, published in his famous work *Essay on the Principle of Populations* has had substantial impact on many fields and, perhaps, was the beginning of the field of demography.

When interest lies in the distance from a specified point to its nearest neighbor in any direction, a circle with radius r is an appropriate measure of area. The parameter λ equals n/A where A represents the total area under consideration and n the total number of observed points. The value $\lambda = n/A$ is the frequency of points per unit area (density over the area A).

The probability that one or more points is found in a circle of radius r is

$$F(r) = 1 - P \text{ (no points occur within radius } r) = 1 - e^{-n\pi r^2/A} \quad (5.9)$$

as long as the spatial distribution of the n points is random. The same probability applies to the nearest neighbor (the minimum distance). That is, the probability of finding one or more points within a circle with radius r is the same as the probability of finding the minimum distance within the same circle. The distribution function $F(r)$ relates the distance r to probabilities associated with nearest-neighbor distance when points are distributed spatially at random. More precisely,

$$P \text{ (nearest-neighbor distance} < r \text{ units)} = 1 - e^{-n\pi r^2/A}. \quad (5.10)$$

Knowledge of the probability function $F(r)$ allows the calculation of various summary statistics associated with nearest-neighbor distances for a sample of randomly distributed points. For example, the expected median distance associated with a sample of n random nearest-neighbor distances is

$$F(r) = 0.5, \text{ which implies that median } (r) = 0.470 \sqrt{\frac{A}{n}}. \quad (5.11)$$

Along the same lines, using a calculus argument, the expected mean distance and variance of the mean are

$$\text{mean } (r) = 0.5 \sqrt{\frac{A}{n}} \quad \text{with} \quad \text{variance } (\bar{r}) = 0.068 \frac{A}{n^2} \quad (5.12)$$

when the n points are distributed randomly over the region of interest with area A. Note that the distribution of r is nearly symmetric because the median is practically equal to the mean. Additionally, the probability distribution $F(r)$ provides a basis for a chi-square goodness-of-fit test when large amounts of data are available. That is, the expected number of nearest-neighbor values between any two distances r_i and r_j $(r_i < r_j)$ is

$$\text{expected number} = n \times P(r_i < \text{nearest-neighbor distance} < r_j)$$
$$= n \times [F(r_j) - F(r_i)]$$

where, as before, n is the total number of points observed. The expected numbers can be compared to the observed numbers with the usual chi-square test [i.e., expression (5.4)].

To illustrate, ten hypothetical points are plotted in Figure 5–2 contained in a total area $A = 15^2 = 225$ square units. These points

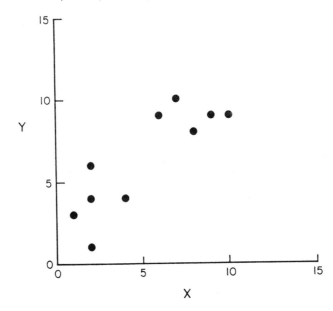

Figure 5–2. Ten hypothetical data points distributed over a square 15 units on a side to illustrate nearest-neighbor calculations

and their nearest-neighbor distances are given in Table 5–4. Figure 5–3 displays the probability distribution $F(r) = 1 - e^{-0.140r^2}$ associated with the 10 hypothetical points in Table 5–4. The expected mean value and variance of the mean calculated for the $n = 10$ nearest-neighbor distances, under the conjecture that the points occur randomly

Table 5–4. Nearest-neighbor example

	Point		Nearest		Distance	
i	X	Y	X'	Y'	r_i^2	r_i
1	1	3	2	4	2	1.414
2	2	1	1	3	5	2.236
3	2	4	1	3	2	1.414
4	2	6	2	4	4	2.000
5	4	4	2	4	4	2.000
6	6	9	7	10	2	1.414
7	7	10	6	9	2	1.414
8	8	8	9	9	2	1.414
9	9	9	10	9	1	1.000
10	10	9	9	9	1	1.000

*Note: $r_i = \sqrt{(x_i - x_i')^2 + (y_i - y_i')^2}$

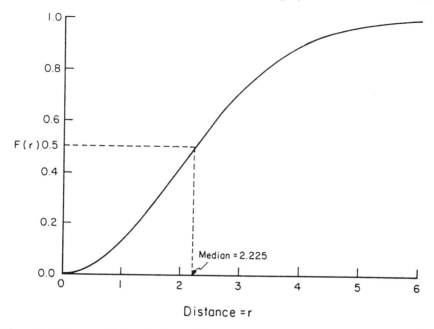

Figure 5–3. The cumulative distribution function from the hypothetical nearest-neighbor data

over the 225 square units of the x/y-plane, are

$$\text{mean }(r) = 0.5\sqrt{\frac{225}{10}} = 2.372 \quad \text{and} \quad \text{variance }(\bar{r}) = 0.068\frac{225}{100} = 0.153. \tag{5.13}$$

The observed mean of the ten nearest-neighbor distances $\bar{r}$ has an approximately normal distribution even for moderate sample sizes and, specifically,

$$\bar{r} = \frac{1}{n}\sum r_i = \frac{15.307}{10} = 1.531, \tag{5.14}$$

gives

$$z = \frac{\bar{r} - \text{mean }(r)}{\sqrt{\text{variance }(\bar{r})}} = \frac{1.531 - 2.372}{\sqrt{0.153}} = -2.150. \tag{5.15}$$

The test statistic z is an observation from a standard normal distribution when no spatial pattern exists. The one-sided p-value associated with $z = -2.150$ is 0.016, indicating that it is not likely that the ten points represent a sample from a random spatial distribution over the 225 square units of area. A one-sided test is most appropriate since small values of z are associated with small values of $\bar{r}$ which only occur when at least some of the observations cluster.

The nearest-neighbor analysis applied to the data shown in Figure 5–1 and given in Table 5–1 confirms the previous Poisson analysis. For $n = 200$ random points distributed on a unit square $(A = 1)$, the expected mean nearest-neighbor distance is $0.5\sqrt{1/200} = 0.0354$ with a standard error of $\sqrt{0.068(1/200^2)} = 0.00130$. The observed mean calculated from the nearest-neighbor distances among the 200 points is $\bar{r} = 0.0351$ producing $z = (0.0351 - 0.0354)/0.00130 = -0.196$, and the associated one-sided p-value of 0.422.

A general problem encountered in spatial analyses is illustrated by the nearest-neighbor data. The determination of the total area (A) is critical to the analysis, but rarely are clear, unequivocal boundaries available to define the relevant area of interest. Boundary determination is complicated because extending boundaries is likely to include noninformative points, which reduces the likelihood of detecting a cluster (decreases power). If an apparent "cluster" occurs in a specific town, it is likely that, when these data are combined with the distribution over the county, the "cluster" will be reduced; further, if the state is included, the "cluster" may disappear altogether. The opposite is also true. If the area of interest is made sufficiently small, only a few cases become a "cluster". Clearly, the boundaries of the area considered, to a large extent, determine whether points cluster. Sometimes "natural" boundaries are appropriate but, by and large, the determination of the total area is fairly subjective. A less important issue that applies to nearest-neighbor analysis also concerns boundary influences. Implicit in the development of the expressions for the expected mean and variance is the assumption, which clearly is violated in practice, that a circle of radius r surrounding a point never intersects a boundary of the study area. Adjustments to the expected mean and variance that partially correct for the problems of edge influences are available [3]. Last, note that nearest-neighbor distances are not independent.

Transformed Maps

Poisson and the nearest-neighbor approaches are not effective in the direct study of spatial distributions of human disease. The spatial pattern of human disease is dominated by the influence of the distribution of the population at risk. For example, Figure 5–4 shows 16 cases of lung cancer (adenocarcinoma) among white women, 55 years and older, in Jefferson and Denver counties, Colorado (1970).

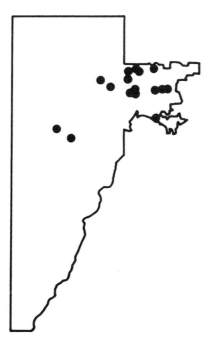

Figure 5–4. Lung cancer incidence cases (adenocarcinoma) among white females age 55 years or older for Jefferson and Denver counties, Colorado (1970) displayed on a geopolitical map

A cluster of cases occurs in the northeast because the vast majority of the population of these two counties lives in the city of Denver which is located in the northeast. Most maps of human disease are so strongly affected by the distribution of the residential population that a direct plot of disease cases is useless. In other words, humans tend to concentrate in specific areas, causing a high frequency of disease in those areas regardless of other factors.

Underlying the Poisson and nearest-neighbor approaches to the analysis of spatial data is the assumption that, if the phenomenon under study occurs at random, the spatial distribution has no pattern. For human populations, a disease can occur at random with respect to risk (every individual is approximately equally likely to contract the disease), but clusters will continue to appear when plotted on a geopolitical map. The reason for this clustering, as mentioned, is a nonuniform distribution of the population at risk over the study area.

One method of depicting and analyzing the spatial distribution of disease, without the interfering influence of the nonuniform population density, involves redrawing the geopolitical boundaries of a map (for a complete description see [4]). A geopolitical map is redrawn so that the density of the individuals at risk is equalized over the area under study. Redrawing a map to equalize population density allows the identification of factors that influence risk because the confounding effect of the population distribution is removed. One such transformed map, called a cartogram, is produced by first dividing the total area into a series of small subdivisions (e.g., census tracts). A computer algorithm is then used to expand the densely populated subareas and contract the sparsely populated subareas until all subdivisions have the appropriate sizes so that they reflect identical densities of persons at risk.

Figure 5–5 is a cartogram of Jefferson and Denver counties constructed with equal population density of white women, age 55 and over, among 179 census tracts. The fundamental feature of the redrawn map is that, when a disease occurs with equal probability among the individuals who make up the population at risk, the distribution of cases on a transformed map will be spatially random. That is, the distribution of the locations of cases will not differ in a systematic way from the uniformly distributed population at risk on a transformed map; only random differences exist. For example, when a disease has no spatial pattern, the location of the population centroid (the center or mean of a two-dimensional distribution) and the centroid of the cases will differ only by chance when located on a density-equalized map (see Figure 5–5). The 16 lung cancer cases plotted in Figure 5–5

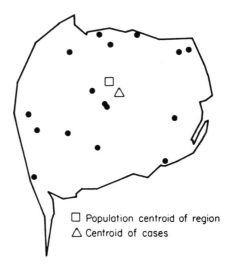

Figure 5–5. Lung cancer incidence cases (adenocarcinoma) among white females age 55 years or older for Jefferson and Denver counties, Colorado (1970) displayed on a density-equalized transformed map

on a density-equalized map show no visual evidence of a spatial pattern once the obvious confounding influence of the spatial distribution of the population at risk is removed. The clustering caused by the high density population of the city of Denver is no longer present, and no other spatial pattern appears to remain. Poisson or nearest-neighbor analysis could be used in conjunction with a transformed map to evaluate statistically the distribution of cases of disease for formal evidence of a spatial pattern.

To illustrate the nearest-neighbor approach using a map transformed to equalize the density of the population at risk, the locations (x_i, y_i) of incidence cases of lymphatic cancer from the city of San Francisco (1973–86) among white residents under the age of 20 are given in Table 5–5.

These $n = 26$ cases include both sexes and are located at the centroid of the census tract of residence on a map of San Francisco transformed so that all individuals under the age of 20 are uniformly distributed over the map (Figure 5–6). Each case generates a nearest-neighbor distance (r_i) also given in the Table 5–5. Cases of disease are artificially placed at the center of the census tract of residence (centroid), because the exact location was not available in the sampled data, only census tract of residence was recorded in the data set. The nearest-neighbor distances of zero are an artifact resulting from considering the location of all cases as occurring at the centroid of the census tract of residence. The expected mean nearest-neighbor distance among 26 points distributed at random on the San Francisco transformed map is mean$(r) = 0.5\sqrt{A/n} = 0.5\sqrt{111.444/26} = 1.035$ kilometers with a variance of

Table 5–5. Locations of cases of lymphatic cancer, San Francisco (1977–86)

i	x_i	y_i	r_i	i	x_i	y_i	r_i
1	3.563	4.250	0.880	15	2.742	3.935	0.880
2	−4.640	−1.317	1.551	16	2.769	−1.877	1.852
3	−3.974	4.083	1.635	17	−2.308	−2.536	0.000
4	−2.506	−0.530	1.269	18	1.095	3.028	1.880
5	−2.075	−5.288	1.305	19	−3.549	0.192	0.000
6	−0.998	4.031	1.393	20	−0.934	2.329	1.534
7	−2.368	3.779	1.189	21	4.331	−0.883	1.852
8	−2.250	−3.994	1.054	22	−2.308	−2.536	0.000
9	0.711	−2.470	2.142	23	−2.308	−2.536	0.000
10	−2.668	2.628	1.189	24	−3.549	0.192	0.000
11	−2.308	−2.536	0.000	25	−3.918	−3.729	1.002
12	−0.826	−0.666	1.685	26	−0.013	1.102	1.534
13	−4.001	−2.730	1.002	—	—	—	—
14	−1.207	−3.840	1.054	—	—	—	—

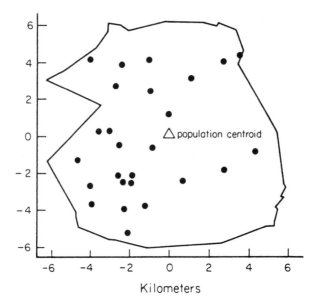

Figure 5–6. Lymphatic cancer incidence cases among white males and females age 20 years or younger displayed on a density-equalized transformed map (San Francisco, California, 1977–86)

variance$(\bar{r}) = 0.068A/n^2 = 0.068(111.444)/26^2 = 0.011$, where $A =$ 111.444 square kilometers (the area of the city of San Francisco). The observed mean calculated from the 26 nearest-neighbor distances is $\bar{r} = 1.072$ kilometers. The comparison of the expected and observed values yields a standard normal value $z = (1.072 - 1.035)/\sqrt{0.011} = 0.352$ and a one-sided p-value of 0.637. The nearest-neighbor analysis shows no evidence of spatial clustering of San Francisco lymphatic cancer cases among individuals under 20 years old.

Spatial Distribution about a Point

An important question concerning spatial distributions arises in a variety of contexts: Is there an excess of disease associated with a point source of exposure? For example, toxic waste dumps and nuclear facilities are often suspected as a cause of local increases in disease incidence. If a point source is associated with a disease, then the observed average distance between the source and the cases is likely to be smaller than a distance calculated under the hypothesis that no spatial association exists. This null hypothesis can be stated in two ways: Disease occurs at random on a density-equalized map or all individuals are at equal risk of disease regardless of their location on a geopolitical map. In the first case clustering may be apparent on a transformed map but the analysis is somewhat complicated ([5], [6]). In the second case the analysis is not complicated, but cases displayed on a geopolitical map are confounded by the distribution of the population at risk.

Spatial disease data are often collected for a specific area where the geographic area can be subdivided into a series of subareas such as census tracts. If the population for each subarea is known and the distance to a point source of exposure calculated, then it is relatively easy to assess statistically the degree of association between a spatial pattern of cases of disease and a specific geographic location. Suppose the point source of exposure is located at a specific point (x_0, y_0). Under the hypothesis that no spatial pattern exists among the n cases, the expected distance from the location of a randomly selected person (x_i, y_i) to the point (x_0, y_0) on a geopolitical map is approximately

$$\text{expected mean distance} = ED \approx \frac{\sum\limits_{i=1}^{k} p_i d_i'}{\sum\limits_{i=1}^{k} p_i}, \tag{5.16}$$

where p_i is the number of persons at risk in the ith subarea, d_i' is the distance from the centroid of the ith subarea to the point of exposure, and k is the number of these areas. The variance of the distribution generating the observed distances, again calculated under the assumption that the cases are distributed randomly, is estimated by

$$\text{variance } (D) \approx \frac{\sum\limits_{i=1}^{k} p_i (d_i' - ED)^2}{\sum\limits_{i=1}^{k} p_i}. \tag{5.17}$$

The average distance $[\bar{d} = (1/n) \sum d_i$, where $d_i = \sqrt{(x_i - x_0)^2 + (y_i - y_0)^2}$ is the distance from the location of the ith case to the point (x_0, y_0) on a geopolitical map] can be calculated between the location of the n observed cases and the location of the point source of exposure. A statistical test of the hypothesis of no association between the location (x_0, y_0) and the spatial distribution of disease results from the comparison of this observed mean value with the null hypothesis generated expectation or

$$z = \frac{\bar{d} - ED}{\sqrt{\text{variance } (D)/n}}, \tag{5.18}$$

where z has an approximate standard normal distribution when no spatial pattern exists associated with the point (x_0, y_0). The test statistic

z is an accurate assessment of observed spatial patterns associated with a specific point when the number of cases is not extremely small (greater than 10 or 15) and the number of subareas used to calculate ED and variance (D) from expression (5.16) and (5.17) is large.

A possible point source of exposure is a large microwave tower located near the center of the city of San Francisco (see Figure 5–7). The location and the distance in kilometers to the tower for $n = 27$ cases of brain cancer found in white individuals less than 20 years old are given in Table 5–6 (also shown in Figure 5–7).

The expected distance to the microwave tower for a random white person less than 20 years old living in San Francisco is approximately $ED = 3.735$ kilometers, and the variance associated with a distribution of random cases is estimated to be variance $(D) = 2.115$ [from expressions (5.16) and (5.17)], based on $k = 148$ San Francisco census tracts. The observed mean distance to the point source (x_0, y_0) for the 27 brain cancer cases is $\bar{d} = 3.379$ kilometers where the microwave tower is located at $(x_0 = -2.0, y_0 = 0.2)$. These 27 cancer cases exhibit an average distance to the point source of about 0.5 kilometers less than the distance expected for a noncase (3.379 versus 3.735). Comparing this observed mean to the expected value yields a standard normal statistic, when the spatial pattern of disease is random, of $z = -1.270$ with a one-sided p-value of 0.102. The p-value indicates that the

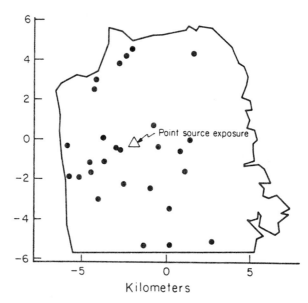

Figure 5–7. Brain cancer incidence cases among white males and females age 20 years or younger displayed on a geopolitical map (San Francisco, California, 1977–86)

Table 5–6. Locations of cases of brain cancer, San Francisco (1977–86)

i	x_i	y_i	d_i	i	x_i	y_i	d_i
1	−1.136	0.718	1.406	15	−4.865	−1.154	2.831
2	−0.163	−3.429	3.818	16	−6.156	−1.854	4.288
3	−2.718	4.185	4.415	17	1.036	−0.013	3.241
4	−3.090	−0.532	0.950	18	0.474	−0.568	2.699
5	−4.103	0.111	1.928	19	−0.141	−5.267	5.470
6	−4.664	2.567	3.705	20	−2.741	4.196	4.429
7	−5.528	−1.899	3.736	21	−2.865	−2.249	2.154
8	−0.842	−0.363	1.367	22	−4.036	−1.093	2.042
9	2.330	−5.074	6.654	23	−4.513	3.042	3.983
10	−1.393	−2.411	2.353	24	−4.849	−1.142	2.812
11	−1.636	−5.274	5.105	25	−6.267	−0.282	4.067
12	−2.732	4.177	4.410	26	1.257	4.304	5.678
13	−3.055	−0.513	0.911	27	0.748	−1.574	3.253
14	−4.346	−3.017	3.541				

pattern of disease observed is somewhat unlikely to have occurred by chance. That is, the spatial distribution of cases (Figure 5–7) in proximity to the microwave tower is possibly associated with factors other than the distribution of the population at risk.

Spatial patterns of disease do not unequivocally identify specific causes. Such factors as differential smoking patterns, socioeconomic differences, and access to medical care are examples of possible explanations of observed spatial patterns. For analyses based on a density-equalized map or a geopolitical map, evidence of a spatial pattern of disease remains subject to the same limitations in interpretation as most pairwise associations. Like most epidemiologic data, spatial patterns of disease are no more than a special type of observational (nonrandomized) data.

Time/Space Analysis

Time/space analysis is characterized by the absence of a measure reflecting the population at risk. Data on the nondiseased population or data consisting of disease rates are not necessary. All that is needed is the time of occurrence and the location of each case for a defined geographic region. Time differences and distances between disease locations form the basis of a time/space analysis. A sample of n observed times and locations is used to generate a series of all possible unsigned differences in time and distance between cases producing $\mathcal{N} = n(n-1)/2$ pairs of time/distance data. Eight hypothetical cases occurring at time t_i and located at (x_i, y_i), shown in Figure 5–8, are

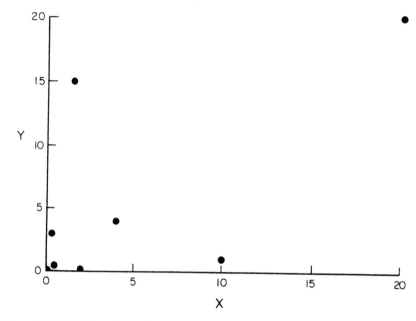

Figure 5–8. Eight hypothetical points distributed over a square 20 units on a side to illustrate time/space clustering calculations

given in Table 5–7. These eight cases generate $N = 8(7)/2 = 28$ possible different pairs of time/distance observations, shown in Table 5–8. As before, the distance between (x_i, y_i) and (x_j, y_j) is $d_{ij} = \sqrt{(x_i - x_j)^2 + (y_i - y_j)^2}$. A plot of the time/distance pairs is displayed in Figure 5–9.

The principle underlying the time/space approach is that cases of disease with common underlying factors will likely be close in time and location, while unrelated cases will tend to be separated by typical

Table 5–7. Data: time/space

i	Time t_i	Location x_i	y_i
1	1.0	0.1	0.1
2	1.4	2.0	0.2
3	2.0	0.3	3.0
4	2.6	4.0	4.0
5	5.0	0.5	0.5
6	7.0	10.0	1.0
7	10.0	1.5	15.0
8	13.0	20.0	20.0

Table 5–8. All pairs: time/distance

	$|t_i - t_j|$	d_{ij}		$|t_i - t_j|$	d_{ij}
1	0.4	1.90	15	3.0	2.51
2	1.0	2.91	16	5.0	9.90
3	1.6	5.52	17	8.0	12.06
4	4.0	0.57	18	11.0	26.02
5	6.0	9.94	19	2.4	4.95
6	9.0	14.97	20	4.4	6.71
7	12.0	28.14	21	7.4	11.28
8	0.6	3.28	22	10.4	22.63
9	1.2	4.29	23	2.0	9.51
10	3.6	1.53	24	5.0	14.53
11	5.6	8.04	25	8.0	27.58
12	8.6	14.81	26	3.0	16.38
13	11.6	26.76	27	6.0	21.47
14	0.6	3.83	28	3.0	19.16

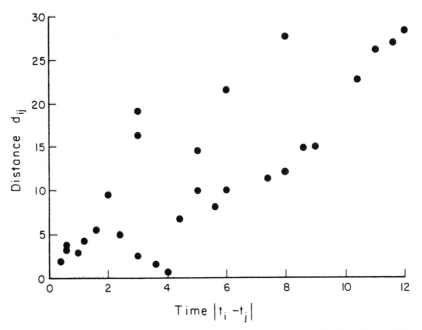

Figure 5–9. The 28 possible pairs of time/space "data" for the eight hypothetical data points

differences in time or distance. Clustering in space only or time only does not provide evidence of an association between cases of disease. For example, cases clustering only because of unequal population densities are not likely to cluster with respect to time when no relationship exists among cases of disease. Figure 5–4 shows a cluster of lung cancer cases due to the high population density of the city of Denver. When all individuals are at equal risk, no reason exists for cases within Denver city limits to occur at times different from those cases that occur outside the city in the less populated areas. Also, in the absence of an association, cases that cluster in time (e.g., seasonality) will not occur closer in distance than would be expected by chance. It is only when cases occur in proximity in both time and location that excess pairs of small time differences and relatively short distances appear together. Infectious disease frequently exhibits classic time/distance clustering where cases arise at similar times and in similar places because of the contagious nature of the disease. Infectious disease serves as a biological model for the time/space approach.

A difficulty in analyzing time/distance data is the increased variability incurred by creating the $N = n(n - 1)/2$ pairs. A simple analysis of time/distance data using a 2×2 table reduces the impact of this variation [7]. Critical values for time and for distance are employed to classify time/distance pairs into four categories. Suppose the critical difference for time is t_0 and the critical distance between cases is d_0, then the time/distance pairs form a typical 2×2 table (Table 5–9).

A two-way table treats all time/distance pairs where at least one value exceeds the critical distance (d_0) or time (t_0) values as equivalent, thereby reducing the variability induced by the formation of the time/distance pairing. Using an approach based on a 2×2 table implicitly makes the assumption that cases occurring beyond t_0 or d_0 are not related, and at least some cases occurring with time and distance measurements less than both t_0 and d_0 potentially provide information on clustering. This approach applies to most sets of spatial data producing a binary variable to assess clustering in time and space—

Table 5–9. Notation for a 2 × 2 table of time/distance pairs

	$t < t_0$	$t \geq t_0$	Total
$d < d_0$	a	b	$a + b$
$d \geq d_0$	c	d	$c + d$
Total	$a + c$	$b + d$	N

Table 5–10. A 2 × 2 table of time/distance pairs for leukemia data

	$t < t_0$	$t \geq t_0$	Total
$d < d_0$	5	20	25
$d \geq d_0$	147	4,388	4,535
Total	152	4,408	4,560

and

	"Close"	Not "Close"	Total
Observed	5	4,555	4,560
Expected	0.833	4,559.167	4,560

binary in the sense that both members of a pair are less than t_0 and d_0 ("close") or not.

In a study of clustering among 96 cases of leukemia [8], the critical distance was set at one kilometer $(d_0 = 1)$ and the critical time set at 60 days $(t_0 = 60)$, producing $N = 96(95)/2 = 4,560$ time/distance pairs distributed as shown in Table 5–10.

The expected number of pairs "clustering" by chance is estimated from the expression $(a + b)(a + c)/N = (25)(152)/4,560 = 0.833$, where time and distance are postulated as unrelated (independent); that is, the expected number of random "close" pairs $= N \times P(\text{time} < t_0$ and distance $< d_0) = N \times P(\text{time} < t_0)P(\text{distance} < d_0)$ which is estimated by

$$\text{estimate expected number} = N \frac{a + b}{N} \frac{a + c}{N}, \qquad (5.19)$$

where the notation for the observations from a 2 × 2 table is given in Table 5–9.

> Aside: The Poisson distribution is used to investigate the likelihood of rare events among a series of unrelated binary outcomes. Rare events, under the hypothesis that each event in the series under investigation occurs independently with equal probability, are assigned Poisson distribution probabilities (in fact, binomial probabilities). In this time/space context, the question is: How likely is the occurrence of five or more "close" pairs among the 4,560 pairs if all pairs occur at random when the expected number of "close" pairs is 0.833? The Poisson distribution gives
>
> $$P(X \geq k) = \sum_{i=k}^{\infty} \frac{e^{-\lambda}\lambda^i}{i!} = 1 - \sum_{i=0}^{k-1} \frac{e^{-\lambda}\lambda^i}{i!} \qquad (5.20)$$

and, specifically,

$$P(X \geq 5) = 1 - (0.4346 + 0.3622 + 0.1509 + 0.0419 + 0.00870$$

$$= 1 - 0.9983 = 0.0017$$

(λ is estimated by $\hat{\lambda} = 0.833$) as the answer. That is, five or more "close" pairs will rarely occur when time and distance are unrelated. The Poisson-derived p-value is useful in evaluating results arising from rare events and provides an alternative to the more common chi-square test for independence which is not accurate when the expected values per cell become small (less than 3 or so).

Using a Poisson distribution, the observed result of five "close" pairs is unlikely under the hypothesis of no association between time and distance. Five pairs with both time and distance less than the critical values ($t_0 = 60$ days and $d_0 = 1$ kilometer), when 0.833 pairs are expected, occur with probability 0.0017 when time and distance are unrelated.

Application of the Poisson distribution is not strictly correct. Time/distance pairs are not independent. The formation of the N time/distance pairs introduces some dependency, because the same observations appear in a number of pairings. This lack of independence, however, has only slight impact on the accuracy of the results when the sample size is large. More important issues involve the loss of information from categorizing two continuous variables and the lack of clear-cut choices for the critical values. A number of other approaches to time/distance data have been proposed that avoid these two problems. For example, a regression analysis using the reciprocal of the time and the reciprocal of the distance has been suggested [9]. Another approach involves a permutation test to evaluate time/distance association [9] which is the topic of the next section.

Permutation Tests

A permutation test is a statistical procedure that applies to numerous situations as well as the study of time/distance data. The application of this technique does not require sophisticated statistical distributions (e.g., t-distribution or F-distribution) but does require the use of a computer when the sample size is more than 10 or so. Before applying a permutation test to time/distance data, the permutation test analogous to the two-sample t-test illustrates the approach.

Analyzing cholesterol levels from the WCGS individuals classified as type-A and type-B with a permutation test allows comparison with

Table 5–11. WCGS data: Cholesterol and behavior type

	Chol	A/B		Chol	A/B
1	344	B	21	169	B
2	233	A	22	226	B
3	291	A	23	175	B
4	312	A	24	276	A
5	185	B	25	242	B
6	250	A	26	252	B
7	263	B	27	153	B
8	246	A	28	183	B
9	246	B	29	234	A
10	224	B	30	137	B
11	212	B	31	181	A
12	188	B	32	248	A
13	250	B	33	252	A
14	197	A	34	202	A
15	148	B	35	218	A
16	268	A	36	202	B
17	224	A	37	212	A
18	239	A	38	325	A
19	239	A	39	194	B
20	254	A	40	213	B

previous t-test results for the same data (Chapter 2). The data (repeated from Table 2–1) on the 40 heaviest WCGS participants are given in Table 5–11. The observed mean cholesterol level of the 20 type-A individuals is $\bar{y}_A = 245.050$ and $\bar{y}_B = 210.300$ for the 20 type-B individuals.

The null hypothesis that behavior type is unrelated to cholesterol level is equivalent to considering the data as if 20 individuals were chosen at random and labeled A while the remaining 20 individuals were labeled B. In fact, when 20 individuals are selected at random from the group of 40, the mean cholesterol level of 20 randomly chosen individuals then estimates the cholesterol level in the group and the mean of the remaining 20 observations also estimates the same mean. Differences between two mean values based on groups of randomly chosen individuals result only from the random sampling process. The behavior type status is unimportant since individuals with behavior type-A and type-B will likely be balanced when comparisons are made between two randomly chosen groups. In principle all possible samples of 20 could be selected from the 40 measured cholesterol levels and used to calculate all possible mean values for 20 randomly sampled and 20 nonsampled individuals. The set of differences between these means is the distribution of the test statistic $\bar{y}_A - \bar{y}_B$ under the null hypothesis that behavior type is unrelated to cholesterol level. Choosing the observations that make up the mean values at random guarantees that the null hypothesis is true. The number of all such differences is too large even for a fast computer (1.4×10^{11} samples) to make this simple calculation. However, it is possible to program a computer to take a large number of random samples of 20 from the data set and calculate a series of mean differences in cholesterol levels between the sampled and nonsampled groups. Such a series of estimates reflects the distribution of differences uninfluenced by any systematic effects that may exist, called a null-distribution. Also special computer programs exist (e.g., *StatXact*) to further refine the estimate of the null-distribution.

A set of 5,000 random samples of 20 from the 40 WCGS individuals (Table 5–11) produces the summary statistics for the values of "$\bar{y}_A - \bar{y}_B$" given in Table 5–12 (Note: The quotes indicate the values generated by random selection).

This null-distribution is determined entirely by the empirical process of repeatedly sampling 20 values from the 40 WCGS observations (5,000 times). A histogram of the observed frequencies of mean differences is shown in Figure 5–10. The null-distribution is essentially symmetric with mean near zero (-0.013). This empirical distribution accurately reflects a *t*-distribution. For example, the *t*-distribution predicts a 95th percentile of 23.927 and the observed percentile is 23.450. The observed mean difference between type-A and type-B individuals is $\bar{y}_A - \bar{y}_B = 245.050 - 210.300 = 34.75$. Again using the computer, it is a simple matter to count the more extreme values in the sample of 5,000. Only 35 randomized mean differences exceeded 34.75, showing that observed differences larger than 34.75 are not

Table 5–12. Summary of 5,000 random samples from the WCGS cholesterol/behavior type data—the distribution of "$\bar{y}_A - \bar{y}_B$"

	Number of Samples	5,000
	Mean value	-0.013
	Variance	211.300
	Standard deviation	14.536
	Minimum value	-45.150
	Maximum value	58.250

Percentiles	1%	5%	10%	90%	95%	99%
Observed value	-33.650	-23.450	-18.550	18.950	23.450	32.750

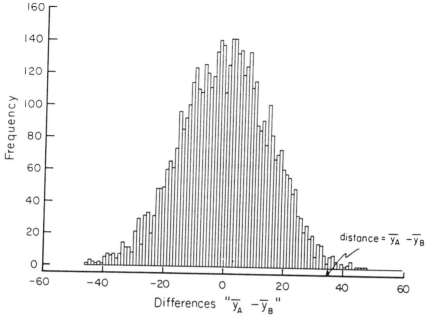

Figure 5–10. The histogram of the null-distribution of "$\bar{y}_A - \bar{y}_B$"

likely when no association exists between behavior type and cholesterol level. The p-value based on estimated null-distribution is $35/5{,}000 = 0.007$, which almost exactly agrees with the previous p-value of 0.00725 ($T = 2.562$) found using the t-distribution and the "shift" model [expression (2.9)].

Of course, when the assumptions underlying a t-test hold, it is easily and directly applied. But when the assumptions do not hold, t-test results become suspect while the permutation test continues to give an accurate p-value under almost all conditions. The t-test is designed for the test statistic $\bar{y}_2 - \bar{y}_1$, but a permutation procedure allows the use of most test statistics. If, for example, the ratio of two mean cholesterol levels is a sensitive measure of the association between behavior type and cholesterol, then a t-test is not possible (ratios do not usually have normal distributions), but a permutation test follows the same pattern. Instead of a sample of random differences, a series of ratios is constructed from randomly sampled data and the observed ratio of $\bar{y}_A/\bar{y}_B$ is evaluated against this series (e.g., the number random ratios that exceed the observed ratio estimates a one-sided p-value). The simplicity and the general applicability of the permutation test makes the approach an important analytic tool.

Time/Space: Permutation Test

A permutation test is well suited to investigate possible patterns of disease in time and space. Since most measures of clustering are statistically complex, a repeated sampling scheme avoids difficult mathematical issues and, at the same time, produces a rigorous evaluation of the degree of time/distance clustering found in collected data.

Parallel to the t-test illustration, the hypothesis of no clustering is equivalent to postulating that the time/distance pairs are formed at random. A total of $N = n(n-1)/2$ observed pairs occur, where each pair contains a time and a distance measurement. There are $N!$ possible sets or permutations of time/distance data, which are the basis for describing probabilities under the null hypothesis because each set is equally likely when no time/space association exists. For samples of seven or more pairs complete enumeration of all possible $N!$ sets of time/distance data is impractical, but again a computer can be programmed to select sets of random pairings. That is, special computer algorithms produce random pairings of distance and time under the hypothesis of no time/space clustering. The repeated calculation of a statistical measure of clustering from these randomized sets of "data" forms an estimate of the null hypothesis generated distribution.

One choice to measure of time/space clustering is

$$c = \sum_{i=1}^{N} (t_i - \bar{t})(d_i - \bar{d}), \tag{5.21}$$

where, as before, t_i is the unsigned difference in time and d_i is the distance between the location of two cases. Subtracting the means, $\bar{t}$ and $\bar{d}$, reduces the magnitude of the product $t_i d_i$ for ease of computation and produces a value likely close to zero when time and distance are unrelated. The test statistic c is large when an excess of "close" time/distance pairs occurs. Therefore, a large value of c indicates a positive association between time and distance where a value in the neighborhood of zero indicates no association. The distribution of c, under the null hypothesis, can be estimated by forming random sets of time/distance pairs and calculating a series of randomized values "c." The distribution of "c" (estimated null-distribution) is then applied to assess the observed value c calculated from the data.

In 1981, chemical solvents were detected in the drinking water supplied to a portion of Santa Clara county, California. A likely source of this contamination was leakage from storage tanks that are part of the electronics manufacturing industry. It was thought that this contamination might be associated with an increase in the number of

Table 5–13. Time/Space: Santa Clara county, 1981–83

Time	Location		Time	Location		Time	Location	
t_i	x_i	y_i	t_i	x_i	y_i	t_i	x_i	y_i
1	156.20	31.43	4	163.34	29.53	3	162.93	29.59
3	159.55	27.02	4	162.03	32.30	33	153.59	31.79
2	156.60	29.45	6	160.67	27.89	9	162.05	30.33
2	158.96	28.84	2	159.47	29.77	18	163.32	28.36
2	161.77	25.48	27	163.30	28.69	3	157.28	29.07
4	159.94	27.95	36	157.69	31.05	6	162.26	26.45
4	156.48	28.35	6	161.43	33.40	6	162.98	27.45
6	155.85	31.44	30	165.17	28.01	2	159.12	30.75
12	157.64	30.98	2	157.99	30.74	2	157.90	29.96
12	162.65	29.14	5	162.07	28.65	4	168.23	21.31
30	163.10	29.81	6	161.75	27.26	6	159.83	28.03
2	159.34	28.18	6	161.73	29.26	8	164.29	25.96
1	154.25	31.37	2	160.44	26.97	12	161.68	26.42
1	161.20	31.60	4	161.78	29.56	27	157.94	29.92
6	156.55	31.68	4	170.72	17.40	24	162.10	31.24
6	170.14	16.62	6	168.28	21.30	24	161.53	26.30

cardiac defects among newborn infants. The data in Table 5–13 (adapted from Shaw [10]) gives the time (months) and the location (geographic coordinates modified to protect confidentiality) of the occurrence of 48 cardiac defects among births during the years 1981, 1982, and 1983 in Santa Clara county.

These $n = 48$ observations produce $N = 48(47)/2 = 1,128$ time/distance pairs. The observed value c calculated from the 1,128 pairs is $c = -1715.06$. To evaluate formally this observed measure of time/space clustering of cardiac defect cases, a series of 5,000 samples each made up of 1,128 randomly paired time/distance observations was computer generated using the values in Table 5–13. A value of "c" was calculated for each set forming an estimated null-distribution. Estimated percentiles from the computer generated null-distribution are given in Table 5–14.

The mean of the null-distribution is 11.8 with a median value of -14.9, which indicates an almost symmetric distribution of values of "c" (see Figure 5–11). If all possible samples were used, then the

Table 5–14. Estimated percentiles of the null-distribution of c generated from the Santa Clara data

Percentile	1%	5%	10%	90%	95%	99%
Observed value	$-3,336.3$	$-2,344.9$	$-1,803.9$	1,851.9	2,375.2	3,409.7

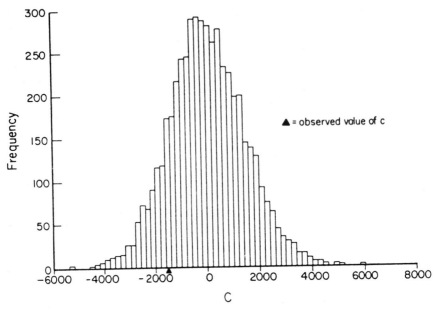

Figure 5–11. The histogram of the null-distribution of "c"

null-distribution would be perfectly symmetric with mean and median equal to zero. The number of null-distribution values of "c" greater than the observed $c = -1,715.06$ is 4,447, giving an estimated one-tail p-value of $4,447/5,000 = 0.889$. Therefore, a greater value of c than the one observed is estimated to occur with a frequency of about 90% when no time/distance association exists. A further analysis of these data might utilize the location of the cases in relation to the contamination. For example, the previously suggested population density-equalized map could be employed (again, [11]).

To summarize, some advantages and disadvantages of a permutation test approach are:

ADVANTAGES

1. No assumptions are necessary about the structure of the sampled population.
2. The process is conceptually simple even for complex measures of associations.
3. Permutation tests apply to almost all usual analytic situations (t-test, correlation analysis, analysis of variance, etc.).
4. Permutation tests are valid for any sample size.
5. The null-distribution can be generated for essentially any test statistic, allowing a wide range of measures of association to be used.

DISADVANTAGES

1. The results are not consistent—the test statistic depends on a series of random samples of observations, meaning that different analyses will produce slightly differing p-values from the same data.
2. The permutation test usually requires a special computer program for application.
3. If the assumptions underlying a data set generate an accurate null-distribution, then a test statistic is easily evaluated (tables and computer programs exist) and is often the statistically optimum technique. For example, if the assumptions generating a t-test hold, then the easily evaluated t-statistic is more powerful than any other approach.

Jackknife Estimation

Jackknife estimation is designed to produce an estimate and its variance and, like the permutation test, usually requires implementation with a computer. Estimating a quantity and at the same time evaluating its precision often involves the assumption that the population sampled has a particular structure. An assumption often made, for example, is that the sample of observations comes from a population with a normal distribution. Clearly data do not always come from populations with normal distributions or even symmetric distributions, which complicates the process of calculating and assessing a summary estimate. A method called a jackknife estimate, because it is so handy, is one way to estimate a quantity and its variance for a wide range of situations without assumptions about the properties of the sampled data. The payment for this flexibility is that the procedure generally requires computer implementation.

A jackknife estimate is calculated from a sample of n independent observations by creating a series of n truncated subsamples. Each subsample consists of $n - 1$ observations formed by deleting a different observation from the sample. The jackknife estimate and its variance are then calculated from these truncated subsamples.

If a summary statistic represented by θ is estimated by $\hat{\theta}$, then the key to a jackknife estimate is a series of n estimates $\hat{\theta}_{(i)}$ derived in the identical manner as the estimate $\hat{\theta}$, but with the ith value deleted from the sample. The mean of the $\hat{\theta}_{(i)}$-values is the jackknife estimate of θ or, in symbols,

$$\hat{\theta} = \frac{\sum_{i=1}^{n} \hat{\theta}_{(i)}}{n} \qquad (5.22)$$

and the variance of this estimate is estimated by

$$\text{variance }(\hat{\theta}) = \frac{(n-1) \sum_{i=1}^{n} (\hat{\theta}_{(i)} - \hat{\theta})^2}{n}. \tag{5.23}$$

Another feature of the jackknife estimate is that an estimate of bias, if any, is also available and given by the expression

$$\text{estimated bias} = (n-1)(\hat{\theta} - \hat{\theta}), \tag{5.24}$$

where $\hat{\theta}$ is the estimated quantity based on the complete set of n observations. Note that this process is relatively simple and remains relatively simple even when the estimate $\hat{\theta}$ is a complicated quantity.

Example

Consider the jackknife estimate of the mean and standard deviation of nine observations (2, 6, 10, 34, 66, 4, 8, 22, 45). The nine truncated subsamples are shown in Table 5–15.

The jackknife mean and its estimated variance are derived from the next to last column in Table 5–15 ($\bar{x}_{(i)}$). That is,

$$\bar{x} = \frac{24.375 + \cdots + 19.000}{9} = 21.889, \quad \text{[expression (5.22)]} \tag{5.25}$$

and the variance of this estimate is estimated by [expression (5.23)]

$$\text{variance }(\bar{x}) = \frac{8[(24.375 - 21.889)^2 + \cdots + (19.000 - 21.889)^2]}{9} = 54.568. \tag{5.26}$$

Table 5–15. The nine subsamples used in the jackknife estimate of the mean and the standard deviation

i	1	2	3	4	5	6	7	8	Sum	$\bar{x}_{(i)}$	$s\hat{d}_{(i)}$
1	6	10	34	66	4	8	22	45	195	24.375	22.309
2	2	10	34	66	4	8	22	45	191	23.875	22.818
3	2	6	34	66	4	8	22	45	187	23.375	23.207
4	2	6	10	66	4	8	22	45	163	20.375	23.188
5	2	6	10	34	4	8	22	45	131	16.375	15.767
6	2	6	10	34	66	8	22	45	193	24.125	22.580
7	2	6	10	34	66	4	22	45	189	23.625	23.026
8	2	6	10	34	66	4	8	45	175	21.875	23.691
9	2	6	10	34	66	4	8	22	152	19.000	21.804

The estimates of the mean and variance in this simple situation are the same as the usual estimates of the mean and variance [i.e., $\bar{x} = \sum x_i/n = 21.889$ and variance$(\bar{x}) = \sum (x_i - \bar{x})^2/[n(n-1)] = 54.568$). Therefore, the estimated bias will always be zero (i.e., estimated bias $= (n-1)(\bar{\bar{x}} - \bar{x}) = 0$.].

The jackknife estimate of the standard deviation, using the last column of Table 5–15 ($s\hat{d}_{(i)}$), follows the same pattern. An estimate of the standard deviation is

$$s\hat{d} = \frac{22.309 + \cdots + 21.804}{9} = 22.043, \tag{5.27}$$

and the variance of this estimate is estimated by

$$\text{variance}(s\hat{d}) = \frac{8[(22.309 - 22.043)^2 + \cdots + (21.804 - 22.043)^2]}{9}$$

$$= 41.578. \tag{5.28}$$

The usual estimate of a standard deviation is easily calculated from the nine observations ($s\hat{d} = \sqrt{\sum (x_i - \bar{x})^2/(n-1)} = 22.161$), but estimates of the variance and the bias of this estimate are not simple. However, an estimate of the variance for the jackknife-estimated standard deviation is easily calculated (41.578) and, in addition, an estimate of the bias is $bias = 8(22.043 - 22.161) = -0.941$. Jackknife estimation applies in the same manner to many situations where expressions for an estimate and its variance are either complicated or unknown.

Applied Example

A map showing incidence cases of oral/pharyngeal cancer in Contra Costa county, California suggests that the spatial distribution is more clustered among females than males (Figure 5–12). The data in terms of the longitude and latitude coordinates of the observed cases are given in Table 5–16.

Several investigators have noted (e.g., [12] and [13]) an excess of lung cancer that might be associated with the oil refining industry located in the northern part of Contra Costa county. Suppose for simplicity that the concentration of refining activity is located at a specific point (longitude $x_0 = 122.3$ and latitude $y_0 = 38.1$; see Figure 5–12). The distance from the point (x_0, y_0) to each case of oral/pharyngeal cancer can be calculated (symbolized by d_i). Mantel [9] suggests that the sensitivity to detect clusters of observations is increased by employing the reciprocal of the distance $(1/d_i)$ rather than

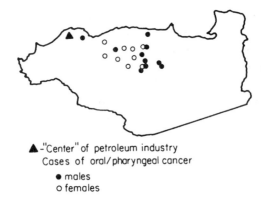

▲ -"Center" of petroleum industry
Cases of oral/pharyngeal cancer

    ● males
    ○ females

Figure 5–12. Oral/pharyngeal cancer incidence cases among white males and females ages 35 to 55 for Contra Costa county, California (1978–81)

Table 5–16. Longitude and latitude location of male and female oral/pharyngeal cancer cases in Contra Costa county (1978–81) among individuals ages 35 to 54

	Female		Male	
i	Longitude	Latitude	Longitude	Latitude
1	121.91	38.15	121.60	38.02
2	121.90	37.88	121.25	38.20
3	122.05	37.93	122.01	37.95
4	122.10	37.95	122.04	37.91
5	122.00	37.85	122.05	37.88
6	122.15	37.88	122.08	37.98
7	122.12	37.80	122.01	37.81
8	122.25	37.78	122.11	38.15
9	122.20	37.95	122.32	37.83
10	—	—	122.31	37.84

using distance (d_i) directly. The transformation $1/d_i$ is a simple function of distance which strongly emphasizes the short distances and minimizes the influence of large distances observed in the sampled data. Following this suggestion, the distance from the "source" of pollution to a cancer case is examined for both males and females with a harmonic mean. A harmonic mean is defined as

$$\bar{h} = \frac{1}{\dfrac{1}{n}\sum_{i=1}^{n}\dfrac{1}{d_i}}, \tag{5.29}$$

where n is the number of cases ($n = 9$ for females and $n = 10$ for males).

Table 5–17. Harmonic mean distances $\bar{h}_{(i)}$ in kilometers

i	1	2	3	4	5	6	7	8	9	10
Female	29.339	28.722	29.936	30.722	28.997	30.061	29.076	29.147	32.147	—
Male	29.694	29.164	31.458	31.361	31.161	32.590	30.503	34.462	31.425	31.570

A complicated expression such as the harmonic mean $\bar{h}$ is easily evaluated with a jackknife estimate because its accompanying variance is readily calculated. Each truncated sample using the data from Table 5–16 produces an estimated harmonic mean $\bar{h}_{(i)}$ based on deleting the ith longitude/latitude pair from the n observations, giving Table 5–17.

Using the series of the $\bar{h}_{(i)}$-values to calculate the jackknife-estimated harmonic mean and the jackknife variance allows an approximate 95% confidence interval to be constructed for the harmonic mean for each sex. Summary statistics are displayed in the Table 5–18.

Comparison of the jackknife estimates ($\bar{h}$-values) shows a smaller mean distance for female cases compared to males. The variability associated with these estimates, however, is considerable, and because the confidence intervals almost completely overlap, no statistical evidence exists that the proximity to the center of the oil refining industry has differing effects on the spatial pattern of risk of oral/pharyngeal cancer between females and males in the age group 35–54.

Jackknife estimation and permutation tests are two examples of a class of modern computer-intensive statistical techniques with two fundamental features. They free the user from employing sometimes unverifiable assumptions, and equally important, these techniques work for many complex statistical measures and not just the handful of measures employed in the past. Most statistical methods in use today were developed before 1950, when computation was done almost

Table 5–18. Summary statistics from the jackknife estimates of mean distances

Statistic	Female	Male
Sample size (n)	9	10
Mean $(\bar{h})$	29.793	31.339
variance $(\bar{h})$	8.327	17.604
SE $(\bar{h})$	2.886	4.195
Bias	−0.269	−0.548
Upper limit (95%)	35.450	39.562
Lower limit (95%)	24.136	23.116

exclusively by hand. Mathematically tractable approaches are no longer necessary, because mathematical tractability has been replaced by high-speed electronic computation, which continues to become less expensive and easier to apply. Thus computer-intensive approaches allow the user to explore complicated issues with methods dictated by epidemiology, unrestricted by traditional techniques and measures. More extensive descriptions of computer-intensive methods are found in [14] and [15].

6 The Two × K Contingency Table and the Two × Two × Two Table

THE TWO × K CONTINGENCY TABLE

A basic tool for epidemiologic investigation is the 2 × 2 table. An important extension is the 2 × K table where the presence or absence of a disease is recorded at K levels of a risk factor. The 2 × K contingency table can be viewed from the perspective of a K-level variable (risk factor) or from the perspective of a binary variable (disease). In terms of analytic approaches, the two perspectives produce a regression or two-sample analysis. Expressed as questions, these perspectives are:

1. Regression: What is the relationship between a K-level risk factor and a binary disease outcome?
2. Two-sample: Does the mean level of the risk factor differ between two disease outcome groups?

These two questions generate rather different descriptions of the data but, as will be seen, produce the same statistical test. Ridit analysis is another technique for analyzing a 2 × K table. All three methods are "distribution-free" because no knowledge or assumptions about the distribution that generates the data are required. A number of texts fully develop the analysis and interpretation of discrete data classified into multi-way tables (e.g., [1], [2], and [3]).

Data on coffee consumption and pancreatic cancer [4] provide a concrete example for the discussion of a 2 × K table. Men ($n = 523$) classified as cases ($Y = 0$; row 1) or controls ($Y = 1$; row 2) and by consumption of 0, 1, 2, and 3 or more cups of coffee per day ($X = j$, $j = 0$, 1, 2, or 3; columns) are shown in Table 6–1. For simplicity, three or more cups consumed per day are coded as 3. The data are given in Table 6–1 (also displayed in Figure 6–1).

The analysis of a 2 × K table is addressed from three points of view. First, a general technique to evaluate the hypothesis of independence or homogeneity is described (Is coffee drinking related in any way to

Table 6–1. Pancreatic cancer and coffee consumption

	$X = 0$	$X = 1$	$X = 2$	$X = 3$	Total
$Y = 0$	9	94	53	60	216
$Y = 1$	32	119	74	82	307
Total	41	213	127	142	523

2 by K table: data

	X=0	X=1	X=2	X=3	total
Y=0	9	94	53	60	216
Y=1	32	119	74	82	307
total	41	213	127	142	523

Independence and homogeneity 2 by K table: notation n_{ij}

	X=1	X=2	X=3	X=4				X=k	total
Y=0	n_{11}	n_{12}	n_{13}	n_{14}	.	.	.	n_{1k}	$n_{1.}$
Y=1	n_{21}	n_{22}	n_{23}	n_{24}	.	.	.	n_{2k}	$n_{2.}$
total	$n_{.1}$	$n_{.2}$	$n_{.3}$	$n_{.4}$	.	.	.	$n_{.k}$	n

2 by K table: notation p_{ij}

	X=1	X=2	X=3	X=4				X=k	total
Y=0	p_{11}	p_{12}	p_{13}	p_{14}	.	.	.	p_{1k}	$p_{1.}$
Y=1	p_{21}	p_{22}	p_{23}	p_{24}	.	.	.	p_{2k}	$p_{2.}$
total	$p_{.1}$	$p_{.2}$	$p_{.3}$	$p_{.4}$	.	.	.	$p_{.k}$	1.0

2 by K table: null hypothesis generated values

	X=1	X=2	X=3	X=4				X=k	total
Y=0	$np_{1.}p_{.1}$	$np_{1.}p_{.2}$	$np_{1.}p_{.3}$	$np_{1.}p_{.4}$	.	.	.	$np_{1.}p_{.k}$	$np_{1.}$
Y=1	$np_{2.}p_{.1}$	$np_{2.}p_{.2}$	$np_{2.}p_{.3}$	$np_{2.}p_{.4}$	.	.	.	$np_{2.}p_{.k}$	$np_{2.}$
total	$np_{.1}$	$np_{.2}$	$np_{.3}$	$np_{.4}$	.	.	.	$np_{.k}$	n

2 by K table: expected values under the hypothesis of independence

	X=0	X=1	X=2	X=3	total
Y=0	16.93	87.97	52.45	58.65	216
Y=1	24.07	125.03	74.55	83.35	307
total	41	213	127	142	523

Figure 6–1. Notation for a $2 \times K$ table

pancreatic cancer?). Second, the relationship between a numeric or coded variable and the binary outcome is explored (Does pancreatic cancer risk increase as the amount of coffee consumption increases?). Last, the mean values of the numeric variable are compared for the two outcomes (Does the mean level of the amount of coffee consumed differ between cases and controls?).

Independence and Homogeneity

The general notation for a $2 \times K$ contingency table is displayed in Table 6–2 (also given in Figure 6–1). The symbol n_{ij} represents the count of observations falling into the ith row and the jth column (e.g., cell frequency $= n_{23} = 74$ for the pancreatic cancer data—second row and third column). The marginal frequencies (sums of the columns or the rows) are represented as $n_{.j}$ and $n_{i.}$. More precisely,

$$n_{.j} = n_{1j} + n_{2j} \quad \text{and} \quad n_{i.} = n_{i1} + n_{i2} + \cdots + n_{ik} = \sum_{j=1}^{k} n_{ij}. \quad (6.1)$$

Underlying a $2 \times K$ contingency table are several sets of probabilities that an observation falls in a specific cell (p_{ij}), the probabilities that $X = j$ $(p_{.j},$ column $= j)$, the probability that $Y = 0$ $(p_{1.},$ row $= 1)$, and the probability that $Y = 1$ $(p_{2.},$ row $= 2)$. In tabular form these probabilities are shown in Table 6–3. Notice that n_{ij} represents a sampled quantity (observed) while p_{ij} represents an unobserved population probability (theoretical).

Table 6–2. Notation for a 2 × K contingency table

	$X = 1$	$X = 2$	$X = 3$	$X = 4$		$X = k$	Total
$Y = 0$	n_{11}	n_{12}	n_{13}	n_{14}	...	n_{1k}	$n_{1.}$
$Y = 1$	n_{21}	n_{22}	n_{23}	n_{24}	...	n_{2k}	$n_{2.}$
Total	$n_{.1}$	$n_{.2}$	$n_{.3}$	$n_{.4}$	...	$n_{.k}$	n

Table 6–3. Notation for the probabilities p_{ij}

	$X = 1$	$X = 2$	$X = 3$	$X = 4$		$X = k$	Total
$Y = 0$	p_{11}	p_{12}	p_{13}	p_{14}	...	p_{1k}	$p_{1.}$
$Y = 1$	p_{21}	p_{22}	p_{23}	p_{24}	...	p_{2k}	$p_{2.}$
Total	$p_{.1}$	$p_{.2}$	$p_{.3}$	$p_{.4}$	...	$p_{.k}$	1.0

Independence

The most basic question asked about data classified into a $2 \times K$ contingency table concerns the statistical independence of the row variable (Y) and the column variable (X). If X and Y are unrelated, then the cell probabilities in the table are completely determined by the marginal probabilities. That is, the probability that $Y = 0$ and $X = j$ simultaneously is $P(Y = 0 \text{ and } X = j) = P(Y = 0)P(X = j) = p_1.p_{.j}$ and similarly, $P(Y = 1 \text{ and } X = j) = P(Y = 1)P(X = j) = p_2.p_{.j}$. Under the hypothesis of independence, the expected cell frequencies based on the marginal probabilities become those displayed in Table 6–4. The expected number of observations in the ith, j^{th} cell is $np_i.p_{.j}$.

Because the cell probabilities (p_{ij}) are theoretical quantities (population parameters), estimates of these values are almost always derived from the collected data. Under the hypothesis of independence, the estimates of p_{ij} (denoted $\hat{p}_{ij}$) are based on the marginal frequencies where

$$\hat{p}_{i.} = \frac{n_{i.}}{n} \quad \text{and} \quad \hat{p}_{.j} = \frac{n_{.j}}{n} \quad \text{giving} \quad \hat{p}_{ij} = \hat{p}_{i.}\hat{p}_{.j}. \tag{6.2}$$

An estimated cell frequency is then $\hat{n}_{ij} = n\hat{p}_{ij} = n\hat{p}_{i.}\hat{p}_{.j}$, which is more succinctly written as $\hat{n}_{ij} = n_{i.}n_{.j}/n$. These estimates are typically calculated for each cell and compared to the observed values using a chi-square statistic to assess the likelihood that variables X and Y are independent. For the pancreatic cancer data, the estimated cell frequencies $(\hat{n}_{ij})$ generated under the hypothesis of independence of coffee consumption and disease status are given in Table 6–5.

Table 6–4. Values generated under the hypothesis of independence

	$X = 1$	$X = 2$	$X = 3$	$X = 4$		$X = k$	Total
$Y = 0$	$np_1.p_{.1}$	$np_1.p_{.2}$	$np_1.p_3.$	$np_1.p_{.4}$	$\cdots$	$np_1.p_{.k}$	$np_1.$
$Y = 1$	$np_2.p_{.1}$	$np_2.p_{.2}$	$np_2.p_3.$	$np_2.p_{.4}$	$\cdots$	$np_2.p_{.k}$	$np_2.$
Total	$np_{.1}$	$np_{.2}$	$np_{.3}$	$np_{.4}$	$\cdots$	$np_{.k}$	n

Table 6–5. Expected values generated under the hypothesis of independence

	$X = 0$	$X = 1$	$X = 2$	$X = 3$	Total
$Y = 0$	16.93	87.97	52.45	58.65	216
$Y = 1$	24.07	125.03	74.55	83.35	307
Total	41	213	127	142	523

A chi-square test statistic summarizes the correspondence between estimated values and the observed data. Specifically,

$$X^2 = \sum_{i=1}^{2} \sum_{j=1}^{4} \frac{(n_{ij} - \hat{n}_{ij})^2}{\hat{n}_{ij}} = \sum_{i=1}^{2} \sum_{j=1}^{4} \frac{(n_{ij} - n_{i.} n_{.j}/n)^2}{n_{i.} n_{.j}/n} = 7.100. \qquad (6.3)$$

The value of X^2 has an approximate chi-square distribution with $k - 1$ degrees of freedom when applied to independent variables classified into a $2 \times K$ contingency table. For the coffee/cancer data, the degrees of freedom are three and the significance probability (p-value) is 0.069. The estimated values generated under the hypothesis that the amount of the coffee consumed and pancreatic cancer risk are unrelated do not reflect the observed data extremely well (Table 6–5 compared to Table 6–1) which supports the inference that some sort of systematic relationship exists between the risk factor and case/control status.

> Aside: The pancreatic cancer case/control data in Table 6–1 can be viewed as $n = 523$ pairs of observations. Each pair has a value X equal to 0, 1, 2, or 3 and a value Y equal to 0 or 1. The association between X and Y is the focus of a chi-square test of independence. A permutation test can also be conducted to assess the association between these two variables. In both cases the null hypothesis postulates that X and Y are unrelated. Using a computer program or specialized software, the 523 values of X can be randomly associated with the 523 values of Y conforming perfectly to the null hypothesis. Furthermore, any test statistic can be calculated from the resulting random sets. A large sample of such summary statistics calculated from these null hypothesis generated "data" characterizes the null-distribution. For the pancreatic cancer data, 5,000 random permutations of X (coffee consumption) and Y (case/control status) were generated and the usual chi-square statistic calculated for each set. Using these 5,000 chi-square values, the likelihood a null-hypothesis generated chi-square value exceeds the observed value of $X^2 = 7.100$ by chance is estimated as $344/5,000 = 0.069$. That is, a total of 344 chi-square values evaluated from the ramdom permutation "data" exceeded the observed value 7.100. As expected for a large sample of data ($n = 525$), the p-value estimated from permutation test is similar to the chi-square statistic calculated from the goodness-of-fit approach to evaluating independence in a contingency table (p-value = 0.069). However, if the data were sparely distributed in the table or n was small, the chi-square statistic [expression (6.3)] will not give accurate p-values, but the permutation test continues to produce a valid significance probability for any sample size.

Homogeneity

Sometimes data classified into a $2 \times K$ table are assessed for homogeneity. The basic issue is the consistency of the probabilities p_j, where p_j is the probability that $Y = 0$ for a specific value of X or $p_j = P(Y = 0 \mid X = j)$. An estimate of p_j is $\hat{p}_j = n_{1j}/n_{.j}$. A null hypothesis is imposed stating that the data come from a series of populations where the probabilities p_j are the same regardless of the level of X and, therefore, the estimates $\hat{p}_j$ differ only because of random variation, or

$$\text{homogeneity hypothesis—}H_0: p_1 = p_2 = p_3 = \cdots = p_k = p.$$

To evaluate H_0 the common value p is estimated from the data $(\hat{p} = n_{1.}/n)$ and compared to each p_j, also estimated from the data $(\hat{p}_j = n_{1j}/n_{.j})$. Again a chi-square statistic is used to assess the deviations of the estimated probabilities $\hat{p}_j$ from the single overall estimated probability $\hat{p}$ generated under the hypothesis of homogeneity. That is,

$$X^2 = \sum_{j=1}^{k} \frac{(\hat{p}_j - \hat{p})^2}{\text{variance } (\hat{p}_j)} = \frac{\sum_{j=1}^{k} n_{.j}(\hat{p}_j - \hat{p})^2}{\hat{p}(1 - \hat{p})} \tag{6.4}$$

has an approximate chi-square distribution with $k - 1$ degrees of freedom when the null hypothesis is true. For the pancreatic cancer data, the test statistic is $X^2 = 7.100$. It is not coincidental that the chi-square value to evaluate independence and the chi-square value to evaluate homogeneity are identical. A little algebra shows that the test for homogeneity and the test for independence produce the same chi-square statistic. If p_j is constant for all levels of X, then the variable Y is not influenced by the variable X, which is another way of saying that X and Y are unrelated. In symbols, the relationship between homogeneity and independence follows:

$$\text{homogeneity} = P(Y = i \mid X = j) = P(Y = i) \quad \text{implies}$$
$$P(Y = i \mid X = j) P(X = j) = P(Y = i) P(X = j) \quad \text{and, therefore,}$$
$$P(Y = i \text{ and } X = j) = P(Y = i) P(X = j) = \text{independence,}$$

which is the relationship that generates the expected values for the chi-square test of independence (Table 6–5).

Regression

When the categorical variable represented as X is numeric, a regression approach identifies a linear association between X and Y in a $2 \times K$ contingency table. The previous chi-square analysis of independence [expression (6.3)] does not require the X-values to be numeric, or even ordered, and applies to most $2 \times K$ tables. However, considerable gains (increased power) are achieved by forming and testing specific hypotheses about the data. One such opportunity occurs when the X variable is numeric or characterized by meaningful numeric values. In this setting, a $2 \times K$ contingency table can be viewed as a set of k pairs of values. An estimated probability is generated for each value of X producing k pairs $(x_j, \hat{p}_j)$ where, as before, $\hat{p}_j$ is the estimated probability that $Y = 0$ associated with each level represented by x_j. For example, the pancreatic cancer data yield the four pairs of values $(0, 0.220)$, $(1, 0.441)$, $(2, 0.417)$, and $(3, 0.423)$ (Figure 6–2), where $\hat{p}_j$ is the proportion of cases for each amount of coffee consumed (x_j).

One approach to analyzing these k pairs of values is to estimate a straight line to represent the $\hat{p}_j$-values and use the slope of the estimated line as a summary of the relationship between X and Y. Analogous to simple linear regression analysis applied to continuous variables, three quantities are necessary to derive the basic statistical measures: the sum of squares for X (S_{xx}), the sum of squares for Y (S_{yy}), and the sum of cross-products for X and Y (S_{xy}). These expressions calculated from a $2 \times K$ contingency table are:

$$S_{xx} = \sum_{j=1}^{k} n_{.j}(x_j - \bar{x})^2, \quad \text{where} \quad \bar{x} = \sum_{j=1}^{k} n_{.j}x_j/n, \tag{6.5}$$

$$S_{yy} = n_{1.}n_{2.}/n, \quad \text{and} \tag{6.6}$$

$$S_{xy} = (\bar{x}_1 - \bar{x}_2) S_{yy}, \quad \text{where} \quad \bar{x}_i = \sum_{j=1}^{k} n_{ij}x_j/n_{i.}. \tag{6.7}$$

These sums of squares are the same as those used in standard simple linear regression analysis but simplify somewhat due to the simpler structure of the data (i.e., Y takes on only two values and there are

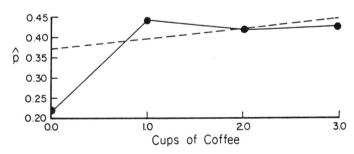

Figure 6–2. Proportion of cases of prostatic cancer for 0, 1, 2, and 3 cups of coffee consumed per day

only k different X-values). Also the quantity $\bar{x}_1$ is the mean for the X-values for which $Y = 0$ based on n_1 observations (row 1) and $\bar{x}_2$ is the mean of the X-values for which $Y = 1$ based on n_2 observations (row 2) with $n = n_1 + n_2$ total observations. It is not necessary to consider the data in terms of a $2 \times K$ contingency table. The means and the sums of squares are the same when the data are viewed as n pairs of values (x_i, y_j) where the cell frequencies are the numbers of identical pairs. The values for the pancreatic cancer data are: $\bar{x}_1 = 1.759$, $\bar{x}_2 = 1.671$, $S_{xx} = 474.241$, $S_{yy} = 126.792$, and $S_{xy} = 11.189$.

The estimated slope of the line summarizing the observed proportions, analogous to simple linear regression, is given by

$$\hat{b}_{y|x} = \frac{S_{xy}}{S_{xx}}, \tag{6.8}$$

and an estimate of the variance of the estimated regression coefficient (the estimated slope) $\hat{b}_{y|x}$ is

$$\text{variance}\,(\hat{b}_{y|x}) = \frac{S_{yy}}{(n-1)\,S_{xx}}. \tag{6.9}$$

To evaluate the magnitude of the estimated slope, a chi-square criterion is typically used. The ratio of the squared estimated slope to its variance has an approximate chi-square distribution with one degree of freedom when a linear function of X is unrelated to p_i. More technically, for the null hypothesis $b_{y|x} = 0$, the test statistic

$$X_L^2 = \frac{\hat{b}_{y|x}^2}{\text{variance}\,(\hat{b}_{y|x})} \quad (L \text{ for linear—see Appendix D}) \tag{6.10}$$

has an approximate chi-square distribution with one degree of freedom. These quantities for the pancreatic cancer data are: $\hat{b}_{y|x} = 0.0236$ and variance $(\hat{b}_{y|x}) = 0.000512$, giving a chi-square value $X_L^2 = 1.087$ (p-value $= 0.297$). No strong evidence exists that coffee consumption has a linear dose response relationship with the proportion of cases of pancreatic cancer (Figure 6–2). The calculation and testing of the slope $\hat{b}$ is frequently referred to as a test for trend in a $2 \times K$ table.

A further refinement of this regression approach is achieved by dividing the total chi-square value X^2 [expression (6.3) or (6.4)] into two parts:

Part 1: Linear $= X_L^2$ has an approximate chi-square distribution with 1 degree of freedom;

Part 2: Nonlinear $= X_{NL}^2 = X^2 - X_L^2$ (NL for nonlinear) has an approximate chi-square distribution with $k - 2$ degrees of freedom;

and clearly, $X_{NL}^2 + X_L^2 = X^2$. The quantity X_{NL}^2 measures the lack of linearity in the relationship between X and p_i. Large values X_{NL}^2 indicate a possible nonlinear association. The partitioning of a chi-square statistic into two meaningful pieces is developed more rigorously in Appendix D.

For the pancreatic cancer data, the previous X^2-value is 7.100 and the linear component is $X_L^2 = 1.087$ (p-value $= 0.297$) giving the nonlinear component as $X_{NL}^2 = 7.100 - 1.087 = 6.013$ with $k - 2 = 4 - 2 = 2$ degrees of freedom (p-value $= 0.049$). This moderately large nonlinear chi-square value (of borderline significance at the 5% level) suggests a nonlinear relationship between cancer risk and the consumption of coffee (note a potential thresholdlike effect of coffee consumption in Figure 6–2). The amount of coffee consumed does not seem to have a consistent influence (linear) on case/control status but risk associated with coffee drinkers may differ from noncoffee drinkers. A summary of the partitioned chi-square statistic is given in Table 6–6.

It is possible that the total chi-square (X^2) test is not significant while the test for linearity (X_L^2) indicates evidence of a linear relationship. This apparent contradiction occurs because the total chi-square test is not extremely powerful and can fail to show heterogeneity of response among the levels of X. A failure to reject this hypothesis does not mean that X and Y are unrelated; it means there is insufficient evidence to declare that X is likely unrelated to Y. A more powerful approach, such as a test for linearity, has a higher probability of detecting a specific relationship.

Two additional properties of a regression approach are worth noting. First, for regression analysis with the roles of X and Y reversed, the estimated slope and estimated variance of the slope differ from the previous values, expressions (6.8) and (6.9). However, the chi-square statistic is the same. That is, with the roles of X and Y reversed, the

Table 6–6. Summary of partitioned chi-square statistic

	Chi-square	Degrees of Freedom	p-value
X_L^2	1.087	1	0.291
X_{NL}^2	6.013	2	0.049
X^2	7.100	3	0.069

chi-square statistic remains unchanged;

$$X_L^2 = \frac{\hat{b}_{x|y}^2}{\text{variance } (\hat{b}_{x|y})}. \tag{6.11}$$

From the illustrative data, $\hat{b}_{x|y} = 0.088$ and variance $(\hat{b}_{x|y}) = 0.00717$, but $X_L^2 = 1.087$ is unchanged.

Second, a correlation coefficient measuring the degree of linear association between X and Y calculated in the usual way is

$$r_{xy} = \frac{S_{xy}}{\sqrt{S_{xx} S_{yy}}} \tag{6.12}$$

based on all n pairs of observations [expression (2.10)]. The point biserial correlation r_{xy} is a number between -1 and $+1$ that expresses the degree of linear association between X and Y, where Y is a binary variable and X takes on any number of values. The correlation between the case/control status and coffee consumption is $r_{xy} = 0.046$. One would expect the correlation coefficient to relate to the test of significance of $\hat{b}_{y|x}$, which also measures the degree of linear association between X and Y. The exact relationship between the two measures of association is $X_L^2 = (n-1)r_{xy}^2$. For the pancreatic cancer data, $X_L^2 = 522(0.046)^2 = 1.087$.

The statistical measure r_{xy} summarizes the association between X and Y by a standardized value. The test statistic X_L^2 allows the regression coefficient to be evaluated in terms of a probability calculated under specific conditions. These two approaches are complementary. A measure of association assesses the strength of a relationship, while a statistical test gives an idea of the likelihood that such an association occurs by chance. The t-test and the point biserial correlation coefficient have an analogous relationship for the continuous case, as noted earlier [expression (2.11)].

A primary goal of analyzing a $2 \times K$ table for trend is to evaluate a dose-response relationship. When risk increases steadily as the dose increases, strong evidence is produced of a direct relationship, even a causal relationship, between a dose variable and an outcome. When risk more or less smoothly increases with increasing dose, it is less plausible that the association results from bias or artifact and more likely that the observed relationship between risk and outcome is "real." The example of coffee consumption and pancreatic cancer shows some evidence of a threshold response. This relationship is less easy to justify from a biologic perspective. Threshold situations, like the one illustrated by the coffee-drinking data, can be indications of bias, particularly bias from a confounding variable.

Two-Sample: Comparison of Two Means

Another logical way to address the question of a relationship between a binary variable and a numeric variable is the comparison of the mean values of the numeric variable calculated at each of the two levels of the binary variable. This two-sample approach to a $2 \times K$ table is based on a t-test style comparison of the mean level of X for the two values of Y. As before, the mean $\bar{x}_1$ is calculated for all values where $Y = 0$ (n_1 observations), and $\bar{x}_2$ is calculated for all values where $Y = 1$ (n_2 observations). A natural measure of the influence of Y is the difference between the two means, $(\bar{x}_2 - x_1)$. In terms of the pancreatic cancer example, the mean level of coffee consumption among the $n_1 = 216$ cases is $\bar{x}_1 = 1.759$ cups per day, and the mean level among the $n_2 = 307$ controls is $\bar{x}_2 = 1.671$. The question arises as to the importance of the observed difference and whether it indicates a non-random increase in coffee drinking among pancreatic cancer patients.

An estimate of the variance of the difference between the mean values is necessary for evaluating the difference $\bar{x}_2 - \bar{x}_1$ and is calculated two ways (parallel to the t-test reviewed in Chapter 2). The first makes no assumptions about variance of the X-values. The variance of each mean value is estimated by

$$\text{variance}\ (\bar{x}_i) = \frac{\sum\limits_{j=1}^{k} n_{ij}(x_j - \bar{x}_i)^2}{n_{i.}(n_{i.} - 1)} \tag{6.13}$$

and the variance of $(\bar{x}_2 - \bar{x}_1)$ is variance $(\bar{x}_2)$ + variance $(\bar{x}_1)$. This variance estimate is used, for example, to construct confidence intervals.

The second method is based on the conjecture or knowledge that the variances in each group are equal. The variance of the difference between two means is then estimated by

$$\text{variance}\ (\bar{x}_2 - \bar{x}_1) = V_p^2 \left(\frac{1}{n_{1.}} + \frac{1}{n_{2.}} \right), \tag{6.14}$$

where V_p^2 is a pooled estimate of the variability of the X-values and is estimated from the sum of squares by

$$V_p^2 = \frac{S_{xx}}{n-1}. \tag{6.15}$$

A t-like statistical test of the difference in mean values is given by

$$z = \frac{\bar{x}_2 - \bar{x}_1}{\sqrt{\text{variance } (\bar{x}_2 - \bar{x}_1)}} = \frac{\bar{x}_2 - \bar{x}_1}{\sqrt{V_p^2\left(\frac{1}{n_1.} + \frac{1}{n_2.}\right)}}, \tag{6.16}$$

where z has an approximate standard normal distribution (mean $= 0$ and variance $= 1$) when $\bar{x}_1$ and $\bar{x}_2$ differ only because of random variation. For the pancreatic cancer data, $\bar{x}_1 = 1.759$, $\bar{x}_2 = 1.671$, and variance $(\bar{x}_2 - \bar{x}_1) = 0.00717$, giving $z = -1.042$ with p-value $= 0.297$. Note that the value $z^2 = (-1.402)^2 = 1.087$ is identical to X_L^2 calculated previously; the regression approach and the comparison of two mean values lead to identical tests of significance in general (i.e., $X_L^2 = z^2$).

The point biserial correlation coefficient (r_{xy}), the regression coefficient $(\hat{b}_{y|x})$ and the mean difference $(\bar{x}_2 - \bar{x}_1)$ are interrelated when calculated from a $2 \times K$ table. For example, each has an expected value of zero when the variables X and Y are unrelated. The three statistics measure the association between the numeric levels of a risk factor and a disease in different ways but, in terms of probability, lead to the same inference.

In the discussion so far the numeric coding of the X-variable has been ignored. The determination of the X-values is important and careful thought should be given to their determination. Some fields almost always use the logarithm of the dose as the measure of X. In yet other situations natural units arise, such as the number of cups of coffee consumed per day. In other cases, rather complicated polynomial expressions are used to determine the values of the "dose variable" [5]. Even a series of X-values made up of zeros and ones can be employed to analyze a threshold response model. The analysis of a dose-response relationship will differ, sometimes considerably, depending on the choice of the X-values. This choice is essentially nonstatistical and rests primarily on subject-matter considerations. It should be noted, however, that when choices for the X-values differ only by their measurement units (i.e., $new - x = ax + b$, where a and b are constants), then no changes occur in the chi-square statistic and the associated p-value. For example, using $X = 0, 2, 4$, and 6 instead of $0, 1, 2$, and 3 will not change the outcome of the statistical analysis.

Additional Example: Childhood Cancer Risk from Prenatal X-ray Exposure

The Oxford Survey of Childhood Cancer [6] provides data on malignancies in children under 10 years of age and information on the

Table 6–7. Numbers of cases and controls by recorded number of maternal x-ray films

Films	0	1	2	3	4	≥5	Unk	Total
Cases	7,332	287	199	96	59	65	475	8,513
Controls	7,673	239	154	65	28	29	325	8,513
Total	15,005	526	353	161	87	94	800	17,026
Proportion	0.489	0.546	0.564	0.596	0.678	0.691	—	—
*Expected**	0.489	0.530	0.572	0.613	0.655	0.696	—	—

*Based on a estimated linear response $\hat{p}_i = 0.489 + 0.0415 x_i$.

mother's exposure to x rays. The data in Table 6–7 (a small part of a large study containing data collected since 1953) show the numbers of prenatal x-rays received by mothers of children with a malignant disease, and a series of controls (healthy children of the same age, sex, and similar areas of residence). The proportion of cases whose mothers were prenatally x-rayed 0, 1, 2, 3, 4, or ≥5 times (x_i) are 0.489, 0.546, 0.564, 0.596, 0.678, and 0.691 ($\hat{p}_i$), respectively (Table 6–7 and plotted in Figure 6–3).

The average number of x-rays received by mothers of cases is $\bar{x}_1 = 0.191$ and for the controls is $\bar{x}_2 = 0.122$ (for simplicity, the values greater than five were coded as 5 for these calculations). The test statistic

$$z = \frac{0.122 - 0.191}{\sqrt{0.415\left(\dfrac{1}{8038} + \dfrac{1}{8188}\right)}} = -6.805 \tag{6.17}$$

indicates that the difference between cases and controls in mean number of maternal x-ray exposures is not likely a result of chance variation (p-value < 0.001).

An additional assessment of the dose-response relationship is

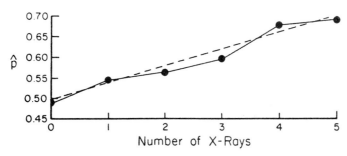

Figure 6–3. Proportion of cases of childhood cancer for exposure to 0, 1, 2, 3, 4, and 5 maternal x-rays during pregnancy

accomplished by partitioning the total chi-square value. The chi-square statistic that measures homogeneity (H_0: the proportion of cases is the same regardless of the degree of maternal x-ray exposure) is $X^2 = 47.286$. A chi-square value of this magnitude indicates the presence of some sort of nonhomogeneous pattern of response (p-value < 0.001). Postulating a linear response between x-ray exposure and the probability of case status allows a description of the "dose" response relationship. The estimated straight line representing the proportion of cases (Table 6–7) has an estimated slope of $\hat{b}_{y|x} = 0.0415$ (estimated standard error $= 0.00609$). The chi-square test to evaluate the null hypothesis that $b_{y|x} = 0$ is

$$X_L^2 = \left(\frac{0.0415}{0.00609} \right)^2 = 46.311, \tag{6.18}$$

which produces the same result as the previous comparison of mean values ($z^2 = (-6.805)^2 = 46.311$). The striking feature of these data is the linearity of the response. This property is formally assessed by partitioning the total chi-square value into linear and nonlinear pieces ($X_{NL}^2 = X^2 - X_L^2 = 47.286 - 46.311 = 0.975$; degrees of freedom $= 4$ makes the p-value $= 0.914$). The extremely small chi-square value measuring nonlinearity verifies the impression of linearity of response clearly seen from the plotted data (Figure 6–3). The partitioned chi-square is summarized in Table 6–8. The linear response provides convincing evidence of a strong risk from prenatal x-rays and the subsequent development of cancer in children.

Ridit Analysis

A chi-square analysis applied to a $2 \times K$ table to investigate independence or homogeneity places no requirements on the k column values (X). To assess a dose-response relationship, the column variable must take on an ordered sequence of numeric values. An intermediate approach involves the analysis of a $2 \times K$ table, where the column variables are ordered but not necessarily numeric. For example,

Table 6–8. Summary of partitioned chi-square

	Chi-square	Degrees of Freedom	p-value
X_L^2	46.311	1	<0.001
X_{NL}^2	0.975	4	0.914
X^2	47.286	5	<0.001

injuries from car accidents can be ordered as none, minor, moderate, severe, critical, and fatal without depending on a numeric value. The impact of such a variable is effectively explored with a statistical summary called a ridit. The rather strange name comes from using the initials "r" for relative, "i" of identified, and "d" for distribution along with "it" to resemble other terms in statistical use, such as logit or probit. Ridit analysis compares one group or a series of groups to a baseline distribution. The ridit was first presented by Bross in an analysis of car seat-belt safety [7], but it is not different from the well-known nonparametric Wilcoxon or Mann-Whitney procedures. A ridit analysis capitalizes on the fact that the columns in the $2 \times K$ table are ordered, producing a more powerful approach than a chi-square test for independence but without the necessity of assigning specific numeric values to levels of X. Additionally, the ridit approach produces a probabilistic-based summary measure, reflecting the magnitude of the differences between two compared groups.

A ridit is the estimated probability that a random individual from a reference group is "to the left" of a random person selected at random from a comparison group. In terms of car accident injuries, if a ridit probability is large, a person from the comparison group is likely to be "worse off" and if the ridit is small, a person from the comparison group is likely to be "better off" than a random person selected from the reference group. If a ridit value is $\hat{P} = 0.25$, for example, the probability is 0.25 that a random individual from the comparison group has a more severe injury than a random individual from the reference group, implying that the comparison group is "better off" than the reference group (more likely to be "to the left" or less likely to be "to the right"). The magnitude of $\hat{P}$ reflects "how much" a specific sample differs from the reference group. A ridit probability of 0.5 implies that no difference exists between the two compared groups. It is equally likely that a random person from the comparison group has a value less or greater than a random person from the reference group. A ridit value greater than 0.5 implies that the comparison group is "to the right," and a value less than 0.5 implies that the comparison group is "to the left" of the reference group. A valuable property of a ridit analysis is that the value $\hat{P}$ can be estimated without knowledge of the specific values of the individuals belonging to the reference and comparison groups.

To estimate a ridit probability, the number of values in the reference group that are less than each value in the comparison group are counted. This number is related to $P = P(X_{\text{reference}} < X_{\text{comparison}})$, where $X_{\text{reference}}$ represents an observed value associated with a random individual selected from the reference group and $X_{comparison}$ represents a random value for an individual selected from the comparison group. A simple example illustrates. Two sets of samples values (X) are:

Comparison group: 0, 4, 12, 24, 62

Reference group: 8, 32, 46, 81.

No value in the reference group is less than 0, no value in the reference group is less than 4, one value in the reference group is less than 12, one value in the reference group is less than 24, and three values in the reference group are less than 62. These counts, symbolized by U_i, are summarized in Table 6–9.

The total count is five values in the reference group $(U = \sum U_i)$ less than each of the members of the comparison group or five of $(5)(4) = 20$ possible paired comparisons are "to the left." These values could also be counted as the number of times values in the comparison group exceed values in the reference group; the answer is still five. The ridit estimate is then $\hat{P} = 5/20$ or 0.25. The estimated probability that a random selection from the reference group is less than a random selection from the comparison group is 0.25. The comparison group is largely "to the left" of the reference group $(\hat{P} < 0.5)$. In general, a ridit probability is $\hat{P} = U/(n_1 n_2)$, where n_1 and n_2 are the respective group sizes. The process of determining a value of U is the basis of the Mann–Whitney nonparametric two-sample test [8]. The value U, as will be illustrated, can be calculated from a set of ordered values (not necessarily numeric) from a $2 \times K$ table.

The same ridit calculation applies to a $2 \times K$ table. A set of data from a 1975 Alameda county health survey illustrates the application of a ridit analysis to a $2 \times K$ table. Surveyed individuals $(n = 165)$ were asked whether they thought that exercise increases life expectancy (reply: yes or no). The same individuals were also asked to report their exercise activities in terms of four categories (none, occasionally, regularly/moderate, and regularly/strenuous), producing Table 6–10.

Table 6–9. U_i counts

	8	32	46	81	U_i
0	0	0	0	0	0
4	0	0	0	0	0
12	1	0	0	0	1
24	1	0	0	0	1
62	1	1	1	0	3
U_i	3	1	1	0	5

Table 6-10. Life expectancy response by reported exercise activity

	None	Occasionally	Moderate	Strenuous	Total
Yes: $Y = 0$	7	7	8	20	42
No: $Y = 1$	25	34	32	32	123
Total	32	41	40	52	165

In terms of a ridit analysis: Is a person selected at random from the "yes" group likely to exercise more than a person selected at random from the "no" group? The amount of exercise is considered as an ordinal variable because it is unlikely that a more accurate measure of physical activity could be obtained with a questionnaire. For the ridit analysis of a $2 \times K$ table, it must be assumed that all individuals within the same column of the table come from the same distribution of values of X. That is, the probability that one value is greater than another within each column is 0.5 regardless of reference/comparison group status. Then, parallel to the previous example, the counts of the numbers of individuals in the reference group ("no" group) whose values are less than each member of the comparison group ("yes" group) leads to an estimate of the ridit probability.

In general, the estimated ridit from a $2 \times K$ table is expressed as

$$\hat{P} = \frac{\sum\limits_{i=1}^{k} [n_{21} + n_{22} + n_{23} + \cdots + (n_{2i}/2)]n_{1i}}{n_{1.}n_{2.}} = \sum\limits_{i=1}^{k} w_i \left(\frac{n_{1i}}{n_{1.}}\right), \quad (6.19)$$

where $[n_{21} + n_{22} + n_{23} + \cdots + (n_{2i}/2)]$ is the number of individuals in the reference group whose values are less than each of the n_{1i} members of the comparison group ("to the left") where

$$w_i = \frac{[n_{21} + n_{22} + n_{23} + \cdots + (n_{2i}/2)]}{n_{2.}}. \quad (6.20)$$

The notation is defined in Table 6-2. The value w_i is the reference weight. If other groups are to be compared to the same reference group, the reference weights remain the same and apply to any number of comparisons.

Specifically, for the survey data, the ridit calculation is shown in Table 6-11. The ridit estimate $\hat{P} = \sum w_i(n_{1i}/n_{1.}) = 0.604$. The interpretation of this estimated ridit probability is that a random person from the "yes" group is likely to exercise a greater amount than a random person from the "no" group. Notice, as expected, that

Table 6–11. Ridit calculation for the Alameda county health survey data

	$n_{1i}/n_1.$	"Number to the Left"	w_i	$w_i(n_{1i}/n_1.)$
None	0.167	25/2	0.102	0.017
Occasionally	0.167	25 + 34/2	0.341	0.057
Moderate	0.190	25 + 34 + 32/2	0.610	0.116
Strenuous	0.476	25 + 34 + 32 + 32/2	0.870	0.414
Ridit	—	—	—	0.604

the ridit weights applied to the reference group itself give a ridit value of exactly 0.5 ($\sum w_i n_{2i}/n_2. = 0.5$).

Like all estimates, an estimate of the variance allows a statistical evaluation of an observed ridit $\hat{P}$. The estimated variance of an estimated ridit is

$$\text{variance } (\hat{P}) = \frac{1}{12n_1.} + \frac{1}{12n_2.}. \tag{6.21}$$

A test statistic is then

$$z = \frac{\hat{P} - 0.5}{\sqrt{\text{variance } (\hat{P})}}, \tag{6.22}$$

which has an approximate standard normal distribution when there is no difference between the comparison and the reference groups (H_0: $P = 0.5$). For the survey data,

$$z = \frac{0.604 - 0.5}{\sqrt{\dfrac{1}{12(42)} + \dfrac{1}{12(123)}}} = 2.020. \tag{6.23}$$

The difference between the ridit value of $\hat{P} = 0.604$ and 0.5 is unlikely to have arisen by chance ($p = 0.043$).

> Aside: As mentioned, the ridit value is no more than another version of the Mann-Whitney or Wilcoxon nonparametric tests. A Wilcoxon rank test consists of ranking data collected from two groups from 1 to $n_0 + n_1$ and using the sum of the ranks of one of the groups as a test statistic, denoted W [8]. The relationship of this measure of "distance" between two groups and the ridit is
>
> $$\hat{P} = \frac{W - \frac{1}{2}n_1(n_1 + 1)}{n_0 n_1},$$
>
> where n_0 is the number of observations in the reference groups and n_1 is the number of observations in the comparison group. The details of this relationship can be found elsewhere [9].

Comparison of Several Groups

An effective comparison of several groups is achieved by plotting a series of statistical summaries along with their confidence intervals. This graphic technique applies to ridit analysis as well as most situations where a number of summary values are compared. The end points of a confidence interval indicate a likely range of a summary value and are an informal way to assess differences among several groups or to compare results from a series of groups to a specific value.

The confidence interval for a ridit is approximately

$$\hat{P} \pm 1.96\sqrt{\text{variance }(\hat{P})}. \tag{6.24}$$

This confidence interval is the usual 95% interval derived under the assumption that $\hat{P}$ has at least an approximate normal distribution. The distribution of the $\hat{P}$ values is not normal, but an approximate confidence interval is still useful for the comparison of a series of ridit values [7].

A data set consisting of counts of white women classified by age, smoking pattern, and socioeconomic status (adapted from [9] and given in Table 6–12) illustrates the use of ridits and confidence intervals as a way to compare a series of $2 \times K$ tables.

The "relative identified distribution" or reference group is arbitrarily chosen as nonsmokers, age 55 or older (column 1, Table 6–12). The data in Table 6–12 can be viewed as five separate 2×5 tables—one reference category and five comparison groups. Using the previous expression (6.19) for $\hat{P}$ gives five estimated ridit values, one for each comparison group. These ridit probabilities, along with their approximate 95% confidence intervals are given in Table 6–13.

The ridits values and confidence intervals are plotted in Figure 6–4. The five comparison groups do not appear to differ from each other

Table 6–12. Numbers of white females by age, smoking pattern, and economic status (I = low)

Status	Nonsmoker Age ≥ 55	Nonsmoker Age < 55	Past Smoker Age ≥ 55	Past Smoker Age < 55	Present Smoker Age ≥ 55	Present Smoker Age < 55
I	37	9	2	1	15	14
II	129	77	6	10	22	84
III	41	38	3	3	12	44
IV	51	17	6	5	17	26
V	14	13	7	6	14	17
Total	272	154	24	25	80	185

Table 6–13. Ridit values for white females classified by age and smoking pattern

| | Nonsmoker | | Past Smoker | | Present Smoker | |
	Age $\geq$ 55	Age < 55	Age $\geq$ 55	Age < 55	Age $\geq$ 55	Age < 55
Ridit	0.5	0.536	0.683	0.639	0.570	0.547
$\sqrt{\text{variance}}$	—	0.029	0.061	0.060	0.037	0.028
P_{lower}	—	0.479	0.562	0.521	0.498	0.493
P_{upper}	—	0.593	0.803	0.757	0.642	0.601

(confidence intervals overlap), but there is some evidence that two and perhaps four of the five groups differ from the reference group (ridit $= P = 0.5$). That is, several groups show statistical evidence that individuals from these groups are likely to have higher socioeconomic status ("to the right") than individuals from the older, nonsmoking reference group (confidence intervals do not contain 0.5 for two age groups and almost excluded 0.5 in two others). The most striking difference occurs for the older, past smokers who have an estimated ridit probability of $\hat{P} = 0.683$ of being in a higher socioeconomic class than a random member of the reference group.

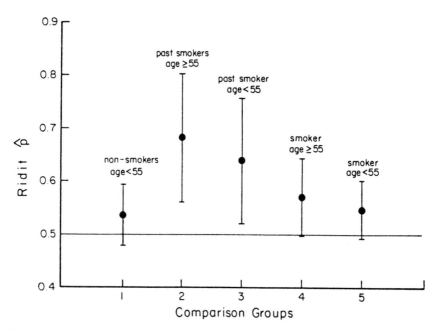

Figure 6–4. Ridit values and their approximate 95% confidence intervals for five smoking and age status comparison groups

THE TWO × TWO × TWO CONTINGENCY TABLE

Another important extension of the 2 × 2 table occurs when a third binary variable is added to the analysis to form a 2 × 2 × 2 table. Classification of three variables, each with two levels, into a 2 × 2 × 2 contingency table is the simplest possible case to study the analysis of an association between a disease and a risk factor in the presence and absence of another variable, frequently a confounding influence. Even this simplest case is somewhat complex. Each variable has two possibilities [disease (D)—no disease $(\bar{D})$, risk factor (F)—no risk factor $(\bar{F})$ and potential confounder present (C)—potential confounder absent $(\bar{C})$] producing eight combinations. The eight combinations reflect five different types of relationships among the three variables. These relationships have a variety of names, but will be referred to as:

1. Complete independence
2. Partial independence
3. Conditional independence
4. No interaction
5. Interaction

The following sections describe these five relationships. Much of the development for the 2 × 2 × 2 table applies to three variables with any number of levels; furthermore, the principles discussed are important for understanding the analysis of categorical data in general. A multiple logistic regression approach (next chapter) can also be applied to multidimensional categorical data. The 2 × 2 × 2 case, therefore, serves as a foundation for understanding a broad range of approaches to discrete data analysis.

Complete Independence

The notation for the eight possible combinations of disease, a risk factor and a possibly confounding variable, each represented by n_{ijk} (i = row, j = column, and k = identifier for each subtable), is given in Table 6–14.

If the variables measuring disease, risk factor and a variable C are completely independent, then the expected counts are a function of only the proportions of each of the three variables in the sampled population. Table 6–15 contains a set of hypothetical data displaying three completely independent binary variables.

Each cell frequency is exactly determined by the marginal frequencies, because the variables are completely independent. For

Table 6–14. Notation: disease by risk factor by $C/\bar{C}$

	C			$\bar{C}$			Total		
	D	$\bar{D}$	Total	D	$\bar{D}$	Total	D	$\bar{D}$	Total
F	n_{111}	n_{121}	$n_{1.1}$	n_{112}	n_{122}	$n_{1.2}$	$n_{11.}$	$n_{12.}$	$n_{1..}$
$\bar{F}$	n_{211}	n_{221}	$n_{2.1}$	n_{212}	n_{222}	$n_{2.2}$	$n_{21.}$	$n_{22.}$	$n_{2..}$
Total	$n_{.11}$	$n_{.21}$	$n_{..1}$	$n_{.12}$	$n_{.22}$	$n_{..2}$	$n_{.1.}$	$n_{.2.}$	n

Table 6–15. Complete independence: disease by risk factor by $C/\bar{C}$

	C			$\bar{C}$			Total		
	D	$\bar{D}$	Total	D	$\bar{D}$	Total	D	$\bar{D}$	Total
F	8	32	40	12	48	60	20	80	100
$\bar{F}$	72	288	360	108	432	540	180	720	900
Total	80	320	400	120	480	600	200	800	1,000

example, the probability associated with the presence of the risk factor is estimated by $P(\text{factor present}) = n_{1..}/n = 100/1,000 = 0.1$, the probability of the disease is given by $P(\text{disease present}) = n_{.1.}/n = 200/1,000 = 0.2$, and the probability associated with the presence of the variable C is estimated by $P(C \text{ present}) = n_{..1}/n = 400/1,000 = 0.4$. An estimate of the cell frequency n_{111} is the product of these three probabilities multiplied by the total sample size, or specifically

$$\hat{n}_{111} = 1,000\left(\frac{100}{1,000}\right)\left(\frac{200}{1,000}\right)\left(\frac{400}{1,000}\right) = 8. \tag{6.25}$$

The estimated value is identical to the observed value because these artificial data exhibit exact complete independence. The other frequencies n_{ijk} in Table 6–15 are also completely determined by the marginal probabilities.

> Aside: An important and, perhaps, subtle issue should be noted. The $P(\text{diseases present}) = 0.2$, for example, does not imply that the chance of acquiring a disease is 2 out of 10 for each person in the population. Disease occurrence behaves in a far more complex fashion. One does not remain free of a disease or become ill by a simple random mechanism analogous to flipping a biased coin [i.e., $P(\text{heads}) = 0.2 = P(\text{disease})$]. A useful interpretation of the phrase "probability of disease" is that if 20% of a population has the disease, then the probability a specific sampled individual will have the disease is 0.2. The disease is present or

absent (not subject to chance). Probability enters the picture because the data are a subset of the population and are subject to sampling variation, which can often be accurately described in terms of probabilities. Chance plays a role in the study of disease because of the nature of the sampling process and is, therefore, part of the foundation underlying the application of statistical models (analyses) to the investigation of disease/risk relationships.

In general, for a three-way table the estimated cell frequency under the hypothesis of complete independence is given by

$$\hat{n}_{ijk} = n\left(\frac{n_{i..}}{n}\right)\left(\frac{n_{.j.}}{n}\right)\left(\frac{n_{..k}}{n}\right). \tag{6.26}$$

The values estimated under the hypothesis of complete independence can be compared to the observed values with the usual chi-square statistic

$$X^2 = \sum_{i=1}^{2}\sum_{j=1}^{2}\sum_{k=1}^{2}\frac{(n_{ijk} - \hat{n}_{ijk})^2}{\hat{n}_{ijk}} \tag{6.27}$$

to evaluate the conjecture of complete independence (an application follows at the end of the chapter; Table 6–29). A consequence of complete independence is that a three-way table serves no useful purpose. All information from completely independent variables is contained in three separate binary classifications, and no new information is obtained by the study or analysis of the tabled frequencies. For the example, the P(disease present) is 0.2 in all parts of Table 6–15, uninfluenced by either the presence or absence of the other two variables (e.g., $P(D|FC) = P(D|F\bar{C}) = P(D|F) = P(D) = 0.2$). No reason, therefore, exists to include the risk factor F or the variable C in the study of a disease when the three variables are completely independent.

Partial Independence

Partial independence occurs when a suspected confounding variable is unrelated (statistically independent) to both disease and risk factor, but an association exists between the disease and the risk factor. Hypothetical data that exhibit perfect partial independence are shown in Table 6–16.

Partial independence means that the joint distribution of the risk factor and disease is the same at both levels of the variable C. When a variable C is not relevant to the relationship between the disease and the risk factor, the subtables formed for each level of the variable

Table 6–16. Partial independence: Disease by risk factor by $C/\bar{C}$

		C			$\bar{C}$	
	D	$\bar{D}$	Total	D	$\bar{D}$	Total
F	45	60	105	255	340	595
$\bar{F}$	15	30	45	85	170	255
Total	60	90	150	340	510	850

labeled C are simply multiples of the table formed by ignoring the variable C.

For the hypothetical data, summing over the two levels of the variable C gives the values in Table 6–17. An estimate of the probability that variable C is present, from Table 6–16, is $P(C \text{ present}) = P(C) = n_{..1}/n = 150/1,000$. The estimated probability $P(C)$ and the values in the summary Table 6–17 generate the values expected for each cell in the $2 \times 2 \times 2$ table under the conjecture of partial independence. For example, the estimated frequency where all three variables are present (n_{111}) is

$$\hat{n}_{111} = 1,000\left(\frac{300}{1,000}\right)\left(\frac{150}{1,000}\right) = 45. \tag{6.28}$$

Again, the fit is perfect for this artificial data, because the variable represented by C is perfectly independent of both risk factor and disease.

In general, for a three-way table the estimated values under the condition of partial independence of variable C are

$$\hat{n}_{ijk} = n\left(\frac{n_{ij.}}{n}\right)\left(\frac{n_{..k}}{n}\right). \tag{6.29}$$

As before, these estimated frequencies can be compared to those observed (n_{ijk} to $\hat{n}_{ijk}$) with a chi-square statistic (again, Table 6–29).

Table 6–17. Variable C ignored: disease by risk factor

	D	$\bar{D}$	Total
F	300	400	700
$\bar{F}$	100	200	300
Total	400	600	1,000

The inference drawn from evidence of partial independence is that the variable C suspected of being a confounder is not a confounder and it can be ignored without biasing the measurement of association between risk factor and disease. That is, the table created by summing the data over the levels of the variable C accurately reflects the disease/risk relationship.

Conditional Independence

A disease and a variable are conditionally independent when the disease is unrelated (statistically independent) to that variable at each level of the risk factor. In this case, the risk factor and disease as well as the risk factor and the variable C are associated. A $2 \times 2 \times 2$ table displaying a set of hypothetical data that exhibit perfect conditional independence of variable C is shown in Table 6–18.

Rearranging these data more directly shows that the disease and the variable labeled C are exactly independent in each of the two subtables (risk factor present and risk factor absent). Specifically, the values in Table 6–19 have an odds ratio of 1.0 in both subtables $(or_{CD|F} = or_{CD|\bar{F}} = 1.0)$.

Based on the exactly conditionally independent "data" (Table 6–18), the estimated value of the cell frequency where all variables

Table 6–18. Conditional independence: disease by risk factor by $C/\bar{C}$

	C			$\bar{C}$		
	D	$\bar{D}$	Total	D	$\bar{D}$	Total
F	30	120	150	10	40	50
$\bar{F}$	45	255	300	75	425	500
Total	75	375	450	85	465	550

Table 6–19. Conditional independence: disease by risk factor by $C/\bar{C}$

	F			$\bar{F}$		
	C	$\bar{C}$	Total	C	$\bar{C}$	Total
D	30	10	40	45	75	120
$\bar{D}$	120	40	160	255	425	680
Total	150	50	200	300	500	800

are present (n_{111}) is

$$\hat{n}_{111} = 200\left(\frac{40}{200}\right)\left(\frac{150}{200}\right) = 30, \tag{6.30}$$

which equals the observed value, because the data are constructed to have exact conditional independence between variable C and disease D.

In general, the estimated cell frequencies under the hypothesis of conditional independence of a disease and a third variable are

$$\hat{n}_{ijk} = n_{i..}\left(\frac{n_{ij.}}{n_{i..}}\right)\left(\frac{n_{i.k}}{n_{i..}}\right). \tag{6.31}$$

Parallel to the partial independence case, the table formed by summing over the variable C also does not change the risk/disease relationship. To illustrate, the conditionally independent values (Table 6–18) summed over the variable C produce Table 6–20. The probability of disease with the factor present is the same when the variable C is present, absent, or ignored. That is, $P(D|FC) = 30/150 = P(D|F\bar{C}) = 10/50 = P(D|F) = 40/200 = 0.2$, showing again that the variable C does not influence the calculation of the probability of disease among individuals with the factor. Consequently, measures of associations relating the risk factor and disease will have identical values in both the subtables and in the combined table $(C + \bar{C})$. Therefore, the variable C is not a confounding influence on the risk/disease relationship when it is conditionally independent of the disease D.

Complete independence, partial independence, and conditional independence with respect to a third variable $(C/\bar{C})$ imply that the variable can be ignored in the study of the association between a risk factor and a disease. Under these conditions a three-variable analysis reduces to, at least, two variables (potential confounder eliminated) allowing a clearer and simpler description of the disease/risk relationship. In other words, the variable C is not a confounder and does not bias the estimation of the association between disease and risk factor.

Table 6–20. Variable C ignored: disease by risk factor

	D	$\bar{D}$	Total
F	40	160	200
$\bar{F}$	120	680	800
Total	160	840	1,000

Confounder Bias in a Two × Two × Two Table

Confounder bias in a 2 × 2 × 2 table, similar to the previous definition (Chapter 2), is the distortion in the risk/disease relationship caused by ignoring the third variable C. The previous three sections demonstrate that a variable must be related to the risk variable and also related to the disease outcome to have a confounding influence. However, the exact way that a variable influences the disease outcome determines whether the variable is a confounder. To cause confounding bias, a variable must be related to the disease after adjustment for all other influences under investigation. That is, the confounding variable must have a direct association with the disease. The case of conditional independence illustrates: If a potential confounding variable and the disease are associated when the risk factor is ignored, but when the confounder/disease association is assessed at each level of the risk factor (i.e., adjusted for the risk factor influence) the association disappears, then the variable labeled C is related to the disease only because of its association with the risk factor (F). When the variable C is not directly related to the disease (conditionally independent), it does not cause confounder bias.

The amount of confounding bias is easily expressed by comparing two measures of the risk/disease association, one taking into account the confounding variable and the other with the confounding variable ignored. The difference measures confounder bias. If this bias is small, then the confounding variable has little or no effect on the study of the risk/disease association in question and can be dropped from the analysis. When this bias is large, the confounding variable should be included in the analysis to produce unbiased estimates of the risk/disease association.

A simple case of confounder bias in a 2 × 2 × 2 table is illustrated by the following hypothetical data in Table 6–21. If the confounding variable is ignored, then these data would appear in the summary (summed over the values of the confounder) 2 × 2 table shown in Table 6–22.

Table 6–21. Disease by risk factor by confounding variable

	C			$\bar{C}$		
	D	$\bar{D}$	Total	D	$\bar{D}$	Total
F	10	10	20	40	20	60
$\bar{F}$	5	20	25	5	10	15
Total	15	30	45	45	30	75

$\widehat{or}_{FD|C} = 4$ and $\widehat{or}_{FD|\bar{C}} = 4$.

Table 6–22. Disease by risk factor

	D	$\bar{D}$	Total
F	50	30	80
$\bar{F}$	10	30	40
Total	60	60	120

$\widehat{or}_{FD} = 5.$

A number of measures of association are available to reflect the risk/disease association, and the amount of confounder bias depends on the measure chosen. Here the odds ratio illustrates the influences of a confounding variable. The odds ratio is $\widehat{or}_{FD|C} = \widehat{or}_{FD|\bar{C}} = 4$, accounting for the influence of the confounding variable C and $\widehat{or}_{FD} = 5$ when the variable C is ignored. The confounder bias, is therefore, simply bias $= 5 - 4 = 1$.

Note that the odds ratios in Table 6–21 are equal in each subtable, when the confounding variable is present and when it is absent (no interaction). If a risk/disease association substantially differs in each subtable (an interaction), then the issue of whether the potential confounding variable can be ignored is answered. Ignoring the variable distorts the risk/disease relationship regardless of whether the variable is a confounder or not. No need exists to consider a summary table combining the two sets of data (subtable C and subtable $\bar{C}$). Interaction in a $2 \times 2 \times 2$ table is the topic of the next section. The issue of when a variable is a nonconfounder is introduced in the context of a $2 \times 2 \times 2$ table, and general considerations exist elsewhere, [10] or [11]. More detail will be added as part of the description of logistic regression (the next two chapters).

Examples

For the following $2 \times 2 \times 2$ table, the odds ratios $or_{CF|D}$ and $or_{CF|\bar{D}}$ are 1.0 (C and F are conditionally independent, but $or_{CF} = 0.667$) where

	C			$\bar{C}$			Total		
	D	$\bar{D}$	Total	D	$\bar{D}$	Total	D	$\bar{D}$	Total
F	4	2	6	8	1	9	12	3	15
$\bar{F}$	3	6	9	6	3	9	9	9	18
Total	7	8	15	14	4	18	21	12	33

and $or_{FD|C} = or_{FD|\bar{C}} = or_{FD} = 4.0$. Because the odds ratios from each subtable are equal to the odds ratio from the combined table, the variable C is not a confounder when the odds ratio is used as a measure of association between risks factor F and disease D.

For the case where $or_{CD|F}$ and $or_{CD|\bar{F}}$ are 1.0 (C and D are conditionally independent but $or_{CD} = 1.667$), the 2 × 2 × 2 table

	C			$\bar{C}$			Total		
	D	$\bar{D}$	Total	D	$\bar{D}$	Total	D	$\bar{D}$	Total
F	12	8	20	3	2	5	15	10	25
$\bar{F}$	2	4	6	4	8	12	6	12	18
Total	14	12	26	7	10	17	21	22	43

produces the odds ratios $or_{FD|C} = or_{FD|\bar{C}} = or_{FD} = 3.0$, again showing that C is not a confounding variable.

But when $or_{CD|F} = or_{CD|\bar{F}} = 2.0$ and $or_{CF|D} = or_{CF|\bar{D}} = 0.6$ (C is related to both F and D), the 2 × 2 × 2 table

	C			$\bar{C}$			Total		
	D	$\bar{D}$	Total	D	$\bar{D}$	Total	D	$\bar{D}$	Total
F	8	2	10	5	5	10	13	7	20
$\bar{F}$	8	4	12	3	6	9	11	20	21
Total	16	6	22	8	11	19	24	17	41

gives the odds ratios for each subtable $or_{FD|C} = or_{FD|\bar{C}} = 4.0$, but $or_{FD} = 1.69$ showing that C is a confounding variable. That is, the measure of association (odds ratio) accounting for C differs from the same measure of association when the variable C is ignored. The example illustrates that the variable C must be directly related to both the disease D and the risk factor F to cause confounding bias.

Interaction

Interaction, in a 2 × 2 × 2 table, is the failure of a measure of association between disease and risk factor to be the same at both levels

Table 6–23. No interaction: disease by risk factor by confounder

		C			$\bar{C}$	
	D	$\bar{D}$	Total	D	$\bar{D}$	Total
F	69	68	137	107	109	216
$\bar{F}$	91	150	241	150	256	406
Total	160	218	378	257	365	622

$\widehat{or}_{FD|C} = 1.675$ and $\widehat{or}_{FD|\bar{C}} = 1.675$.

of the third variable. Hypothetical data with essentially no interaction as measured by an odds ratio are given in Table 6–23.

The odds ratio is chosen as the measure of association and $or_{FD|C} = or_{FD|\bar{C}} = 1.675$, showing the same value in both subtables, no interaction. Additionally, if no interaction between risk factor and disease exists, then the confounder/risk factor and the confounder/disease subtables also show no interaction. Specifically, for the odds ratio,

$$\text{if} \quad or_{FD|C} = or_{FD|\bar{C}}, \quad \text{then} \quad or_{FC|D} = or_{FC|\bar{D}} \quad \text{and} \quad or_{CD|F} = or_{CD|\bar{F}}. \quad (6.32)$$

Estimation

A useful view of interaction comes from calculating a value δ that is added to or subtracted from each data value in a $2 \times 2 \times 2$ table so that the marginal frequencies are unchanged (see the role of δ in Table 6–24) and no interaction exists in the two subtables. The value of δ, thereby, measures the magnitude of the interaction. If $\delta = 0$, then no interaction exists (which is the case for the hypothetical data in Table 6–23). The degree to which δ differs from zero measures the amount of interaction in a $2 \times 2 \times 2$ table.

Rather than discuss the calculation of δ in general, a set of data from an Alameda county health survey (1975) concerning the knowledge of hypertension illustrates the interaction measure δ. Data

Table 6–24. Role of δ: disease by risk factor by confounder

		C			$\bar{C}$	
	D	$\bar{D}$	Total	D	$\bar{D}$	Total
F	$n_{111} + \delta$	$n_{121} - \delta$	$n_{1.1}$	$n_{112} - \delta$	$n_{122} + \delta$	$n_{1.2}$
$\bar{F}$	$n_{211} - \delta$	$n_{221} + \delta$	$n_{2.1}$	$n_{212} + \delta$	$n_{222} - \delta$	$n_{2.2}$
Total	$n_{.11}$	$n_{.21}$	$n_{..1}$	$n_{.12}$	$n_{.22}$	$n_{..2}$

Table 6–25. Perceived hypertension by answer by race

	White			Black		
	Yes	No	Total	Yes	No	Total
"Hypertension"	17	7	24	26	17	43
No "hypertension"	15	12	27	13	27	40
Total	32	19	51	39	44	83

$\widehat{or}_{FD|C} = 1.943$ and $\widehat{or}_{FD|\bar{C}} = 3.176$.

collected on answers to two questions along with the race of the respondent are shown in Table 6–25 where

"Risk factor": Answer to the question—Do you think you have elevated blood pressure? ("hypertension"—H or $\bar{H}$),

"Disease": Answer to the question—Can the symptoms of hypertension be detected without a medical examination and a blood pressure reading? (yes or no); and

Confounder: Race of the respondent (white or black).

A calculation of the factor δ quantifies the amount of interaction (failure of the odds ratio to be identical for the white and black respondents). Specifically, the value δ is calculated from Table 6–26.

To find the δ-value so that the odds ratio is identical for both whites and blacks, the odds ratio when the confounder is present (white) is equated to the odds ratio when the confounder is absent (black) or

$$\frac{(17 + \delta)(12 + \delta)}{(7 - \delta)(15 - \delta)} = \frac{(26 - \delta)(27 - \delta)}{(13 + \delta)(17 + \delta)}. \tag{6.33}$$

A series of trial-and-error iterations yields the solution δ that must be added to and subtracted from the values in each of the eight cells to produce a set of "data" with exactly no interaction as measured by the odds ratio. For the survey data, $\delta = 0.866$. The estimated "data"

Table 6–26. Perceived hypertension by answer by race

	White			Black		
	Yes	No	Total	Yes	No	Total
"Hypertension"	$17 + \delta$	$7 - \delta$	24	$26 - \delta$	$17 + \delta$	43
No "hypertension"	$15 - \delta$	$12 + \delta$	27	$13 + \delta$	$27 - \delta$	40
Total	32	19	51	39	44	83

Table 6–27. No interaction: perceived hypertension by answer by race

	White			Black		
	Yes	No	Total	Yes	No	Total
"Hypertension"	17.866	6.134	24	25.134	17.866	43
No "hypertension"	14.134	12.866	27	13.866	26.134	40
Total	32	19	51	39	44	83

$\widehat{or}_{FD|C} = 2.651$ and $\widehat{or}_{FD|\bar{C}} = 2.651$.

and summary odds ratio under the no-interaction hypothesis are given in Table 6–27.

These estimated values $\hat{n}_{ijk}$ can be compared to n_{ijk} with the usual chi-square statistic to assess the fit of the no-interaction conjecture (Table 6–29). Also the estimate of an odds ratio from these no-interaction "data" (i.e., $\widehat{or} = 2.651$) is an excellent summary value under the hypothesis that the risk/disease relationship is the same in both subtables, and the two observed odds ratios differ only because of sampling variation. Development of other measures of interaction will be taken up in the next chapter. If measures of association other than the odds ratio are used, the value of δ will differ, but the process of finding δ is similar and produces an analogous interpretation.

If no interaction exists (or nearly so), then it is meaningful to assess the influence of a possible confounding variable on the measure of association chosen. If an interaction exists, then as mentioned, confounding is not an issue. Continuing the "hypertension" example, the summary odds ratio when race (confounder) is considered is 2.651. The odds ratio calculated from the table where white and black respondents are combined (ignoring race) is 2.496. The comparison of these two odds ratios directly estimates the amount of confounder bias associated with race when it is assumed that no interaction is present. Whether this bias occurred by chance is not much of an issue, and a statistical test is not a relevant addition to the analysis. If substantial confounder bias exists in the collected data, strategies must be adopted to provide an unbiased description of the influence of a risk factor regardless of whether the bias is "real" or "random." For the perceived hypertension data, the race variable confounds the relationship between "hypertension" and the answer to the question about symptoms (2.651 versus 2.496). The summary table ignoring race is not very useful and, to repeat, it is unimportant whether this bias arose by chance or not.

Table 6–28. Hits against left- and right-handed pitching

	Player A			Player B			Summary		
	Left	Right	Total	Left	Right	Total	Player A	Player B	Total
Hits	50	40	90	10	38	48	90	48	138
Outs	150	60	210	40	62	102	210	102	312
Total	200	100	300	50	100	150	300	150	450

Interaction addresses the question of "summarization." If no interaction exists, then summary values are possibly a useful description of an association. Furthermore, if the variable is a nonconfounder, then a combined table simplifies the analysis. If an interaction is present in a data set, then ignoring this fact (adding the frequencies over the levels of another variable when an interaction is present) produces a table that, at best, is not very meaningful and, at worst, deceptive. Examples of "data" can be created where rather anomalous results occur when interaction is ignored. A famous example is called Simpson's paradox [12]. Another example concerns two baseball players who bat against both left-handed and right-handed pitching with the results shown in Table 6–28.

Player A's batting average is $90/300 = 0.300$, where player B's batting average is $48/150 = 0.320$. Is B a better hitter than A? Note that player A hits better than player B against left-handed pitching ($50/200 = 0.250$ versus $10/50 = 0.200$). Player A also out-hits player B against right-handed pitching ($40/100 = 0.400$ versus $38/100 = 0.380$). The true worth of the two players is reflected in the subtables rather than the summary table. This example serves as a reminder that when interaction is present summary tables or measures of association derived from summary tables do not reflect accurately the issues under study. The concept of interaction takes on more precise meaning in the context of a logistic regression analysis and is discussed further in the next two chapters.

Summary

It is worth noting the hierarchal ordering of the five statistical relationships among a potential confounding variable, a risk factor, and a disease outcome. If the values classified into a $2 \times 2 \times 2$ table are completely independent, then necessarily the variables are partially independent, conditionally independent, and no interaction exists in

Table 6–29. Perceived hypertension by answer by race—expected values under four models

C	D	F	Count	Complete	Partial*	Conditional**	No Interaction	Data
White	"yes"	H	n_{111}	13.511	16.366	19.380	17.866	17
White	"yes"	$\bar{H}$	n_{211}	13.511	10.657	12.620	14.134	15
White	"no"	H	n_{121}	11.989	9.134	7.238	6.134	7
White	"no"	$\bar{H}$	n_{221}	11.989	14.843	11.762	12.866	12
Black	"yes"	H	n_{112}	21.989	26.634	23.620	25.134	26
Black	"yes"	$\bar{H}$	n_{212}	21.989	17.343	15.380	13.866	13
Black	"no"	H	n_{122}	19.511	14.866	16.762	17.866	17
Black	"no"	$\bar{H}$	n_{222}	19.511	24.157	27.238	26.134	27

* = Partial independence of race.
** = "Hypertension" and race are independent at each level of the answers "yes" and "no."

all subtables. Additionally, if the data are partially independent, then the data also must be conditionally independent and no interaction exists. Last, conditional independence implies that no interaction exists. In other words, complete independence is a special case of partial independence, partial independence is a special case of conditional independence, and conditional independence is a special case of no interaction.

An important issue pertaining to a $2 \times 2 \times 2$ table remains: Which of the four possible models is the "right" description of a set of sampled data? The chi-square statistic $\sum\sum\sum (n_{ijk} - \hat{n}_{ijk})^2/\hat{n}_{ijk}$ serves to summarize the fit of the four models, where $\hat{n}_{ijk}$ is estimated under (i) complete independence, (ii) partial independence, (iii) conditional independence, and (iv) no interaction structures for all eight cells in the $2 \times 2 \times 2$ table. The data and the estimated cell frequencies as well as a chi-square goodness-of-fit statistic for each statistical model are given in Table 6–29 based on the perceived hypertension data (Table 6–25).

Summary

	Complete	Partial*	Conditional**	No Interaction
X^2	10.745	4.582	1.367	0.430
Degrees of freedom	4	3	2	1
p-value	0.030	0.205	0.505	0.512

* = Partial independence of race.
** = "Hypertension" and race are independent at each level of the answers "yes" and "no."

Table 6–30. The odds ratios for the five descriptions of data in a 2 × 2 × 2 table

Model	$or_{FD|C}$	$or_{FD|\bar{C}}$	or_{FD}	$or_{FC|D}$	$or_{FC|\bar{D}}$	or_{FC}	$or_{DC|F}$	$or_{DC|\bar{F}}$	or_{DC}
Complete	1.00	1.00	1.00	1.00	1.00	1.00	1.00	1.00	1.00
Partial	2.50	2.50	2.50	1.00	1.00	1.00	1.00	1.00	1.00
Conditional	2.50	2.50	2.50	1.00	1.00	1.15	1.90	1.90	1.90
No interaction	2.65	2.65	2.50	0.70	0.70	0.83	2.07	2.07	1.90
Data	1.94	3.18	2.50	0.57	0.93	0.83	1.59	2.60	1.90

The four descriptions of the data produce specific patterns of any measure of association. The odds ratio, for example, applied to the expected values (Table 6–29) derived from the Alameda county health survey data for the four basic models produce the values in Table 6–30. Note that since complete independence, partial independence, and conditional independence are special cases of no interaction, the odds ratio are identical in all pairs of subtables (e.g., $or_{FD|C} = or_{FD|\bar{C}}$). The values in Table 6–30 emphasizes that a choice of a model to represent the data is also a choice of a pattern of the measures of association.

The more complex the model (fewer degrees of freedom), the better the fit of the estimated values to the data. These four analyses, like most statistical investigations, involve a trade-off between simplicity of the statistical structure and increasing goodness-of-fit (the chi-square values get smaller). For statistical models in general, increased complexity leads to greater flexibility of the mathematical structure which, in turn, leads to less unexplained variation. Although the chi-square measure is useful in the process of deciding on a statistical structure, it does not provide an unequivocal answer. The primary role of the chi-square criterion is to identify those statistical structures that are imcompatible with the data. The ultimate choice of the "right" model to represent the relationships among the variables in collected data should be based on biological or physical considerations supported by statistical analysis.

7 The Analysis of Contingency Table Data: Logistic Model I

Epidemiologic data often occur as a series of counts resulting from tabulating discrete variables or tabulating continuous variables made discrete. Converting continuous variables to categorical variables simplifies the interpretation and is usually based on traditional cut points (at a cost of statistical power, as already noted). For example, individuals are considered hypertensive or not hypertensive depending on whether their systolic blood pressure exceeds 140 mm Hg, and smokers are categorized into a series of intervals based on 0,1–20, 21–30, and ≥ 30 cigarettes reported smoked per day. The end-result is a multidimensional table of counts. A table is certainly a useful summary of collected data, but, in addition, it is important to explore the sometimes complex relationships found in a table.

An example of a multidimensional table describing three risk factors and a disease outcome from the Western Collaborative Study (WCGS—see Appendix A) data is shown in Table 7–1.

This table consists of counts of coronary heart disease (CHD) events and the number of individuals at risk classified by behavior type, blood pressure, and smoking exposure. Clearly, increased risks are incurred by increasing amounts smoked, by being in a high blood pressure category, or by having a type-A behavior pattern. However, a number of questions are not easily answered. Among them are:

1. Does smoking have a threshold influence or does risk increase more or less consistently as the number of cigarettes smoked increases?
2. What is the influence of blood pressure and smoking on the behavior/disease relationship?
3. Do these three risk factors influence the frequency of CHD events in an independent way?
4. If these risk factors are not independent, how do they act together to influence the probability of a coronary event?
5. What is the relative influence of each of these factors on the risk of coronary heart disease?

Table 7-1. Coronary disease by behavior type by systolic blood pressure by smoking: a summary

Blood Pressure	Behavior Type	Smoking Frequency—Cigarettes per Day			
		0	1–20	21–30	≥30
≥140 mm	A	29/184 = 0.158	21/97 = 0.216	7/52 = 0.135	12/55 = 0.218
≥140 mm	B	8/179 = 0.045	9/71 = 0.127	3/34 = 0.088	7/21 = 0.333
<140 mm	A	41/600 = 0.068	24/301 = 0.080	27/167 = 0.162	17/133 = 0.128
<140 mm	B	20/689 = 0.029	16/336 = 0.048	13/152 = 0.086	3/83 = 0.036

The inability to answer elementary questions about risk/disease relationships in a satisfactory way stems, to a large extent, from lack of data. If hundreds of thousands of individuals were classified into a table with more categories, the answers to most questions about the role of the risk factors and disease would be clear. The "thinness" of the data requires a more sophisticated approach in the form of a statistical model. When several variables are investigated, a table often fails to summarize the data adequately and a need arises to deal yet more efficiently with the relationships among the categorical variables. Additionally, human disease is, almost always, a relatively rare event causing sparse cell frequencies in tabulated data (e.g., only three events occur in the low blood pressure, heavy smoking, type-B category among the more than 3,000 observations), making it important that any analytic procedure account for the impact of sampling variation. The logistic model is one way to describe succinctly and efficiently, as well as analyze quantitatively, the relationships between a set of risk factors and a disease outcome. The use of a multivariable model to analyze data classified into a multidimensional table is the topic of this chapter; the extension to include continuous risk variables is the topic of the following chapter. Logistic regression is by no means the only approach to the analysis of risk/disease relationships but is one that is frequently used and demonstrates both the strengths and weaknesses of multivariate data analysis techniques applied to epidemiologic data.

The Simplest Case

A 2×2 table provides the simplest application of a logistic model to the relationships among contingency table variables. To start, the variables to be studied are the presence ($D = 1$) and absence ($D = 0$) of a disease investigated at two levels of a risk factor ($F = 1$, risk factor present and $F = 0$, risk factor absent). The general notation (repeated) for a contingency table applies and is specifically shown in Table 7–2.

There are many ways to analyze such tables. A chi-square analysis is the most common approach for assessing statistical significance.

Table 7–2. Notation for a 2×2 contingency table

	Disease: $D = 1$	No Disease: $D = 0$	Total
Factor present: $F = 1$	n_{11}	n_{12}	$n_{1.}$
Factor absent: $F = 0$	n_{21}	n_{22}	$n_{2.}$
Total	$n_{.1}$	$n_{.2}$	n

Other methods based on conditional probabilities such as $P(D|F)$ and $P(\bar{D}|F)$ are also used to describe the risk/disease relationship.

Yet another choice is to employ the odds as a measure of association between a risk factor and a disease calculated from data recorded in a 2×2 table. The odds of disease among those individuals without the risk factor is the ratio of $P(D|F=0)$ to $P(\bar{D}|F=0)$ and can be compared to the odds among those with the risk factor, $P(D|F=1)/P(\bar{D}|F=1)$. A statistically strategic measure is the logarithm of the odds, called the log-odds or logit. One motivation for employing a log-odds measure of risk is its utility for detecting multiplicative effects among risk factors. Taking the logarithms of an odds changes a ratio measure into a linear measure of risk. Linear measures are far simpler to understand and to analyze statistically.

A baseline measure of disease risk on a log-odds scale is an estimate of the log-odds when the risk factor is absent, or

$$\hat{a} = \log\left(\frac{\hat{P}(D|F=0)}{\hat{P}(\bar{D}|F=0)}\right) = \log\left(\frac{n_{21}/(n_{21}+n_{22})}{n_{22}/(n_{21}+n_{22})}\right) = \log(n_{21}/n_{22}) \quad (7.1)$$

so that

$$\hat{a} \quad \text{is an estimate of } a \quad \text{where} \quad a = \text{log-odds} = \log\left(\frac{P(D|F=0)}{P(\bar{D}|F=0)}\right). \quad (7.2)$$

A measure of particular interest is an estimate of the increase or decrease in the log-odds due to the presence of the risk factor measured relative to the baseline value or

$$\hat{b} = \log(n_{11}/n_{12}) - \log(n_{21}/n_{22}) \quad (7.3)$$

so that

$$\hat{b} \quad \text{is an estimate of } b \quad \text{where} \quad b = \log\left(\frac{P(D|F=1)}{P(\bar{D}|F=1)}\right) - \log\left(\frac{P(D|F=0)}{P(\bar{D}|F=0)}\right). \quad (7.4)$$

Also note that

$$e^b = \frac{P(D|F=1)/P(\bar{D}|F=1)}{P(D|F=0)/P(\bar{D}|F=0)} = \quad \text{or} \quad (7.5)$$

is the odds ratio measure of association from a 2×2 table.

The two quantities (a, b) form the simplest possible linear model. That is, log-odds $= a + bF$, where $F = 0$ or $F = 1$ so that

$$\text{when} \quad F = 0, \quad \text{then} \quad \text{log-odds} = \log(n_{21}/n_{22}) = \hat{a} \quad (7.6)$$

and

$$\text{when} \quad F = 1, \quad \text{then} \quad \text{log-odds} = \log(n_{11}/n_{12}) = \hat{a} + \hat{b}. \quad (7.7)$$

The value $\hat{b}$ estimates, on the log-odds scale, the change in risk of disease associated with the presence of the risk factor (F) relative to the absence of the same factor $(\bar{F})$. The risk factor in the context of a linear model has other names—sometimes called the predictor variable, the explanatory variable, or the independent variable. A log-odds measure is not a particularly intuitive way to assess the risk/disease association, but it has tractable mathematical properties and relates directly to the odds ratio measure of risk which is a natural measure of association when data are analyzed using a logistic regression model.

Consider a 2×2 table (Table 7–3) from the WCGS data describing the relationship between behavior type (risk factor) and a coronary event (disease outcome).

From these data,

$$\hat{a} = \log(79/1{,}486) = -2.934 \quad \text{and} \quad \hat{a} + \hat{b} = \log(178/1{,}411) = -2.070.$$

The estimated change in the log-odds of CHD associated with type-A individuals (risk factor present) relative to type-B individuals (risk factor absent—baseline) is $\hat{b} = -2.070 - (-2.934) = 0.864$ (Figure 7–1). Since $\hat{b} = \log(n_{11}n_{22}/n_{12}n_{21}) = \log(\widehat{or})$, then $e^{\hat{b}} = n_{11}n_{22}/n_{12}n_{21}$ which is the usual estimate of the odds ratio calculated from a 2×2 table (Appendix A). For the behavior type data (Table 7–3) the odds ratio estimate is $\widehat{or} = e^{0.864} = 2.373$. The odds of a coronary event is, therefore, 2.373 times greater for a type-A individual than for a type-B individual. This odds ratio can also be calculated directly from the tabled data where $\widehat{or} = (178)(1{,}486)/(1{,}411)(79) = 2.373$.

When the number of parameters estimated equals the number of observed log-odds values in a table of data, the results of using a model to describe associations and making direct calculations are identical. When a logistic model approach and direct calculations produce identical results, the model is said to be saturated. The two-parameter logistic model applied to a 2×2 table is an example of a saturated model.

The two primary ways to evaluate the influence of sampling variation on the estimate $\hat{b}$ are a significance test and a confidence interval.

Table 7–3. CHD by A/B

	CHD	No CHD	Total
Type-A	178	1,411	1,589
Type-B	79	1,486	1,565
Total	257	2,897	3,154

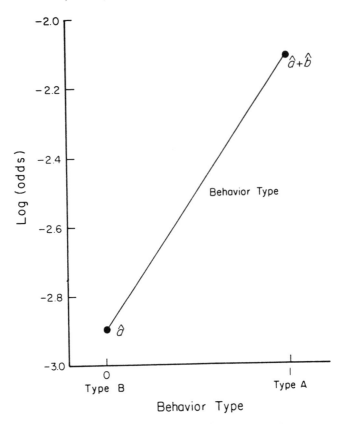

Figure 7–1. Log-odds associated with CHD risk by behavior type

Aside: The relative merits of a confidence interval versus a significance test have been occasionally discussed, even debated (e.g., [1], [2], and [3]). The confidence interval and the two-sided significance tests are in reality similar and rarely give contradictory results. The confidence interval conveys more information in the sense that the interval width gives some idea of the range of parameter possibilities (power). A confidence interval is expressed in the same units as the estimated quantity, which is sometimes helpful. A significance test reported in isolation tends to reduce conclusions to two choices ("significant" or "not significant") which, perhaps, emphasizes the role of chance variation too simply. For example, estimates can be "significant" (chance not a plausible explanation) because a large number of observations are involved, but the results do not reflect an important biological or physical measurement. However, a confidence interval approach is complicated when more than one estimate is involved.

In many cases, as will be seen, several estimates can be assessed simultaneously with a significance test where the analogous confidence region is difficult to construct and to interpret. Of course, a significance test and a confidence interval can both be presented. However, if one approach must be chosen, a confidence interval usually allows a simple and more comprehensive assessment of the influence of random variation on a single estimated quantity.

Lack of precision, incurred when a sample represents a fraction of the population, must be taken into account to assess realistically a factor's influence on the risk of a disease. To evaluate the impact of random variation associated with the estimate $\hat{b}$, both a significance test and a confidence interval require an estimate of the variance of $\hat{b}$, which is estimated by

$$\text{variance}(\hat{b}) = \frac{1}{n_{11}} + \frac{1}{n_{12}} + \frac{1}{n_{21}} + \frac{1}{n_{22}}. \tag{7.8}$$

For the behavior type data (Table 2–3), the estimated variance associated with $\hat{b} = 0.864$ is

$$\text{variance}(\hat{b}) = \frac{1}{178} + \frac{1}{1,411} + \frac{1}{79} + \frac{1}{1,486} = 0.020. \tag{7.9}$$

Aside: For reasons beyond the scope of this text, the variance of the logarithm of the number of observations in a specific cell of a table is approximately variance $[\pm \log(n_{ij})] \approx 1/n_{ij}$. This estimate of the variance is based on the assumption that the number of observations occurring in a specific cell, at least approximately, represents an independent sample from a Poisson distribution. Risk measures based on the log-odds can be broken into a sum of independent terms of the form $\pm \log(n_{ij})$ and, therefore, the variance of these risk measures is a sum of the variances associated with each of these terms. For example, since $\hat{a} = \log(_{21}/n_{22}) = \log(n_{21}) - \log(n_{22})$, then the estimated variance of $\hat{a}$ is

$$\text{variance}(\hat{a}) = \text{variance}[\log(n_{21})] + \text{variance}[-\log(n_{22})] = 1/n_{21} + 1/n_{22}. \tag{7.10}$$

The estimated variance of the estimated coefficient $\hat{b}$ [expression (7.8)] follows the same pattern.

To test the null hypothesis that the risk factor is unrelated to the disease outcome ($H_0: b = 0$), the test statistic

$$X^2 = \frac{\hat{b}^2}{\text{variance}(\hat{b})} \tag{7.11}$$

has an approximate chi-square distribution with one degree of freedom when the null hypothesis is true. The quantity X^2 is frequently called Wald's test. A statistical test of $b = 0$ is equivalent to testing a number of other hypotheses including: odds ratio $= 1.0$, $P(D|F) = P(D|\bar{F})$ or $P(F|D) = P(F|\bar{D})$. These expressions all indicate the same property, namely that the disease outcome and the risk factor are unrelated; more technically, disease outcome and risk factor are statistically independent, or $P(D|F) = P(D)$. For the WCGS data, $X^2 = (0.864)^2/0.020 = 37.985$ yielding a p-value <0.001 indicating that the A/B behavior type is associated with CHD incidence.

An approximate $(1 - \alpha)\%$ confidence interval based on the estimate $\hat{b}$ has the bounds

$$\text{upper bound} = \hat{b} + z_{1-\alpha/2}\sqrt{\text{variance }(\hat{b})} \tag{7.12}$$

and

$$\text{lower bound} = \hat{b} - z_{1-\alpha/2}\sqrt{\text{variance }(\hat{b})} \tag{7.13}$$

since $\hat{b}$ has an approximate normal distribution for moderate or large samples of observations. The value $z_{1-\alpha/2}$ is, as usual, the $(1 - \alpha/2)$-percentile from a standard normal distribution. A $(1 - \alpha)\%$ confidence interval for the odds ratio $or = e^b$ is then $(e^{\text{lower}}, e^{\text{upper}})$. The approximate 95% confidence interval based on $\hat{b} = 0.864$ from the behavior type data is $(0.589, 1.139)$. The approximate 95% confidence interval for the odds ratio or is then $(e^{0.589} = 1.803, e^{1.139} = 3.123)$, indicating the precision of the estimate $\widehat{or} = e^{0.864} = 2.373$.

Using a linear model to represent the log-odds is related to describing the probabilities from a 2×2 table with a logistic function. The logistic function, which has historically been used in a variety of contexts to study biological phenomena, is formally

$$f(x) = \frac{1}{1 + e^{-x}}. \tag{7.14}$$

The function $f(x)$ is an "s-shaped" curve where large negative values of x yield $f(x)$ near 0, large positive values of x yield $f(x)$ near 1, and a value of $x = 0$ produces $f(0) = 0.5$. The logistic curve produces values that are always greater than 0 and less than 1, which makes it ideal for representing probabilities, which are also bounded between 0 and 1.

In symbols, the logistic probabilities applied to a 2×2 table are

$$P(D|F = 0) = \frac{1}{1 + e^{-a}} \quad \text{and} \quad P(D|F = 1) = \frac{1}{1 + e^{-(a+b)}}, \tag{7.15}$$

where a and b are the quantities previously defined in terms of log-odds.

In other words, the same parameters (a, b) describe the relationships within a contingency table using either the log-odds or logistic probabilities as measures of risk. A logistic relationship among the probabilities from a 2×2 table implies a linear relationship among the log-odds and vice-versa. To illustrate,

$$\text{log-odds} = \log\left(\frac{P(D|F=1)}{P(\bar{D}|F=1)}\right) = \log\left(\frac{1/(1+e^{-(a+b)})}{e^{-(a+b)}/(1+e^{-(a+b)})}\right) \quad (7.16)$$

$$= \log(e^{a+b}) = a + b.$$

The odds ratio is most easily interpreted when the frequency of the disease is low (less than 0.1 in both the risk-factor and non-risk factor groups) since, in this case, the estimated odds ratio is approximately equal to a simpler measure of association between risk factor and disease called the relative risk [i.e., $or \approx$ relative risk $= P(D|F)/P(D|\bar{F})$]. Relative risk is a natural measure of risk to apply to prospective data when one group is "exposed" and another is "unexposed" and is discussed in detail elsewhere (e.g., [4] and [5]). However, the odds ratio is a valid measure of association regardless of the frequency of the outcome variable.

A summary of the logistic regression analysis of the association between behavior type and coronary disease in the WCGS data is shown in Table 7–4. The logistic probabilities are estimated as $\hat{P}(D|F=0) = 0.050$ and $\hat{P}(D|F=1) = 0.112$, which can be calculated from the logistic function using estimates $\hat{a}$ and $\hat{b}$ and expression (7.15) or directly from the data, again indicating that the logistic model is saturated when applied to a 2×2 table.

The Two × Two × Two Table

When an association is detected in a 2×2 table, a natural question is: How is this relationship influenced by other variables? The WCGS data show a strong association between behavior type and coronary

Table 7–4. CHD by A/B—two-parameter model

Variable	Term	Estimate	Std. Error	p-value	$\widehat{or}$
Constant	$\hat{a}$	−2.934	0.115	—	—
A/B	$\hat{b}$	0.864	0.140	<0.001	2.373

-2 Log Likelihood $= 1740.334$ (see Appendix E); number of model parameters $= 2$.

Table 7-5. CHD by A/B by systolic blood pressure

	Blood Pressure ≥ 140			Blood Pressure < 140		
	CHD	No CHD	Total	CHD	No CHD	Total
Type-A	69	319	388	109	1,092	1,201
Type-B	27	278	305	52	1,208	1,260
Total	96	597	693	161	2,300	2,461

$$or_1 = 2.227 \qquad or_2 = 2.319$$

disease, but an important question remains: Could this association be, at least in part, due to the influence of other risk factors? For example, systolic blood pressure level is related to coronary disease as well as behavior type and could influence the observed association. A $2 \times 2 \times 2$ contingency table sheds some light on the influence of another variable on the relationship under investigation. To illustrate, the role of systolic blood pressure as a possible confounding influence on the relationship between behavior type and coronary disease is explored from a $2 \times 2 \times 2$ (Table 7-5). Another version of these data in terms of the log-odds is given in Table 7-6.

The influence of behavior type is measured by $\hat{b}_1 = \hat{l}_{11} - \hat{l}_{12} = 0.801$ for individuals with blood pressure ≥ 140 and by $\hat{b}_2 = \hat{l}_{21} - \hat{l}_{22} = 0.841$ for blood pressure < 140. These two quantities do not differ from the log-odds measure previously described for a 2×2 table but are calculated twice, once in each blood pressure subtable. In the case of a $2 \times 2 \times 2$ table, measures of risk associated with blood pressure can also be estimated in each of the two behavior categories. The two log-odds measures of blood pressure risk are $\hat{c}_1 = \hat{l}_{11} - \hat{l}_{21} = 0.773$ for type-A individuals and $\hat{c}_2 = \hat{l}_{12} - \hat{l}_{12} = 0.813$ for type-B individuals. The failure of these two measures ($\hat{b}$'s or $\hat{c}$'s) to be equal in each of the subtables brings up a fundamental concern. One of two possible situations exists:

1. The influence of the risk factor under study is the same in both subtables, and the observed differences arise only because of the influence of random variation (no interaction), or
2. The influence of the risk factor under study is different in each subtable (interaction present).

The first possibility suggests that the two estimates should be combined to produce a single summary measure of the association between risk factor and disease. The second indicates quite the opposite.

Table 7–6. CHD by A/B systolic blood pressure: a summary

Blood Pressure	Behavior Type	CHD	No CHD	Log-Odds	Notation
≥ 140	A	69	319	-1.531	l_{11}
≥ 140	B	27	278	-2.332	l_{12}
< 140	A	109	1,092	-2.304	l_{21}
< 140	B	52	1,208	-3.145	l_{22}

As noted before, if a variable behaves differently in each subtable, then a combined estimate of the influence will conceal or exaggerate the difference and likely be misleading—interactions restrict "summarization."

In symbolic terms, for a $2 \times 2 \times 2$ table, an interaction measure using log-odds is

$$\text{interaction} = b_1 - b_2 = (l_{11} - l_{12}) - (l_{21} - l_{22}) = l_{11} - l_{12} - l_{21} + l_{22} \tag{7.17}$$

or, similarly,

$$\text{interaction} = c_1 - c_2 = (l_{11} - l_{21}) - (l_{12} - l_{22}) = l_{11} - l_{12} - l_{21} + l_{22}. \tag{7.18}$$

The expression $l_{11} - l_{12} - l_{21} + l_{22}$ quantifies the amount of interaction associated with two risk factors on a log-odds scale and is occasionally used as the definition of interaction. An estimate of the magnitude of the interaction associated with behavior type and blood pressure is

$$\hat{b}_1 - \hat{b}_2 = \hat{c}_1 - \hat{c}_2 = \hat{l}_{11} - \hat{l}_{12} - \hat{l}_{21} + \hat{l}_{22}$$

$$= -1.531 + 2.332 + 2.304 - 3.145 = -0.040.$$

An important issue is whether the data provide evidence of a nonrandom ("real") interaction. Testing the null hypothesis that $l_{11} - l_{12} - l_{21} + l_{22} = 0$ is equivalent to testing the hypothesis that $b_1 = b_2$ or $c_1 = c_2$. A statistical test to evaluate the magnitude of the estimated interaction effect requires an expression for the variance. Along the lines discussed for the 2×2 contingency table, the variance of the estimated interaction effect is estimated by

$$\text{variance (interaction)} = \sum_{i=1}^{2} \sum_{j=1}^{2} \sum_{k=1}^{2} \frac{1}{n_{ijk}}, \tag{7.19}$$

where n_{ijk} represents a cell frequency in the $2 \times 2 \times 2$ table (notation in Table 6–14). For example, the estimated interaction effect associated with blood pressure and behavior type is -0.040, and the estimated variance associated with this estimate is

$$\text{variance (interaction)} = \frac{1}{69} + \frac{1}{319} + \frac{1}{27} + \frac{1}{278} + \frac{1}{109} + \frac{1}{1{,}092} + \frac{1}{52} + \frac{1}{1{,}208}$$

$$= 0.088. \tag{7.20}$$

The test statistic

$$X^2 = \frac{(l_{11} - \hat{l}_{12} - \hat{l}_{21} + \hat{l}_{22})^2}{\text{variance (interaction)}} \tag{7.21}$$

has an approximate chi-square distribution with one degree of freedom when no interaction exists and provides a rigorous assessment of the importance of the estimated interaction effect. Continuing the WCGS example, the chi-square statistic of $X^2 = (-0.040)^2/0.088 = 0.018$ with a p-value $= 0.892$ formally indicates no evidence of an interaction between the risk factors blood pressure and behavior type in the analysis of CHD risk.

A linear model underlying the log-odds approach to describing relationships in a $2 \times 2 \times 2$ table is

$$l_{11} = a + b_2 + c_2 + d,$$

$$l_{12} = a + c_2,$$

$$l_{21} = a + b_2, \quad \text{and} \tag{7.22}$$

$$l_{22} = a,$$

where d represents the magnitude of the interaction effect (i.e., $d = l_{11} - l_{12} - l_{21} + l_{22}$). The values b_2 and c_2 represent the direct effects of behavior type and blood pressure as defined earlier. Notice the parameters b_1 and c_1 are redundant since $b_1 = b_2 + d$ and $c_1 = c_2 + d$ (four parameters uniquely establish four log-odds values; see Figure 7–2). The coefficient a represents a constant baseline level of risk.

Another view of the parameter d is

$$d = b_1 - b_2 = c_1 - c_2, \quad \text{or} \quad e^d \frac{or_1}{or_2}, \tag{7.23}$$

where or_1 is the odds ratio from the first 2×2 subtable and or_2 is the odds ratio from the second 2×2 subtable. For the blood pressure and behavior type data, $\widehat{or}_1 = 2.227$ and $\widehat{or}_2 = 2.319$ yielding $e^d = 0.960$ and again $\hat{d} = -0.040$. When $d = 0$ ($e^0 = 1.0$), the odds ratios are identical in both subtables; otherwise the magnitude of e^d reflects the degree of interaction in terms of the ratio of odds ratios.

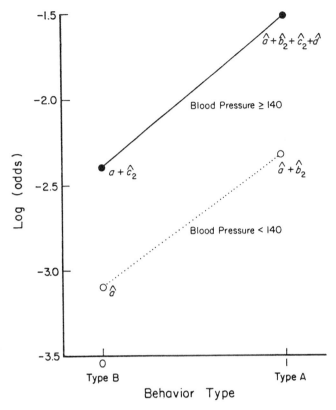

Figure 7–2. Log-odds associated with CHD risk by behavior type and by systolic blood pressure (<140 and ≥ 140)

Table 7–7 summarizes the estimates of these four components and describes the relationship of coronary disease to the variables blood pressure, and behavior type in terms of the logistic model [expression (7.22)].

The application of the logistic model to a $2 \times 2 \times 2$ table can be geometrically interpreted as two straight lines on a log-odds scale, each depicting the influence of the risk factor at each level of the other variable.

Table 7–7. CHD by A/B by systolic blood pressure—four-parameter model

Variable	Term	Estimate	Std. Error	p-value	$\widehat{or}$
Constant	$\hat{a}$	−3.145	0.142	—	—
A/B	$\hat{b}_2$	0.841	0.174	<0.001	2.319
Blood Pressure	$\hat{c}_2$	0.814	0.246	<0.001	2.256
Interaction	$\hat{d}$	−0.040	0.297	0.892	0.960

-2 Log Likelihood $= 1,709.934$; number of model parameters $= 4$.

The parameter d reflects the degree to which these two lines are not parallel. Figure 7–2 shows the lines representing the change in CHD risk associated with behavior type for the two levels of blood pressure estimated from the WCGS data. It should be noted that the same estimated odds ratios (last column in Table 7–7) could have been calculated directly from the tabled data, indicating that the model [expression (7.22)] is saturated. For example, $\hat{b}_2 = 0.841$ gives $\widehat{or} = e^{b_2} = 2.319$, which is identical to $\widehat{or}_2 = (109)(1,208)/(52)(1,092) = 2.319$. Four log-odds values means a four-parameter logistic model is saturated.

When no interaction exists (i.e., $d = 0$; that is, $or_1 = or_2$), an additive logistic model (nonstaturated) represents the relationships in a $2 \times 2 \times 2$ table, again in terms of the log-odds

$$
\begin{aligned}
l_{11} &= a + b + c, \\
l_{12} &= a + c, \\
l_{21} &= a + b, \quad \text{and} \\
l_{22} &= a.
\end{aligned}
\tag{7.24}
$$

This statistical structure is additive because the log-odds associated with possessing both risk factors (l_{11}) is exactly the sum of the influences from each risk factor. Note also that $d = l_{11} - l_{12} - l_{21} + l_{22} = 0$ by definition of the additive model. The values b and c take the place of the previous values b_1, b_2, c_1, and c_2 (i.e., $b_1 = b_2 = b$ and $c_1 = c_2 = c$). An iterative procedure [expression (6.33)] or a computer program is necessary to estimate the values of a, b, and c from a $2 \times 2 \times 2$ table. Using such a program, the maximum likelihood estimates (see Appendix E for a description) from the WCGS data are $\hat{a} = -3.136$, $\hat{b} = 0.827$, and $\hat{c} = 0.786$. The expected values generated by the model and the log-odds based on these estimates are given in Table 7–8. For example, $\hat{l}_{11} = -3.136 + 0.827 + 0.786 = -1.523$ and $388/(1 + e^{1.523}) = 69.46$ CHD events are expected among individuals who are type-A with high blood pressure when these two variables have an additive influence on risk.

The additive (no-interaction) model requires that the influence of

Table 7–8. CHD by A/B by systolic blood pressure: expected values based on the additive model

Blood Pressure	Behavior Type	CHD	No CHD	Log-Odds	Notation
≥ 140	A	69.46	318.54	-1.523	$\hat{l}_{11}$
≥ 140	B	26.54	278.46	-2.350	$\hat{l}_{12}$
< 140	A	108.54	1,092.46	-2.309	$\hat{l}_{21}$
< 140	B	52.46	1,207.54	-3.136	$\hat{l}_{22}$

the risk factor be exactly the same in both subtables or $b_1 = b_2 = b$ and $c_1 = c_2 = c$. The odds ratio associated with behavior type is $\widehat{or}_{A/B} = e^{\hat{b}} = e^{0.827} = 2.286$, which is an evaluation of the CHD risk associated with behavior type adjusted for the influence of blood pressure. A type-A individual has odds of a coronary event 2.286 times greater then a type-B individual in both blood pressure status groups (≥ 140 or < 140). Similarly, $\widehat{or}_{bp} = e^{\hat{c}} = e^{0.786} = 2.195$ is the estimated odds ratio reflecting CHD risk of individuals with blood pressure equal to or exceeding 140 relative to those with values less than 140 for both behavior types. Also the product $\widehat{or}_{A/B}\,\widehat{or}_{bp} = (2.286)(2.195) = 5.018$ is a measure of the CHD risk associated with simultaneously possessing both risk factors (type-A with blood pressure ≥ 140) relative to an individual with neither risk factor (type-B with blood pressure < 140). In terms of the additive model, the estimated difference in log-odds associated with possessing both risk factors relative to possessing neither factor is $l_{11} - l_{22} = \hat{a} + \hat{b} + \hat{c} - \hat{a} = 1.613$, and the odds $ratio = e^{\hat{b}+\hat{c}} = e^{1.613} = 5.018$. In general, the odds ratio derived from a logistic regression coefficient, when no interaction is present, is a measure of the contribution of a specific factor or factors to the risk of disease, adjusted for the influences of other risk factors in the model. A summary of the no-interaction model is given in Table 7–9.

A comparison of the estimated values from the additive (no-interaction) model in Table 7–9 with the corresponding values in Table 7–7 (saturated model) shows no important differences occur when the interaction term is deleted from the model. The influence of interaction can be formally evaluated by contrasting the likelihood statistics (see Appendix E) associated with each model. For statistical reasons, it is much more convenient to work with the logarithm of the likelihood values multiplied by a -2. When the logarithm of a likelihood value is multiplied by -2 the resulting value will be called the likelihood statistic and symbolized by L. A likelihood statistic is a relative measure of the goodness-of-fit of a specific model and produces a measure of goodness-of-fit with an approximate chi-square

Table 7–9. CHD by A/B by systolic blood pressure—three-parameter model

Variable	Term	Estimate	Std. Error	p-value	$\widehat{or}$
Constant	$\hat{a}$	-3.136	0.124	—	—
A/B	$\hat{b}$	0.827	0.138	<0.001	2.286
Blood pressure	$\hat{c}$	0.786	0.141	<0.001	2.195

-2 Log Likelihood $= 1709.954$; number of model parameters $= 3$.

distribution. The likelihood statistic decreases with each parameter added to a model. This reduction is likely to be small when the added parameter is unrelated to the disease under study and substantial if the added parameter is related to the disease. The difference between two likelihood statistics can be used, therefore, to assess the comparative strengths of two models to "explain" the data.

For the WCGS data the two likelihood statistics are $L_{d=0} = 1,709.954$ for the no-interaction model (the parameter d set equal to zero) and $L_{d \neq 0} = 1,709.934$ for the saturated model (the parameter d not equal to zero) showing that the descriptive power of the logistic model is essentially unchanged by assuming that no interaction exists (i.e., $d = 0$). The difference between two likelihood statistics has an approximate chi-square distribution when the difference observed arises from random variation alone. The degrees of freedom are equal to the difference in the number of parameters necessary to describe each model. Using this chi-square test verifies that setting $d = 0$ in the logistic model has essentially no impact ($L_{d=0} - L_{d \neq 0} = 1,709.954 - 1,709.934 = 0.020$ with one degree of freedom produces a p-value of 0.888). Contrasting likelihood statistics to evaluate the descriptive worth of two competing models is an important statistical tool and is used repeatedly in the following sections.

When there is no interaction, the factors influencing the outcome act additively on the log-odds scale and multiplicatively on the odds scale. No interaction, therefore, means that each factor contributes to the risk of disease separately and the overall odds ratio can be expressed as a product of a series of specific odds ratios each strictly associated with a risk factor (i.e., $or = \prod or_i$); or, conversely, the overall risk can be factored into a set of individual component parts (or_i). Under these additive conditions, risk factors are said to have "independent" influences on the risk of disease.

To evaluate the role of systolic blood pressure, the logistic model with blood pressure not included is helpful. The additive model with the parameter c set to zero is summarized in Table 7–4. The difference in the likelihood statistics for the model including blood pressure and the model excluding blood pressure reflects the contribution of the blood pressure variable to the additive model describing the risk of coronary disease. That is, $L_0 = 1,740.344$ (blood pressure excluded) and $L_1 = 1,709.954$ (blood pressure included) gives $L_0 - L_1 = 30.390$ with one degree of freedom producing a p-value < 0.001, showing that blood pressure is important in the description of CHD risk. The comparison is uninfluenced by behavior type since this variable is maintained in both models. A likelihood approach to evaluating a single variable is not basically different from the statistical test of a parameter $c = 0$. As indicated earlier, a squared estimated coefficient divided by its variance (the Wald statistic—$X^2 = \hat{c}^2/\text{variance}(\hat{c}) = 32.4$ with a p-value < 0.001) has an approximate chi-square distribution with one degree of freedom when the expected value of the coefficient is zero. The usefulness of employing likelihood statistics to evaluate hypotheses stems from the fact that combinations of risk factors can be assessed simultaneously by comparing models containing several risk factors with a model excluding these factors, resulting in a rigorous statistical test.

A Note on the Power to Detect Interaction Effects

The power of a statistical test to detect an interaction can be relatively low compared to tests of direct effects. In terms of the WCGS data, the probability of identifying a blood pressure/behavior type interaction is less than the probability that such variables as blood pressure and behavior type will be identified as important risk factors. In a $2 \times 2 \times 2$ contingency table, the reason for a relatively less powerful test is easily seen. Recall that the variance of the estimated measure of interaction is

$$\text{variance (interaction)} = \sum\sum\sum \frac{1}{n_{ijk}}, \tag{7.25}$$

where n_{ijk} represents a cell frequency in the $2 \times 2 \times 2$ table. From the previous example [expression (7.20)] the estimated measure of an interaction associated with blood pressure and behavior type is -0.040, and the estimated variance of this estimate is

$$\text{variance (interaction)} = \frac{1}{69} + \frac{1}{319} + \frac{1}{27} + \frac{1}{278} + \frac{1}{109} + \frac{1}{1,092} + \frac{1}{52} + \frac{1}{1,208}$$

$$= 0.088.$$

This variance involves all eight cells of the contingency table, and its value is primarily determined by the cells with the lowest frequency, in this case 27 and 52. Therefore, the variance of the interaction is necessarily larger than $1/27 = 1/52 = 0.057$. Since the measure of an interaction involves all cells in the table, the variance is largely determined by the cells with the fewest observations, which can lead to unreliable estimates (large variances) of the interaction measure and an accompanying loss of statistical power. Estimates of the direct effects do not necessarily involve the low-frequency cells producing more reliable estimates (lower variances) and increased power. In more complex situations the investigation of interactions also suffers from problems of low power for much the same reasons as illustrated in the $2 \times 2 \times 2$ case. Failure of a statistical test to reject the null hypothesis of no interaction provides some justification for employing an additive model, but the power of this test is often low. Therefore, an analysis based on the proposition that the risk factors are additive simplifies the interpretation but also is potentially biased.

It is important to detect interaction effects when they exist. It is not critical to eliminate interaction terms from the logistic model when the data can support an additive model. In terms of assessing the null hypothesis of no interaction (H_0), a type I error (rejecting H_0 when H_0 is true) is not as important as a type II error (accepting H_0 when H_0 is not true) when it comes to testing for an interaction. For a test of the interaction, it is a good idea to increase the level of significance (say, $\alpha = 0.2$) to increase the power. Increasing α to attain more statistical power (decreasing the type II error) is a conservative strategy in the sense that relatively minor losses occur, such as some loss of efficiency and increased complexity of the model, if interaction terms are unnecessarily included in the model. Mistaken elimination of interaction effects, however, can substantially disrupt the validity of any conclusions ("wrong model bias").

Interactions can also occur among combinations of more than two variables. A failure of interaction effects to be the same at levels of other variables is called a second-order interaction (the interactions interact). These higher-order interactions are rarely considered in epidemiological applications, for at least three reasons. Like the two-factor interactions, the estimation of higher-order interactions is unreliable without large sample sizes and well-distributed data (no low-frequency categories). These interactions are also usually highly correlated (close to collinear) with lower-order terms of the logistic model, which also makes estimation unreliable. Higher-order interactions are usually difficult to interpret and experience indicates that they add little to the description of many risk/disease investigations.

Some argue that one solution to the "issue" of interactions is to find a measurement scale to minimize their effects. A better goal is a clear understanding of the nature of the interaction which, therefore, allows deeper insight into the way the variables investigated are related to each other as well as to a disease outcome.

The Two $\times$ *K* Table

A $2 \times K$ table can be effectively analyzed using a log-odds measure of risk. As before, underlying the log-odds approach is the assumption

Table 7-10. CHD by smoking—a 2 × K table

Cigarettes/Day	0	1–20	21–30	> 30	Total
CHD	98	70	50	39	257
No CHD	1,554	735	355	253	2,897
Total	1,652	805	405	292	3,154

that risk factor influences act as series of multiplicative effects. The previous approach to a 2 × K table describes a series of proportions with a straight line (Chapter 6), implying a linear relationship between the levels of the risk factor and the probability of disease. The WCGS data relating coronary heart disease to the amount smoked ($k = 4$ levels) are given in Table 7–10.

A logistic model that exactly duplicates (saturated model) the information contained in a 2 × K contingency table in terms of log-odds (l_i; $i = 1, 2, \ldots, k$) is, for $k = 4$,

$$l_0 = a, \quad l_1 = a + b_1, \quad l_2 = a + b_2, \quad \text{and} \quad l_3 = a + b_3 \quad (7.26)$$

or

$$\text{log-odds} = a + b_1 x_1 + b_2 x_2 + b_3 x_3, \quad (7.27)$$

where x_1, x_2, and x_3 are three binary variables $(0, 1)$, called dummy variables or design variables, identifying each level of the categorical risk factor. For example, the design variables $x_1 = 0$, $x_2 = 1$, and $x_3 = 0$ produce a value log-odds $= l_2 = a + b_2$, which reflects the risk from smoking 21 to 30 cigarettes per day. The values $x_1 = x_2 = x_3 = 0$ establish a baseline of comparison (i.e., log-odds $= l_0 = a$ and reflects the CHD risk among nonsmokers).

Aside: In Chapter 6 it was noted that the values of the k-level variable in a 2 × K table can have at least three forms—numeric, ordered, and nominal. Each variable type suggests a specific analytic approach. In using a logistic model to analyze categorical data similar issues arise. Categories that can be characterized numerically generate values that are typically used directly in the regression analysis, implying a specific relationship among the values. However, nominal categorical values have no specific ordering and usually no logical numeric coding is possible. A nominal variable is incorporated into a logistic regression equation with a binary indicator variable. For example, if two races are being considered, say white and black, one is coded 0 and the other 1. The logistic regression coefficients and the odds ratios are then relative to the variable coded zero. If the odds ratio is 2 and whites are coded as 0 and blacks as 1, then the odds are two times greater among blacks than whites.

The principle of using an indicator variable can be extended. If more than two categories are present (e.g., whites, black, Hispanics, and Asians), then a series of indicator or design variables is used. For k categories, $k - 1$ indicator variables, each taking on the values 0 or 1, allow the analysis to include a series of nominal variables in a regression model. Again a baseline category is established by setting the associated $k - 1$ design variables equal to zero. The members of other categories are identified by a single design variable that takes on the value 1 while the remaining design variables are set to zero. For example, if blacks, Hispanics, and Asians are to be compared relative to the whites, then for $k = 4$,

$$\text{Whites: } x_1 = 0, x_2 = 0, \quad \text{and} \quad x_3 = 0;$$

$$\text{Blacks: } x_1 = 1, x_2 = 0, \quad \text{and} \quad x_3 = 0;$$

$$\text{Hispanics: } x_1 = 0, x_2 = 1, \quad \text{and} \quad x_3 = 0;$$

$$\text{Asians: } x_1 = 0, x_2 = 0, \quad \text{and} \quad x_3 = 1.$$

Like the binary case, the resulting logistic regression coefficients and the odds ratios measure the role of each category relative to the category with all design variables set equal to zero. Any number of categories can be identified with this scheme, allowing the assessment of risk using a logistic model without requiring a numeric value or even requiring that the categories be ordered. Many software analysis sytems set up a series of design variables automatically.

An artificial data set illustrating design variables to identify four racial categories is given in Table 7–11. Twelve observations f_i (3 whites, 4 blacks, 2 Hispanics, and 3 Asians) make up the "data" set.

Table 7–11. Illustration of the use of design variables to establish membership in four racial categories

Race	Observation	x_1	x_2	x_3
Black	f_1	1	0	0
White	f_2	0	0	0
Asian	f_3	0	0	1
White	f_4	0	0	0
Black	f_5	1	0	0
Black	f_6	1	0	0
Hispanic	f_7	0	1	0
Asian	f_8	0	0	1
White	f_9	0	0	0
Asian	f_{10}	0	0	1
Black	f_{11}	1	0	0
Hispanic	f_{12}	0	1	0

Design variables are a way of incorporating categorical variables into multivariable models and are essentially a mathematically convenient method to describe tabular data. For example,

$$\text{log-odds} = a + b_1 x_1 + b_2 x_2 + b_3 x_3$$

produces the same results as analyzing the outcome variable classified into a table with four categories. The estimated odds ratios, for example, are the same whether calculated directly from the table or from the estimated coefficients $\hat{b}_i$.

The model describing four categories of smoking exposure and CHD risk is not restricted in any way, so the saturated linear model can produce any pattern of log-odds necessary to describe the relationship of disease response to the differing levels of the risk factor. A logistic model that does not imply a particular ordering in the l_i-values is said to be unconstrained. Estimates of the unconstrained model parameters are (notation is given in Table 6–2)

$$\hat{a} = \log(n_{11}/n_{21}), \quad \hat{b}_1 = \log(n_{12}/n_{22}) - \hat{a}$$

$$\hat{b}_2 = \log(n_{13}/n_{23}) - \hat{a}, \quad \text{and} \quad \hat{b}_3 = \log(n_{14}/n_{24}) - \hat{a} \tag{7.28}$$

giving the estimates from the WCGS smoking exposure data shown in Table 7–12.

The odds ratios $(\widehat{or}_{0i} = e^{\hat{b}_i})$ measure the multiplicative risk for each smoking category relative to a baseline (nonsmokers). For example, smoking more than 30 cigarettes a day produces an odds 2.445 $(e^{0.894})$ times greater than the odds among nonsmokers. The odds ratios associated with increasing levels of smoking show an increasing risk of CHD (increasing from 1.5 to 2.2 to 2.4; see Table 7–12 and Figure 7–3). This pattern is a property of the data and not the model; any pattern, as mentioned, could have emerged from this unconstrained logistic regression model.

One reason to construct a $2 \times K$ table is to explore the question of whether a risk factor has a specific pattern of influence on the risk of

Table 7–12. CHD by smoking

Variable	Term	Estimate	Std. Error	p-value	$\widehat{or}$
Constant	$\hat{a}$	−2.764	0.104	—	—
Smoking (1–20)	$\hat{b}_1$	0.412	0.163	<0.001	1.510
Smoking (21–30)	$\hat{b}_2$	0.804	0.183	<0.001	2.233
Smoking (>30)	$\hat{b}_3$	0.894	0.201	<0.001	2.445

−2 Log Likelihood = 1751.695; number of model parameters = 4.

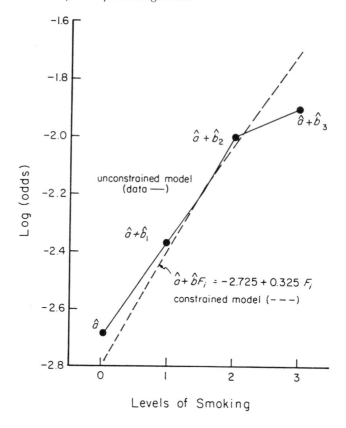

Figure 7–3. Log-odds associated with CHD risk by amount smoked (unconstrained and constrained models)

disease. Does the risk, for example, of a coronary event increase in a specific pattern with increases in the level of smoking? Multiplicative relationships translate into additive relationships of logarithms. In terms of a logistic model, the log-odds are then generated by an additive relationship described by the straight line

$$\text{log-odds} = l_i = a + bF_i, \tag{7.29}$$

where F_i represents one of the k numeric levels of the risk factor and l_i represents the log-odds resulting from the ith level of the risk factor. The choices of the F_i-values brings a degree of subjectivity to the analysis that influences the results. For the WCGS example, the values $F_0 = 0$, $F_1 = 1$, $F_2 = 2$, and $F_3 = 3$ are chosen to reflect the four smoking levels. Other equally spaced F_i-values reflecting each category would give the same analysis (i.e., same p-values and likelihood statistics but different values of a and b). For example, using the levels of 0, 10, 20, and 30 cigarettes per day would not change the analytic results. For this straight-line model the log-odds must follow a linearly increasing or decreasing pattern, making the model constrained.

Computer-generated (maximum likelihood) estimates for the parameters of the constrained model from the smoking data are $\hat{a} = -2.725$ and $\hat{b} = 0.325$ (Figure 7–3). The log-odds increases by an amount 0.325 between each of the four smoking categories. The likelihood statistic reflecting the fit of the two-parameter constrained model is $L_0 = 1,753.045$ (degrees of freedom = 2). The previous unconstrained saturated model yields a likelihood statistic of $L_1 = 1,751.695$ (degrees of freedom = 4). The difference in likelihood statistics has an approximate chi-square distribution with two degrees of freedom when the models being compared differ strictly because of sampling variation ($L_0 - L_1 = 1.350$, p-value = 0.509). The comparison shows that using a single line to represent the smoking/CHD relationship does not differ in any important way from the saturated, unconstrained model (again see Figure 7–3). The straight-line model adequately and more simply describes the relationship between smoking and CHD using two parameters. Consequently, smoking levels can be usefully represented as increasing the risk of a CHD event in a multiplicative pattern. Note that

$$\hat{l}_i = \hat{a} + \hat{b}F_i \quad \text{implies} \quad \widehat{or}_{0i} = (e^{\hat{b}})^{F_i}, \tag{7.30}$$

where $\widehat{or}_{0i}$ represents the odds ratio associated with the ith level of the risk factor relative to a baseline. For the smoking data then,

$$\widehat{or}_{0i} = (e^{\hat{b}})^{F_i} = (e^{0.325})^{F_i} = (1.384)^{F_i}, \tag{7.31}$$

where the baseline is the nonsmoking group ($F_0 = 0$) and the estimated odds ratios for the values of F_i are shown in Table 7–13. The linear constrained model translates into logistic probabilities (Table 7–13) since

$$\hat{p}_i = \frac{1}{1 + e^{-(\text{log-odds})}} = \frac{1}{1 + e^{-\hat{l}_i}} = \frac{1}{1 + e^{-(\hat{a} + \hat{b}F_i)}} = \frac{1}{1 + e^{-(-2.725 + 0.325F_i)}}. \tag{7.32}$$

which provides an alternative expression of the relationship between

Table 7–13. CHD by smoking: straight-line model

Levels	$F = 0$	$F = 1$	$F = 2$	$F = 3$
Odds ratio ($\widehat{or}_{0i}$)	1.000	1.384	1.916	2.651
$\hat{p}_i$	0.062	0.083	0.112	0.147

smoking exposure and CHD risk. For example, based on a linearly constrained model, smoking 30 or more cigarettes a day produces an odds of a CHD event 2.651 times greater than the odds among nonsmokers and a probability of a CHD event of 0.147. Of course these two estimated values are related—

$$\widehat{or}_{03} = \frac{\beta_3/(1-\beta_3)}{\beta_0/(1-\beta_0)} = \frac{0.147/0.853}{0.062/0.938} = 2.651.$$

The Two × Two × *K* Table

When a logistic model is used to explore the relationships in a set of data, there are two typical ways to begin: the simplest model or the most complex model. In the first case, variables are added to the model until a useful description is achieved ("forward"). In the second case, variables are removed from the most complex model until a simpler but satisfactory statistical structure is found ("backward"). In this section the most complicated (most parameters) model serves as a starting point for analyzing the risk of a disease at k levels of a categorical risk factor at two levels of another variable, a $2 \times 2 \times K$ table. The most complicated model (saturated model) for $k = 4$ levels of one variable and two levels of another is given by

$$\text{log-odds} = a + b_1 x_1 + b_2 x_2 + b_3 x_3 + cC + d_1 C x_2 + d_2 C x_2 + d_3 C x_3, \quad (7.33)$$

where x_i is, as before, a design variable indicating the categories of a four-level risk factor while $C = 1$ produces the log-odds when the another factor is present and $C = 0$ produces the log-odds when that factor is absent. The terms $d_i C x_i$ measure the interaction between the k-level risk factor and the two-level risk factor. In this context, an interaction is the failure of the four categorical variables to have the same relationship with the outcome variable for both levels of variable C. All direct influences and all possible interactions are included in this statistical structure, yielding an eight-parameter saturated model. To be concrete, let x_i indicate smoking level using four smoking categories and C indicate the two levels of behavior type (B coded 0 and A coded 1). The WCGS data for the four smoking levels and the two behavior categories are given in Table 7–14. A logistic model applied to this $2 \times 2 \times 4$ table produces the following estimates for the eight parameters of the saturated logistic model (Table 7–15).

The saturated model is a starting point, but the results are not much different from the data themselves since the contingency table produces

Table 7–14. CHD by smoking by A/B

	Type-A				
Cigs/Day	0	1–20	21–30	≥30	Total
CHD	70	45	34	29	178
No CHD	714	353	185	159	1,411
Total	784	398	219	188	1,589
	Type-B				
Cigs/Day	0	1–20	21–30	≥30	Total
CHD	28	25	16	10	79
No CHD	840	382	170	94	1,486
Total	868	407	186	104	1,565

Table 7–15. CHD by A/B by smoking (saturated)—eight-parameter model

	Term	Estimate	Std. Error	p-value	$\widehat{or}$
Constant	$\hat{a}$	−3.401	0.192	—	—
Smoking (1–20)	$\hat{b}_1$	0.675	0.282	0.017	1.963
Smoking (21–30)	$\hat{b}_2$	1.038	0.324	0.001	2.824
Smoking (>30)	$\hat{b}_3$	1.160	0.384	0.003	3.191
AB	$\hat{c}$	1.079	0.229	<0.001	2.941
Interaction	$\hat{d}_1$	−0.412	0.347	0.235	0.662
Interaction	$\hat{d}_2$	−0.410	0.395	0.299	0.664
Interaction	$\hat{d}_3$	−0.540	0.452	0.232	0.583

−2 Log Likelihood = 1,713.694; number of model parameters = 8.

eight log-odds values and the model employs eight parameters. Although a saturated model is not a useful summary of a set of data, it produces a baseline against which to compare the efficacy of reduced models (models with fewer parameters) that are simpler representations of the relationships under study. One such reduced model postulates no interactions exist between the k-level factor (smoking exposure) and the dichotomous factor (behavior type). That is, when the two risk factors do not interact, the model becomes

$$\text{log-odds} = a + b_1 x_1 + b_2 x_2 + b_3 x_3 + cC. \qquad (7.34)$$

Note that this model is a special case of the saturated model, formed by setting the interaction coefficients to zero $(d_1 = d_2 = d_3 = 0)$ making the relationship of the log-odds to the k-level categorical

Table 7–16. CHD by A/B by smoking (no-interaction)—five-parameter model

Variable	Term	Estimate	Std. Error	p-value	$\widehat{or}$
Constant	$\hat{a}$	−3.223	0.139	—	—
Smoking (1–20)	$\hat{b}_1$	0.401	0.164	0.014	1.493
Smoking (21–30)	$\hat{b}_2$	0.761	0.185	<0.001	2.141
Smoking (≥30)	$\hat{b}_3$	0.775	0.203	<0.001	2.170
AB	$\hat{c}$	1.815	0.141	<0.001	2.259

−2 Log Likelihood = 1,716.069; number of model parameters = 5.

variable and the variable C additive. The maximum likelihood estimates of the five parameters of the no-interaction model are given in Table 7–16.

Geometrically, the additive model is represented by two parallel lines (Figure 7–4). The pattern is not constrained to either increase

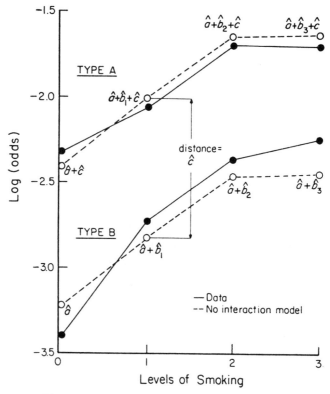

Figure 7–4. Log-odds associated with CHD risk by amount smoked and by behavior type (unconstrained and additive model)

or decrease with increasing levels of smoking, but risk associated with type-A and type-B individuals differs by a constant amount (measured by c in the model) on a log-odds scale for all four levels of smoking exposure. That is, the pattern of risk associated with smoking exposure is exactly the same for both type-A and type-B individuals. The adjusted odds ratio measuring the impact of behavior type and CHD risk is $e^{\hat{c}} = e^{0.815} = 2.259$—independent of smoking exposure.

Formally, the difference between the saturated model and the no-interaction model is evaluated by comparing the respective likelihood statistics $(L_0 - L_1 = 1,716.069 - 1,713.694 = 2.375$ with three degrees of freedom producing the p-value $= 0.498)$. The comparison shows no persuasive evidence that smoking exposure and behavior type interact implying that smoking exposure and behavior type risk factors are usefully represented as additive influences on CHD risk measured on a log-odds scale (multiplicatively on an odds scale). For example, the A-type $(C = 1)$ individuals who smoke more than 30 cigarettes per day $(x_1 = 0, x_2 = 0, x_3 = 1)$ have an estimated odds ratio of $\widehat{or} = e^{(\hat{b}_3 + \hat{c})} = (2.170)(2.259) = 4.904$ relative to B-type individuals $(C = 0)$ who are nonsmokers $(x_1 = x_2 = x_3 = 0)$. Figure 7–4 constrasts the no-interaction model with the data (saturated model).

A further step in building an appropriate model to understand the relationships of the three variables recorded in the $2 \times 2 \times K$ contingency table is to postulate a model that is linearly constrained. When the influence from the k-level factor is linearly related to the risk of disease, the model becomes

$$\text{log-odds} = a + bF_i + cC + dF_iC, \qquad (7.35)$$

where F_i is an observed numeric value representing the ith level of a risk factor. Note that the interaction term F_iC is included. Continuing the analysis of the smoking/behavior type data, as before, $F_i = 0, 1, 2,$ or 3 represents levels of smoking exposure and C is again a binary variable $(0, 1)$ representing the dichotomous risk-factor behavior type (B and A).

Geometrically, this model [expression (7.25)] represents the log-odds from a $2 \times 2 \times K$ contingency table as two straight lines with different slopes and intercepts: one line for each level of the dichotomous variable C. In terms of the example, a straight line for type-A individuals and a straight line for type-B individuals reflect the log-odds risk of disease associated with the four levels of smoking.

Table 7–17. CHD by A/B by smoking (constrained with interaction)

Variable	Term	Estimate	Std. Error	p-value	$\widehat{or}$
Constant	$\hat{a}$	−3.305	0.164	—	—
Smoking	$\hat{b}$	0.423	0.108	<0.001	1.527
AB	$\hat{c}$	1.005	0.198	<0.001	2.733
Interaction	$\hat{d}$	−0.190	0.130	0.144	0.827

−2 Log Likelihood = 1,715.859; number of model parameters = 4.

Explicitly this statistical structure is

$$\text{when} \quad C = 0 \text{ (type-B)}, \qquad \text{then} \quad \text{log-odds} = a + bF_i,$$

and

$$\text{when} \quad C = 1 \text{ (type-A)}, \quad \text{then} \quad \text{log-odds} = (a + c) + (b + d)F_i = A + BF_i.$$
$$(7.36)$$

These two linear relationships do not differ in principle from the straight-line logistic model used in the previous section to analyze the $2 \times K$ contingency table since these data can be viewed as two separate $2 \times K$ contingency tables. The estimates for the four parameters of the constrained, interaction model are given in Table 7–17.

Using the estimated parameters, estimated equations for the two straight lines are:

$$\text{log-odds} = \hat{a} + \hat{b}F_i = -3.305 + 0.423F_i \quad \text{(for type-B individuals)}$$

and

$$\text{log-odds} = \hat{A} + \hat{B}F_i = -2.300 + 0.233F_i \quad \text{(for type-A individuals)}.$$

Contrasting this constrained model with the unconstrained model ($L_0 - L_1 = 1,715.859 - 1,713.694 = 2.165$ with four degrees of freedom produces a p-value of 0.705) shows that two different straight lines describing the response in CHD risk from increased levels of smoking exposure for each behavior type are an excellent summary (Figure 7–5).

A further refinement of this constrained statistical structure is possible by postulating that the response to the k-level risk factor is the same at both levels of the dichotomous risk factor. This no-interaction model is achieved by setting $d = 0$ in the previous model [expression (7.35)], giving an additive three-parameter expression or

$$\text{log-odds} = a + bF_i + cC. \qquad (7.37)$$

Again, the data are described by two straight lines, one for each level of the dichotomous risk factor, but the lines have identical slopes,

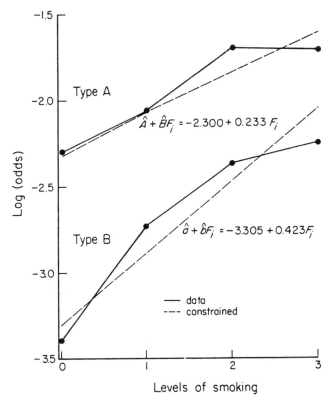

Figure 7–5. Log-odds associated with CHD risk by amount smoked and by behavior type (constrained model)

namely b. Using this model, estimates of the three parameters are given in Table 7–18.

The comparison of the likelihood statistics from the two constrained models shows that describing the WCGS data (Table 7–14) with two parallel lines is not misleading and provides an adequate description of CHD risk $(L_0 - L_1 = 1,717.972 - 1,715.859 = 2.113$ with one degree of freedom, producing p-value $= 0.146)$. This three-parameter

Table 7–18. CHD by A/B by smoking (constrained with no interaction)

Variable	Term	Estimate	Std. Error	p-value	$\widehat{or}$
Constant	$\hat{a}$	−3.171	0.129	—	—
Smoking	$\hat{b}$	0.290	0.060	<0.001	1.336
AB	$\hat{c}$	0.080	0.141	<0.001	2.244

−2 Log Likelihood = 1,717.972; number of model parameters = 3.

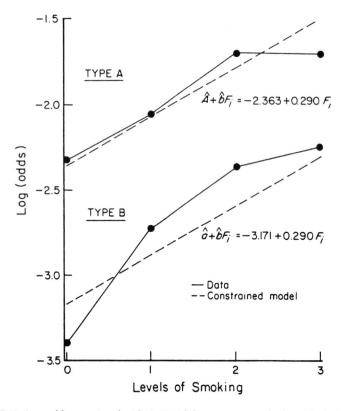

Figure 7–6. Log-odds associated with CHD risk by amount smoked and by behavior type (constrained and additive model).

description of the relationships among smoking, behavior type, and CHD allows a particularly simple expression for the multiplicative role of these factors in the risk of coronary disease (Figure 7–6). The two estimated parallel lines are:

$$\text{log-odds} = \hat{a} + \hat{b}F_i = -3.171 + 0.290F_i \quad \text{(for type-B individuals)}$$

and

$$\text{log-odds} = \hat{a} + \hat{c} + bF_i = -2.363 + 0.290F_i \quad \text{(for type-A individuals)}.$$

The additive constrained model translates into odds ratios:

$$\text{for} \quad C = 0 \ (\text{type-B}), \quad \widehat{or}_{0i} = (1.336)^{F_i}$$

and

$$\text{for} \quad C = 1 \ (\text{type-A}), \quad \widehat{or}_{0i} = 2.244(1.336)^{F_i}, \tag{7.38}$$

where $\widehat{or}_{0i}$ is again the odds ratio associated with the ith level of smoking

Table 7–19. CHD by smoking by behavior type: parallel straight-line model

Levels	$F = 0$	$F = 1$	$F = 2$	$F = 3$
Type-A $(\widehat{or}_{0i})$	2.244	2.998	4.008	5.356
Type-B $(\widehat{or}_{0i})$	1.000	1.336	1.786	2.387

relative to the nonsmokers with type-B behavior. This structure gives the odds ratio estimates shown in Table 7–19. These estimated odds ratios succinctly summarize the role of behavior type and smoking in the risk of a coronary event.

Trend in the Odds Ratios

To a large extent the analysis of trend in a set of odds ratios is contained in the previous discussion, but it is worth focusing specifically on this aspect of logistic regression analysis. Data on smoking and CHD along with a series of odds ratios estimated under different conditions are given in Table 7–20. The directly calculated odds ratios and the odds ratios estimated from the logistic model do not substantially differ. The model

$$\text{log-odds} = a + bF_i \tag{7.39}$$

summarizes, as before, the trend in the odds ratios and produces the model estimated values of $\widehat{or}$ based on $\hat{b} = 0.325$. Both the direct and model estimates show a definite increasing trend in the odds ratios with increasing levels of smoking but fail to take into account influences from other possibly confounding variables. For example, a variable such as blood pressure may have an impact on the observed trend attributed to increased smoking. To account for the influence of blood pressure, a term is added to the logistic model so that the model becomes

$$\text{log-odds} = a + bF_i + dD, \tag{7.40}$$

Table 7–20. Odds ratios: smoking and CHD

F_i	0	1	2	3
CHD	98	70	50	39
No CHD	1,554	735	355	253
$\widehat{or}$ direct	1.0	1.510	2.233	2.445
$\widehat{or}$ model	1.0	1.384	1.916	2.651
$\widehat{or}$ adjusted	1.0	1.378	1.900	2.620

where $D = 0$ (blood pressure < 140) and $D = 1$ (blood pressure ≥ 140). The extended model yields an estimate of the coefficient associated with the trend in disease risk from smoking exposure adjusted for the influence of blood pressure, $\hat{b}' = 0.321$. Comparison of the estimated regression coefficients shows that blood pressure measured as a binary variable has little influence on the increasing risk of coronary event associated with the amount smoked (i.e., $\hat{b} = 0.325$ and $\hat{b}' = 0.321$, adjusted). The lack of difference in these coefficients is, of course, reflected in the similarity of the estimates of the odds ratios (Table 7–20; last two lines). A formal test of trend is the usual Wald test of the coefficient b. A chi-square statistic for trend is, then, $X^2 = [\hat{b}/S_{\hat{b}}]^2$ and X^2 has a chi-square distribution with one degree of freedom when no trend exists ($H_0 : b = 0$).

Adjustment for the influence of any number of variables follows the same pattern. The impact of each variable is accounted for by the logistic model, and the coefficient for trend reflects the pattern of a series of adjusted odds ratios when corresponding risk variables are included in the model. More exactly, the model

$$\text{log-odds} = a + bF_i + cC + dD + \cdots \qquad (7.41)$$

yields an estimate of b adjusted for the influence of the other variables in the expression and produces an unconfounded description of the trend in risk associated with the variable represented by F_i.

Design variables add tremendous flexibility to an analytic model. In the context of investigating a dose/response pattern (a special type of trend analysis), the category with zero dose is sometimes treated separately. A design variable added to a regression model allows estimation of a dose/response relationship among those exposed separated from those unexposed. For example, estimates of trend in disease risk among workers exposed to ionizing radiation can be separated from those among individuals receiving no dose. This separation is easily accomplished using a logistic model with a design variable C and a quantitative dose variable F_i where

$$\text{log-odds} = a + bF_i + cC. \qquad (7.42)$$

The coffee and pancreatic cancer data in Table 6–1 provide an illustration; where again, the "dose" variable $F_i = 0, 1, 2,$ and 3 represents cups of coffee consumed each day and $C = 1$ for noncoffee drinkers, and $C = 0$ for coffee drinkers. Employing these two variables in the logistic model 7.42 allows the estimated dose response to be calculated for coffee drinkers only. The estimated coefficient measuring

Table 7–21. Trend in risk from coffee drinking with zero dose individuals separated

Variable	Term	Estimate	Std. Error	p-value	$\widehat{or}$
Constant	$\hat{a}$	1.269	0.376	—	—
Coffee	$\hat{b}$	0.042	0.109	0.703	1.042
No coffee	$\hat{c}$	−1.061	0.437	0.015	0.346

−2 Log Likelihood = 701.578; number of model parameters = 3.

trend is $\hat{b} = 0.042$ (Table 7–21) and reflects the response among coffee drinkers (exposed individuals), disregarding noncoffee drinkers. The data show no evidence of a relationship between the case status and the amount of coffee consumed among coffee drinkers (p-value = 0.703).

The estimated coefficient $\hat{c} = -1.061$ show evidence that the non-coffee drinkers are distinct from the coffee drinkers (p-value = 0.015). Parallel results were observed in Chapter 6 based on a chi-square approach. Incidentally, if an estimate for the trend is calculated including the noncoffee drinkers ($c = 0$) the estimate of b is quite different (i.e., $\hat{b}' = 0.097$), illustrating the importance of carefully considering the role of the unexposed individuals in an analysis of trend.

The Multi-Way Table

Any number of categorical variables can be used to form a contingency table. This section describes a logistic model employed to summarize relationships among three discrete risk variables and a disease outcome. Interest is again focused on defining the role of behavior type (2 levels) in the risk of a coronary event while accounting for the influences from smoking ($k = 4$ levels) and blood pressure (2 levels). As before, the blood pressure variable is defined as a binary variable based on systolic measurements (<140 and ≥ 140). These three risk variables produce the $2 \times 4 \times 4$ contingency table of WCGS data in Table 7–22. These data, in a slightly different format, are given at the beginning of the chapter (Table 7–1).

The 16 parameters of the saturated model can be estimated from the data in Table 2–22. The likelihood statistic serves as a point of comparison for reduced models. The likelihood statistic is the minimum possible since a saturated model produces a goodness-of-fit measure at its minumum. For the WCGS data, this minimum is likelihood statistic = $L_1 = 1,667.136$ with 16 degrees of freedom.

Table 7–22. CHD by smoking by A/B by blood pressure

	Type-A and Blood Pressure ≥ 140				
Cigs/Day	0	1–20	21–30	≥ 30	Total
CHD	29	21	7	12	69
No CHD	155	76	45	43	319
Total	184	97	52	55	388

	Type-A and Blood Pressure < 140				
Cigs/Day	0	1–20	21–30	≥ 30	Total
CHD	41	24	27	17	109
No CHD	599	277	140	116	1,092
Total	600	301	167	133	1,201

	Type-B and Blood Pressure ≥ 140				
Cigs/Day	0	1–20	21–30	≥ 30	Total
CHD	8	9	3	7	27
No CHD	171	62	31	14	278
Total	179	71	34	21	305

	Type-B and Blood Pressure < 140				
Cigs/Day	0	1–20	21–30	≥ 30	Total
CHD	20	16	13	3	52
No CHD	669	320	139	80	1,208
Total	689	336	152	83	1,260

A basic question to be addressed is: To what extent can the 16-parameter saturated model be simplified and still maintain a faithful but simpler representation of the relationships among the four variables (A/B, smoking, blood pressure, and CHD)? A "minimum" model that accounts for influences from the three risk factors involves four parameters, no interaction among the risk factors, and smoking exposure constrained to produce the same linear response in CHD risk for the four levels of the other two risk variables. This four-parameter logistic model is

$$\text{log-odds} = a + bF_i + cC + dD, \tag{7.43}$$

where F_i is one of the four coded levels of smoking (again, $F_i = 0, 1,$ 2, and 3), $C = 0$ or 1 indicates the behavior type (B, A) and $D = 0$ or

Table 7–23. CHD by A/B by smoking by blood pressure (no interaction and constrained)

Variable	Term	Estimate	Std. Error	p-value	$\widehat{or}$
Constant	$\hat{a}$	−3.365	0.136	—	—
Smoking	$\hat{b}$	0.286	0.060	<0.001	1.331
A/B	$\hat{c}$	0.769	0.142	<0.001	2.157
Blood Pressure	$\hat{d}$	0.779	0.139	<0.001	2.179

−2 Log Likelihood = 1,688.422; number of model parameters = 4.

1 indicates the level of blood pressure (<140, ≥ 140). The estimates of the four parameters for this model are given in Table 7–23. This reduced model produces a likelihood statistic of $L_0 = 1,688.422$.

Geometrically the model represents the data as four parallel straight lines on a log-odds scale (one for each of four blood pressure/behavior type categories), each describing the same linear increase in CHD risk from increased smoking levels. The distance between these lines measures the differing influences of blood pressure and behavior type on the risk of a coronary event. The four parallel lines along with the data (saturated model) are shown in Figure 7–7.

The utility of this four-parameter model compared to the saturated model can be evaluated by contrasting likelihood statistics (reduced versus saturated; $L_0 - L_1 = 1,688.422 - 1,667.138 = 21.284$ with 12 degree of producing a p-value = 0.046). This much simpler statistical structure is not an extremely accurate reflection of the relationships among the risk factors and the log-odds associated with a coronary event. The increase in the likelihood statistic illustrates the typical trade-off between lack of fit and simplicity of the model—simpler models fit less well. Although the simpler model is not ideal, it gives an approximate measure of the magnitude of the influences of the three risk factors on CHD as if they had independent effects, producing Table 7–24.

The odds ratios in Table 7–24 are derived from combinations of the parameter estimates $\hat{b}$, $\hat{c}$, and $\hat{d}$ using the relationship

$$\widehat{or} = e^{\hat{b}F_i + \hat{c}C + \hat{d}D} = (1.331)^{F_i}(2.157)^C(2.179)^D, \qquad (7.44)$$

and expresses the risk associated with the 15 different levels of the risk factors relative to the baseline category (nonsmokers, type-B with blood pressure <140—or $= 1$). Note that the highest risk is about 11 times the baseline when each factor has a separate (multiplicative) influence on the odds ratio. Type-A individuals with blood pressure

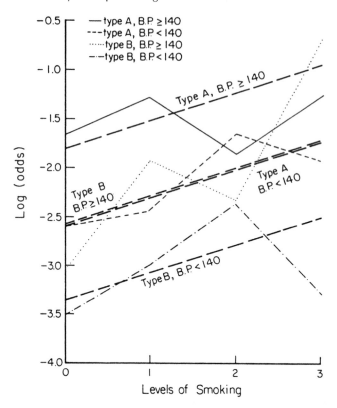

Figure 7–7. Log-odds associated with CHD risk by systolic blood pressure (<140 and ≥140), by amount smoked and by behavior type (constrained and additive model).

<140 have about the same influence of risk as type-B individuals with blood pressure ≥140, which is expected since the logistic model coefficients $\hat{c}$ and $\hat{d}$ are about equal. Table 7–24 addresses the questions suggested by the analogous table presented at the beginning of the chapter (Table 7–1) using the three estimated parameters and a logistic model.

Table 7–24. CHD by A/B by systolic blood pressure: odds ratios

Blood Pressure	Behavior Type	$F = 0$	$F = 1$	$F = 2$	$F = 3$
≥140	A	4.702	6.259	8.331	11.090
≥140	B	2.179	2.901	3.861	5.140
<140	A	2.158	2.872	3.823	5.089
<140	B	1.000	1.331	1.772	2.358

Goodness-of-Fit: Discrete Case

For contingency table data, the goodness-of-fit of a logistic model can be expressed in typical fashion by generating a series of expected values based on the model $(\hat{n}_k)$ and comparing these values to the observed counts (n_k) using a chi-square statistic. The expected value in each cell in the table results from a combination of model parameters. These parameters generate a logistic probability that produces exactly the frequency of CHD events expected under the model when multiplied by a marginal frequency. The data on blood pressure (2 levels), behavior type (2 levels), and smoking exposure (4 levels) produce the following 32 $(k = 1, 2, \ldots, 32)$ expected frequencies based on the four-parameter logistic model (Table 7–25 using [expression (7.43)]. The logistic probabilities are estimated using

$$\hat{p}_{\text{disease}} = \frac{1}{1 + e^{-(\text{log-odds})}} = \frac{1}{1 + e^{-(\hat{a} + \hat{b}F_i + \hat{c}C + \hat{d}D)}}$$

$$= \frac{1}{1 + e^{-(-3.365 + 0.286F_i + 0.769C + 0.779D)}} \tag{7.45}$$

and $\hat{n}_k$ is either $n\hat{p}_{\text{disease}}$ individuals with CHD events or $n\,(1 - \hat{p}_{\text{disease}})$ individuals with no occurrences of CHD where n is the total number of individuals in a category, combining the diseased and nondiseased individuals. For example, $\hat{n}_4 = n\hat{p}_{\text{disease}} = (n_D + n_{\bar{D}})\hat{p}_{\text{disease}} = 55(0.277) = 15.239$ is the number of expected CHD events and $\hat{n}_8 = 55 - 15.239 = 39.761$ is the number of expected individuals without CHD among $n = 55$ study subjects who are type-A individuals with blood pressures greater than or equal to 140 and who smoke more than 30 cigarettes per day. The corresponding observed values are $n_4 = 12$ and $n_8 = 43$. The remaining expected and observed values are similarly calculated. A chi-square goodness-of-fit statistic (the sum of the last column) yields $X^2 = 22.126$ (12 degrees of freedom) and a p-value of 0.036. The four-parameter model, as seen in Table 7–25 (columns 8 or 9), is a reasonable representation of the data for most cells. Only a few categories are seriously misrepresented by the additive, constrained logistic model $(\hat{p}_{\text{disease}})$. The similarity between the classic chi-square approach and the comparison of the likelihood statistics is typical (22.126 versus 21.284 both with degrees of freedom of 12). The two methods are likely to be similar for large sample sizes and usually do not substantially differ even when applied to moderately small data sets.

Table 7–25. Goodness-of-fit—various summaries

Outcome	Type	B.P.	F_i	n_k	$\hat{n}_k$	$n_k - \hat{n}_k$	$\dfrac{n_k - \hat{n}_k}{\hat{n}_k^{1/2}}$	$(n_k - \hat{n}_k)^2 / \hat{n}_k$
CHD	A	≥ 140	0	29	25.722	3.278	0.646	0.418
CHD	A	≥ 140	1	21	17.251	3.749	0.903	0.815
CHD	A	≥ 140	2	7	11.625	−4.625	−1.357	1.840
CHD	A	≥ 140	3	12	15.239	−3.239	−0.830	0.689
No CHD	A	≥ 140	0	155	158.278	−3.278	−0.261	0.068
No CHD	A	≥ 140	1	76	79.749	−3.749	−0.420	0.176
No CHD	A	≥ 140	2	45	40.375	−4.625	0.728	0.530
No CHD	A	≥ 140	3	43	39.761	3.239	0.514	0.264
CHD	A	< 140	0	41	42.027	−1.027	−0.158	0.025
CHD	A	< 140	1	24	27.428	−3.428	−0.655	0.428
CHD	A	< 140	2	27	19.663	7.337	1.655	2.738
CHD	A	< 140	3	17	20.062	−3.062	−0.684	0.467
No CHD	A	< 140	0	559	557.973	1.027	0.043	0.002
No CHD	A	< 140	1	277	273.572	3.428	0.207	0.043
No CHD	A	< 140	2	140	147.337	−7.337	−0.604	0.365
No CHD	A	< 140	3	116	112.938	3.062	0.288	0.083
CHD	B	≥ 140	0	8	12.422	−4.422	−1.255	1.574
CHD	B	≥ 140	1	9	6.411	2.589	1.023	1.046
CHD	B	≥ 140	2	3	3.968	−0.968	−0.486	0.236
CHD	B	≥ 140	3	7	3.141	3.859	2.177	4.741
No CHD	B	≥ 140	0	171	166.578	4.422	0.343	0.117
No CHD	B	≥ 140	1	62	64.589	−2.589	−0.322	0.104
No CHD	B	≥ 140	2	31	30.032	0.968	0.177	0.031
No CHD	B	≥ 140	3	14	17.859	−3.859	−0.913	0.834
CHD	B	< 140	0	20	23.018	−3.018	−0.629	0.396
CHD	B	< 140	1	16	14.778	1.222	0.318	0.101
CHD	B	< 140	2	13	8.771	4.229	1.428	2.039
CHD	B	< 140	3	3	6.256	−3.256	−1.302	1.694
No CHD	B	< 140	0	669	665.982	3.018	0.117	0.014
No CHD	B	< 140	1	320	321.222	−1.222	−0.068	0.005
No CHD	B	< 140	2	139	143.229	−4.229	−0.353	0.125
No CHD	B	< 140	3	80	76.744	3.256	0.372	0.138
Total	—	—	—	3154	3154	0.0	0.0	22.126

SUMMARIZING A SERIES OF TWO × TWO TABLES

As already noted, one way to deal with the counfounding influence of a variable is to stratify the data into a series of more or less homogeneous groups based on values of the confounding variable (discussed in Chapter 2 and again in Chapter 9). This process can produce a series of 2 × 2 tables (one table per stratum). For example, a series of strata formed on the basis of age might each contain individuals classified by the presence or absence of a coronary event as well as behavior type (A or B). To combine properly information from a series of 2×2 tables, three issues are important:

1. Interaction: Is the association between risk factor and disease the same for all tables (strata)?
2. Association: If the association is the same, is it substantial? (not likely a result of random variation)
3. Estimation: If the association is the same and it is not likely random, then what is the magnitude of the risk/disease association?

These issues have been traditionally addressed without using a multivariable statistical model. Ways to begin to answer these questions are briefly reviewed in the following sections, and, additionally, the parallel multivariate logistic model approach is presented.

Test of Homogeneity

A single summary of the relationship within a series of 2×2 tables only makes sense when the relationship summarized is the same for all tables (no interaction). In terms of an odds ratio, if a series of 2×2 tables reflects the same degree of association between risk factor and disease outcome (random fluctuations from a common overall value), then a single summary odds ratio serves as an accurate measure of that association. A method by Woolf [6] is one way to assess homogeneity among a series of odds ratios. The null hypothesis conjectures that the odds ratio estimates calculated from each of k tables differ only because of random variation

$$H_0: or_1 = or_2 = \cdots or_k = or,$$

where or_i is the odds ratio associated with the ith specific 2×2 table. To develop a test statistic to evaluate this hypothesis, instead of the odds ratios themselves, the logarithms of the odds ratios are used since the transformation produces estimates with approximately normal distributions (see Appendix C). The estimate of the odds ratio from each table ($\widehat{or}_i$) can have several forms (again see Appendix C). Here the odds ratio is estimated by

$$\widehat{or}_i = \frac{(a_i + \frac{1}{2})(d_i + \frac{1}{2})}{(b_i + \frac{1}{2})(c_i + \frac{1}{2})}. \tag{7.46}$$

A summary odds ratio ($\widehat{or}_W$) derived from a weighted average of the logarithms of the stratum-specific odds ratios ($\widehat{or}_i$), is

$$\widehat{\log(or_W)} = \frac{\sum\limits_{i=1}^{k} w_i \log(\widehat{or}_i)}{\sum\limits_{i=1}^{k} w_i} \quad \text{and} \quad \widehat{or}_W = e^{\widehat{\log(or_W)}} \tag{7.47}$$

(W for Woolf, who first presented the estimate) with the weights w_i given by

$$w_i = \frac{1}{\text{variance}\,[\log(\widehat{or}_i)]} = \left(\frac{1}{a_i + \frac{1}{2}} + \frac{1}{b_i + \frac{1}{2}} + \frac{1}{c_i + \frac{1}{2}} + \frac{1}{d_i + \frac{1}{2}}\right)^{-1}. \quad (7.48)$$

The intuitive rationale for these weights is that reliable estimates (small variance) should have relatively large weight and unreliable estimates (large variance) should have relatively small weight in determining the overall summary value.

The question of whether the individual odds ratios (or_i) systematically differ from the overall odds ratio (or) is addressed by the Woolf test for homogeneity using the chi-square test statistic

$$X_W^2 = \sum_{i=1}^{k} w_i[\log(\widehat{or}_i) - \widehat{\log(or_W)}]^2. \quad (7.49)$$

The test statistic X_W^2 has an approximate chi-square distribution with $k - 1$ degrees of freedom when the 2×2 tables are homogeneous with respect to the odds ratios (H_0 is true). Large chi-square values indicate that the odds ratios are not likely to be the same in all or some of the k strata.

The WCGS data once again illustrate. Table 7–26 shows study participants divided into five age groups to examine the relationship between behavior type and CHD. These data consist of five separate 2×2 tables, which generate an odds ratio measure of association between behavior type and CHD for each strata (Table 2–27—column 2). Using the example data, $\widehat{\log(or_W)} = 0.773$ ($\widehat{or}_W = e^{0.773} = 2.166$) and

$$X_W^2 = 6.966(0.695 - 0.773)^2 + \cdots + 6.811(1.023 - 0.773)^2 = 0.773. \quad (7.50)$$

Table 7–26. WCGS: age by behavior type by CHD

	Type-A		Type-B		
	CHD	No CHD	CHD	No CHD	Total
Age	a_i	b_i	c_i	d_i	n_i
≥ 40	20	241	11	271	543
40–44	34	462	21	574	1,091
45–49	49	337	21	343	750
50–54	38	209	17	184	448
≥ 55	37	162	9	114	322
Total	178	1,411	79	1,486	3,154

Table 7–27. WCGS: odds ratios by age

Age	$\widehat{or}_i$	$\log(\widehat{or}_i)$	variance $[\log(\widehat{or}_i)]$	w_i
<40	2.004	0.695	0.144	6.966
40–45	1.993	0.690	0.079	12.594
45–49	2.343	0.852	0.073	13.776
50–54	1.937	0.661	0.093	10.717
≥55	2.781	1.023	0.147	6.811
Total	2.373	0.864	—	—

The test of homogeneity ($X_W^2 = 0.773$ with four degrees of freedom; p-value $= 0.942$) shows no reason to believe that the odds ratios differ among the five age categories—no evidence of an interaction.

Test of Association

A second step in summarizing a series of k separate 2×2 tables is to assess the association between the risk factor and disease, using the data from all k tables. One such test is called the Mantel–Haenszel chi-square test [7] (William Cochran suggested a similar test in an earlier paper [8]). The approach argues that the cell frequencies in each 2×2 table can be estimated from the marginal frequencies if the risk factor and disease are independent (null hypothesis). That is, for each stratum the observed value a_i should equal $\hat{A}_i$, except for random variation, where $\hat{A}_i$ is calculated under the hypothesis of independence and, as before [expression (5.20) or (6.2)], the estimated cell frequency is

$$\hat{A}_i = \frac{(a_i + c_i)(a_i + b_i)}{n_i}. \tag{7.51}$$

The variance of a_i is estimated by

$$\text{variance }(a_i) = \frac{(a_i + b_i)(a_i + c_i)(b_i + d_i)(c_i + d_i)}{n_i^2(n_i - 1)}. \tag{7.52}$$

The Mental–Haenszel chi-square test statistic compares $\sum a_i$ with $\sum \hat{A}_i$ and is

$$X_{MH}^2 = \frac{\left(\sum\limits_{i=1}^{k} a_i - \sum\limits_{i=1}^{k} \hat{A}_i\right)^2}{\sum\limits_{i=1}^{k} \text{variance }(a_i)} \tag{7.53}$$

(MH for Mantel–Haenszel, see Appendix D).

The Mantel–Haenszel chi-square statistic combines information from each table resulting in a test statistic that measures the overall association between risk factor and disease outcome as long as the odds ratios are homogeneous (no interaction). The value X^2_{MH} has an approximate chi-square distribution with one degree of freedom when risk factor and disease are unrelated in all k strata. Continuing the WCGS example, since $\sum a_i = 178$ and $\sum \hat{A}_i = 134.684$, then $X^2_{MH} = (178 - 134.684)^2/57.444 = 32.663$ (p-value < 0.001), producing strong evidence that behavior type and CHD are associated within each of the five age strata.

Estimation of a Common Odds Ratio

The third step in summarizing a series of 2×2 tables is to estimate the common measure of association. A popular estimate that provides an overall measure of association is the Mantel–Haenszel summary odds ratio [7] given by

$$\widehat{or}_{MH} = \frac{\displaystyle\sum_{i=1}^{k} \frac{a_i d_i}{n_i}}{\displaystyle\sum_{i=1}^{k} \frac{b_i c_i}{n_i}}. \tag{7.54}$$

When a series of odds ratios is homogeneous, then $\widehat{or}_{MH}$ estimates the common value. For the age and behavior type data, the Mantel–Haenszel summary odds ratio is

$$\widehat{or}_{MH} = \frac{\dfrac{(20)(271)}{543} + \cdots + \dfrac{(37)(114)}{322}}{\dfrac{(241)(11)}{543} + \cdots + \dfrac{(162)(9)}{322}} = 2.214. \tag{7.55}$$

The estimated odds ratio 2.214 summarizes, using information from each age stratum ("adjusted for the influence of age"), the risk of CHD associated with the two behavior types. The Woolf summary odds ratio $\widehat{or}_W = 2.166$ [expression (7.47)] is also an estimate of the odds ratio common to the k separate 2×2 tables.

> Aside: The Mantel–Haenszel estimate combines a series of ratios into a single summary estimate. A summary ratio is usually constructed from a weighted average of each of a series of k ratios where
>
> $$\text{mean ratio} = \bar{r} = \frac{\sum w_i \dfrac{y_i}{x_i}}{\sum w_i},$$

The choice of the weights w_i determines the properties of the resulting summary ratio.

The simplest choice of weights is $w_i = 1.0$, giving

$$\text{mean ratio} = \bar{r} = \frac{1}{k} \sum \frac{y_i}{x_i},$$

where k ratios are averaged to form a single estimate. A more sophisticated estimate is based on the weights $w_i = x_i$. That is, the "worth" of each ratio is proportional to the value x_i giving

$$\text{mean ratio} = \bar{r} = \frac{\sum y_i}{\sum x_i}.$$

This form is a common way ratios are combined from k sources of data.

If the weights are chosen so the $w_i = x_i^2$, then

$$\text{mean ratio} = \bar{r} = \frac{\sum x_i y_i}{\sum x_i^2}$$

which is an estimate of the slope of a straight line (least squares estimate) through the origin.

The weights that yield the Mantel–Haenszel estimate of the odds ratio are $w_i = b_i c_i / n_i$ from each of the k individual 2×2 tables since

$$\text{mean ratio} = \widehat{or}_{MH} = \frac{\sum w_i \widehat{or}_i}{\sum w_i} = \frac{\sum \dfrac{b_i c_i}{n_i} \dfrac{a_i d_i}{b_i c_i}}{\sum \dfrac{b_i c_i}{n_i}} = \frac{\sum \dfrac{a_i d_i}{n_i}}{\sum \dfrac{b_i c_i}{n_i}}.$$

This choice of weights produces an efficient and useful summary estimate of the odds ratio. Other choices are possible and have other properties. For example, Woolf's estimate [expression (7.47)] is also a weighted mean of a series of ratios each from k individual 2×2 tables.

Logistic Regression Approach

The Woolf test for interaction, the Mantel–Haenszel test for association, and the Mantel–Haenszel summary odds ratio have analogous measures derived from a logistic regression approach. In most situations, the results are similar from these rather different approaches.

Four basic logistic models relating CHD outcome to the risk factors age and behavior type (Table 7–26) are:

1. Model (saturated):

$$\text{log-odds} = a + b_1 x_1 + b_2 x_2 + b_3 x_3 + b_4 x_4 + cC + d_1 C x_1 + d_2 C x_2$$
$$+ d_3 C x_3 + d_4 C x_4.$$

The variable C represents type-A (when $C = 1$) and type-B (when $C = 0$) behavior; x_1, x_2, x_3, and x_4 represent design variables to account for the five age categories. The likelihood statistic associated with this saturated ten-parameter model is $L_1 = -2$ Log Likelihood $= 1,702.156$. Three relevant reduced models and parameter estimates follow:

2. Additive model (behavior type and age—no interaction):

$$\text{log-odds} = a + b_1x_1 + b_2x_2 + b_3x_3 + b_4x_4 + cC$$

Variable	Term	Estimate	Std. Error	p-value	$\widehat{or}$
Constant	$\hat{a}$	-2.461	0.192	—	—
Age	$\hat{b}_1$	-0.112	0.232	0.629	0.894
Age	$\hat{b}_2$	0.510	0.225	0.023	1.665
Age	$\hat{b}_3$	0.793	0.236	<0.001	2.211
Age	$\hat{b}_4$	0.921	0.246	<0.001	2.512
A/B	$\hat{c}$	0.793	0.141	<0.001	2.210

$L_2 = -2$ Log Likelihood $= 1,703.010$; number of model parameters $= 6$.

3. Model (age only):

$$\text{log-odds} = a + b_1x_1 + b_2x_2 + b_3x_3 + b_4x_4$$

Variable	Term	Estimate	Std. Error	p-value	$\widehat{or}$
Constant	$\hat{a}$	-2.894	0.192	—	—
Age	$\hat{b}_1$	-0.132	0.231	0.569	0.877
Age	$\hat{b}_2$	0.531	0.224	0.018	1.700
Age	$\hat{b}_3$	0.838	0.234	<0.001	2.311
Age	$\hat{b}_4$	1.013	0.246	<0.001	2.753

$L_3 = -2$ Log Likelihood $= 1,736.578$; number of model parameters $= 5$.

4. Model (behavior type only):

$$\text{log-odds} = a + cC$$

Variable	Term	Estimate	Std. Error	p-value	$\widehat{or}$
Constant	$\hat{a}$	-2.934	0.115	—	—
A/B	$\hat{c}$	0.864	0.140	<0.001	2.373

$L_4 = -2$ Log Likelihood $= 1,740.344$; number of model parameters $= 2$.

Summary results from applying these four models to the WCGS data are shown in Table 7–28.

To test for possible interaction effects (different odds ratios among

Table 7–28. Comparison of models

Model	L_i	Log Likelihood	$\hat{c}$	Std. Error	$\widehat{or}$	Parameters
A/B + age + interactions	L_1	1,702.156	0.715	0.386	2.045	10
A/B + age	L_2	1,703.010	0.793	0.141	2.210	6
Age only	L_3	1,736.578	—	—	—	5
A/B only	L_4	1,740.344	0.864	0.140	2.373	2

some or all of the five age categories), likelihood statistics from two models are contrasted. The likelihood statistic calculated from the saturated model $(L_1 = 1,702.156)$ is compared to the likelihood statistic from the model with the interaction terms ignored $(L_2 = 1,703.010)$ producing a difference of $L_2 = L_1 = 0.854$, which measures the lack of homogeneity among the five odds ratios. The contrast of the fit of the logistic models shows no evidence of an interaction (p-value = 0.931). This result is similar to the Woolf homogeneity chi-square value and these two approaches are likely to be similar in general, particularly where each stratum contains a moderate or a large number of observations.

A Mantel–Haenszel-like test of the association between behavior type and CHD can also be conducted in the context of a logistic model. The difference between the model containing the risk factors behavior type and age (model 2) and the model containing only age (model 3) measures the degree of association between behavior type and CHD outcome while accounting for the influence of age. These models produce a difference in likelihood statistics analogous to the test statistic X^2_{MH}. The difference $L_3 - L_2$ has a chi-square distribution with one degree of freedom when the risk variable is unrelated to the outcome. Both the Mantel–Haenszel chi-square and the logistic model approaches require that no interactions exist among the k tables. For the age/behavior type data, $L_3 - L_2 = 1,736.578 - 1,703.010 = 33.568$ (p-value < 0.001), which is not very different from the value X^2_{MH} calculated to assess the same association. Like the tests of the interaction effects, these two tests of association will usually be similar.

Last, when a series of 2×2 tables shows no interaction, the strictly additive logistic model (model 2) produces an estimate of the strength of the behavior/disease association unbiased by any confounding influences from age. For the WCGS data, $\hat{c}$ is 0.793 and the estimated odds ratio is $\widehat{or} = e^{0.793} = 2.210$, which is almost identical to $\widehat{or}_{MH} = 2.214$. Both estimates are a measure of the relative role of A/B behavior type in determining the risk of CHD adjusted for the influence of age.

The logistic model odds ratio estimate from the additive model and the Mantel–Haenszel summary odds ratio estimate will usually be similar. Note that both estimates require homogeneity of the odds ratios (no interactions) among the k tables to summarize usefully the behavior-type/CHD association. The maximum likelihood estimate $\widehat{or} = e^{\hat{c}}$ from the additive logistic model is very slightly more efficient (smaller variance) than $\widehat{or}_{MH}$. A summary comparing the nonmodel and logistic approaches is given in Table 7–29.

Table 7–29. Two approaches for summarizing k separate 2×2 tables

	No Model	Logistic Model
Homogeneity	$X_W^2 = 0.773$	$X^2 = 0.854$
Association	$X_{MH}^2 = 32.663$	$X^2 = 35.568$
Odds ratio	$\widehat{or}_{MH} = 2.214$	$\widehat{or} = 2.210$

8 The Analysis of Binary Data: Logistic Model II

Three basic features of the logistic regression model are: the appropriateness of binary outcome variables, estimation of adjusted odds ratios, and the effective analysis of both continuous and discrete risk factors. This chapter focuses on the last property. The logistic model capitalizes on the actual measurements to attain the maximum amount of information from a measured risk factor, whether the variable is discrete or continuous. There is no need to distribute continuous data into a series of sometimes arbitrary categories. A logistic model allows analysis of risk factors measured in their original units, producing a less arbitrary and more powerful analysis.

Simple Logistic Regression

The logistic model, as before, is based on either the log-odds of disease or the probability of disease. The log-odds is required to be a linear function of the risk factor magnitude or

$$\text{log-odds} = l_x = a + bx$$

and, necessarily,

$$p_x = \frac{1}{1 + e^{-l_x}} = \frac{1}{1 + e^{-(a+bx)}}, \tag{8.1}$$

where l_x represents the logarithm of the odds of disease occurrence for a specific value x of the risk factor. The coefficient b measures the change (additive) in risk of disease associated with a one unit change in the risk factor on the log-odds scale; e^b measures the change (multiplicative) in the risk of disease associated with a one unit change in the risk factor on the odds scale. Expression (8.1) is functionally the same as the model used in the purely discrete case [expression (7.1)], but when the risk factor represented by x is a continuous variable, the application and interpretation of the logistic model takes on a somewhat different character.

To illustrate logistic regression using a binary disease outcome and a single continuous risk factor, a person's body weight (x) is assessed as a risk factor for coronary heart disease. Computer estimates (maximum likelihood estimates) of the logistic parameters a and b from the $n = 3,154$ WCGS participants are given in Table 8–1. The estimated models relating body weight and the risk of a coronary event are then

$$\hat{l}_x = -4.215 + 0.0104x \quad \text{or} \quad \hat{p}_x = \frac{1}{1 + e^{-(4.215 + 0.0104x)}}, \quad (8.2)$$

where $\hat{p}_x$ is the estimated probability of a CHD event from a level x of a risk factor based on parameter estimates $\hat{a} = -4.215$ and $\hat{b} = 0.0104$.

For example, the estimated log-odds associated with a CHD event for a 200-pound man $(x = 200)$ participating in the WCGS is $\hat{l}_{200} = -2.135$ based on the linear log-odds form of the logistic model. The estimated probability of a CHD event is $\hat{p}_{200} = (1 + e^{2.135})^{-1} = 0.106$ based on the estimated logistic model [expression (8.2)]. This probability refers to about 7.5 years of WCGS data collection and represents about 14.1 cases per 1,000 persons over one year (a more typical unit of time).

The importance of the variable x in influencing the probability of disease can be statistically evaluated in the usual way, using the estimated standard error $(S_{\hat{b}})$ of the estimated coefficient $\hat{b}$. That is, the Wald test statistic

$$X^2 = \left(\frac{\hat{b}}{S_{\hat{b}}}\right)^2 = \left(\frac{0.0104}{0.003}\right)^2 = 12.018 \quad (8.3)$$

has an approximate chi-square distribution with one degree of freedom when the risk factor is unrelated to the disease. The variance estimate $S_{\hat{b}}^2$ is typically a by-product of the maximum likelihood estimation process. Formally, this chi-square statistic provides a test of the null hypothesis that the coefficient represented by b is zero (i.e., $H_0: b = 0$). The logistic regression coefficient $\hat{b} = 0.0104$ shows clear evidence of

Table 8–1. Logistic regression: CHD by weight

Variable	Term	Estimate	Std. Error	p-value	$o\hat{r}$
Constant	$\hat{a}$	−4.215	0.512	—	—
Weight	$\hat{b}$	0.0104	0.003	<0.001	1.010

−2 Log Likelihood = 1,768.938; number of model parameters = 2.

an association (p-value < 0.001) between body weight and the probability of a coronary event.

The odds ratio associated with the risk factor ($e^{b} = \widehat{or}$) measures the increase in odds for a one unit change in the risk factor. For the weight/CHD example (Table 8–1), $\hat{b} = 0.0104$ and the estimated odds ratio is then $\widehat{or} = e^{0.0104} = 1.0104$. At first glance it might be concluded that this odds ratio is essentially 1.0 and not biologically meaningful, but it is important to keep in mind that the coefficient measures risk in the units associated with the risk factor (in the WCGS case, pounds). The odds ratio e^{b} reflects the multiplicative increase in risk for a one unit change in the risk factor or, in terms of the illustrative data, a one pound gain of weight multiplies the odds of coronary disease by a factor of 1.0104. For example, if a person gains 20 pounds in weight, the risk of a coronary event increases $20\hat{b}$ on the log-odds scale and increases the odds of a CHD event by a factor of $e^{20\hat{b}} = (1.0104)^{20} = 1.231$. In general, a t unit increase in the risk factor from level x_0 to level $x_1 = x_0 + t$ produces a change in the odds to $\text{odds}_1 = \text{odds}_0 (e^{b})^{t}$ making the odds ratio for an increase of t units $\text{odds}_1/\text{odds}_0 = e^{bt}$.

An important property of the simple logistic model is seen at this point. The change in risk of disease associated with an increase in a risk factor is the same regardless of the level of the risk factor. A 300-pound man multiplies his risk by a factor of 1.231 for a 20-pound gain in weight as does a 150-pound man. The fact that the log-odds is a linear function of the risk variable is a mathematical property of the simple logistic model and may or may not be biologically reasonable. More complicated logistic models can be formulated to reflect nonlinear relationships. For the risk factor weight, it is perhaps more realistic to postulate that a gain of 20 pounds would increase the risk for a 300-pound man less than the risk for a 150-pound man. Such a logistic model is easily created, and an example of a nonlinear logistic model is presented [expression (8.14)].

An approximate 95% confidence interval for the regression coefficient ($\hat{b} \pm 1.96 S_{\hat{b}}$) is almost always helpful in evaluating the strength of an association. Based on the estimate $\hat{b} = 0.0104$, the confidence interval for b is $(0.005, 0.016)$. The approximate 95% confidence interval for the odds ratio is then $(e^{\text{lower}}, e^{\text{upper}}) = (1.005, 1.016)$. For a gain of 20 pounds, similarly, the 95% confidence interval for the odds ratio is $(e^{20[\hat{b} \pm 1.96 S_{\hat{b}}]}) = (1.095, 1.385)$ based on the estimated odds ratio $\widehat{or} = e^{20\hat{b}} = 1.231$.

The analysis of weight and CHD risk illustrates another point that is generally true for a logistic model applied to human disease data. The range of the logistic probabilities is rather restricted and almost

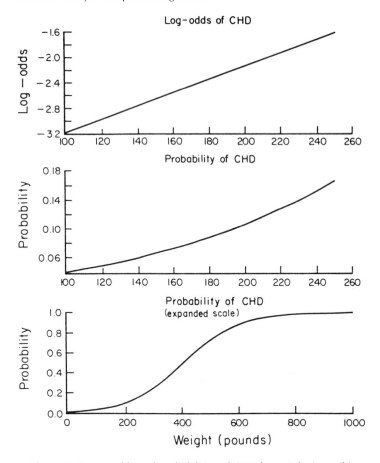

Figure 8–1. Log-odds and probabilities of CHD by weight (pounds)

linear. For example, if $x = 100$ pounds, then $p_x = 0.040$, if $x = 150$, then $p_x = 0.066$, and if $x = 200$ pounds, then $p_x = 0.106$ showing the rate of increase in the probability of disease over this range as more or less linear (see Figure 8–1). A probability of disease greater than 0.1 is not likely for most epidemiologic data since low-frequency diseases are usually studied and the associated risk factors do not strongly influence the frequency.

A related and traditional approach to assessing observed differences between two groups is a *t*-test. In terms of body weight and its influence on CHD, the mean weight of individuals who developed coronary heart disease can be compared with those who did not. The relevant data are given in Table 8–2.

The difference of a little less than 5 pounds in mean weight between these two groups is small in biological terms but is not likely produced

Table 8–2. Example t-test: Weight by CHD

	Sample Size	Mean	Standard Error
CHD	257	174.463	21.010
No CHD	2897	169.554	21.574
Difference	—	4.909	1.401

t statistic $= 3.503$; p-value < 0.001.

by sampling variation (p-value < 0.001). The logistic regression approach and the two-sample procedure show essentially the same strength of association between body weight and CHD ($t = 3.503$ from the t-test and $z = \sqrt{12.018} = 3.467$ from the logistic analysis). The basic difference is that the t-test requires the values represented by x be normally distributed, where the logistic approach requires the log-odds to have a linear relationship with the risk factor x. The logistic model, however, is a more sophisticated structure based on postulating a specific relationship between risk factor and disease. The simple logistic model is naturally extended to include any number of risk factors.

The Bivariate Logistic Regression

The single risk factor model is readily modified to include a second risk factor. A logistic model in terms of log-odds of disease including a value of x of one risk factor and a value of y for the other risk factor is

$$\text{log-odds} = a + bx + cy. \tag{8.4}$$

To illustrate this bivariate model where x and y represent risk variables with independent effects, the variable x represents the age of an individual, the variable y represents the number of cigarettes smoked by that individual, and again, the occurrence or nonoccurrence of CHD among the 3,154 WCGS participants is the disease outcome. The number of cigarettes smoked is not a strictly continuous variable and is recorded with considerable digit preference (Figure 8–2). Since neither property affects the use of smoking exposure in a logistic model, the analysis is based directly on reported number of cigarettes smoked. Estimates for the bivariate model parameters where $x = $ age (years) and $y = $ number of cigarettes smoked per day (as reported) are given in Table 8–3.

As shown in Figure 8–3 (top, left), this logistic model defines the relationship between smoking and the risk of disease by straight lines

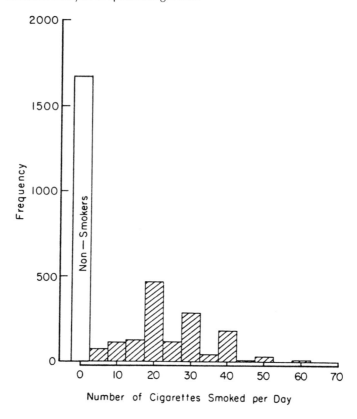

Figure 8–2. Histogram of the frequency of cigarettes smoked (cigarettes per day)

Table 8–3. CHD by smoking and age—no interaction model

Variable	Term	Estimate	Std. Error	p-value	$\widehat{or}$
Constant	$\hat{a}$	−6.360	0.563	—	—
Age	$\hat{b}$	0.0764	0.011	<0.001	1.079
Smoking	$\hat{c}$	0.0239	0.004	<0.001	1.024

−2 Loglikelihood = 1,705.860; number of model parameters = 3.

with slope $\hat{c}$. The influence of age is to increase the overall level of risk by an amount $\hat{b}x$. The lines in Figure 8–3 show the increase in the risk of disease from smoking for the individuals ages $x = 40$, $x = 50$, and $x = 60$. These lines are parallel since the model dictates a linear influence of smoking with the same slope (c) for each value of age (no interaction).

The question immediately arises as to whether the additive model is an adequate representation of the relationship between age, smoking,

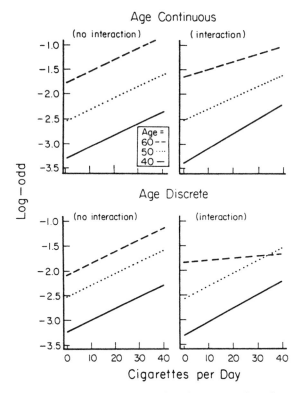

Figure 8–3. Four logistics models describing the relationship of smoking exposure to the risk of CHD for 40, 50, and 60 years of age

and CHD risk. To explore the possibility of an interaction between two continuous risk factors, an interaction model is postulated. Such a model, again in terms of log-odds, is

$$\text{log-odds} = a + bx + cy + dxy. \tag{8.5}$$

The coefficient d measures the influence of any interaction effects. If d is inconsequential, then the interaction term can be ignored and the additive model provides a potentially useful summary of the data. A statistical test of the coefficient d presents no new issues; Wald's statistic $X^2 = (\hat{d}/\hat{S}_d)^2$ has an approximate chi-square distribution with one degree of freedom when no interaction exists (i.e., H_0: $d = 0$). It is reasonable to delete the interaction term (set $d = 0$) from the model when its influence cannot be differentiated clearly from chance variation (p-value > 0.20, say). The parameter estimates for the interaction model [expression (8.5)] from the WCGS smoking and age data are given in Table 8–4.

Table 8–4. CHD by smoking and age—interaction

Variable	Term	Estimate	Std. Error	p-value	$\widehat{or}$
Constant	$\hat{a}$	−6.884	0.776	—	—
Age	$\hat{b}$	0.0872	0.016	<0.001	1.091
Smoking	$\hat{c}$	0.0580	0.035	0.093	1.060
Interaction	$\hat{d}$	−0.0071	0.007	0.310	0.999

−2 Loglikelihood = 1,704.878; number of model parameters = 4.

Figure 8–3 also shows the interaction model (top, right) where the risk from smoking increases at a different rate depending on the subject's age. Again, age $x = 40$, $x = 50$, and $x = 60$ are displayed. The magnitude of the interaction influence measured by $\hat{d}$ is evaluated by $X^2 = (-0.0071/0.007)^2 = 1.029$ producing a p-value of 0.310.

An analogous statistical test compares the likelihood statistics generated by the two models (additive versus interaction). That is, the model including the interaction term yields a likelihood statistic of $L_1 = 1,704.878$, and when the possibility of an interaction is excluded ($d = 0$), the likelihood statistic increases to $L_0 = 1,705.860$. The difference has an approximate chi-square distribution with one degree of freedom ($L_0 - L_1 = 1,705.860 - 1,704.878 = 0.982$ and the p-value is 0.322) when $d = 0$. The similarity of the two tests of $d = 0$ is expected, particularly for data sets with a large number of observations.

Instead of treating age as a continuous variable, age can be divided into three categories (set at 35–44, 45–54, and ≥ 55 years) to illustrate the logistic model with both continuous (smoking) and categorical (age) risk variables. The three age categories are identified by two binary variables, x_1 and x_2. These two design variables indicate three unordered age strata, and the additive logistic model is

$$\text{log-odds} = a + b_1 x_1 + b_2 x_2 + cy. \tag{8.6}$$

Note that $x_1 = 0$ and $x_2 = 0$ indicate the age stratum 35 to 44 years, which serves as baseline for comparisons; $x_1 = 1$ and $x_2 = 0$, the age stratum 45 to 54 years, and $x_1 = 0$ and $x_2 = 1$, the age stratum ≥ 55 years. The estimates of the four model parameters are given in Table 8–5.

The interaction model is a bit more complicated but not different in principle from the previous interaction models and is given by

$$\text{log-odds} = a + b_1 x_1 + b_2 x_2 + cy + d_1 x_1 y + d_2 x_2 y. \tag{8.7}$$

The WCGS data produce the six estimated parameters for the interaction model given in Table 8–6.

Table 8–5. CHD by smoking and age (discrete)—no interaction

Variable	Term	Estimate	Std. Error	p-value	$\widehat{or}$
Constant	$\hat{a}$	− 3.245	0.137	—	—
Age 45–54	$\hat{b}_1$	0.708	0.150	<0.001	2.029
Age ≥ 55	$\hat{b}_2$	1.153	0.201	<0.001	3.168
Smoking	$\hat{c}$	0.0235	0.002	<0.001	1.024

−2 Loglikelihood = 1,710.557; number of model parameters = 4.

Table 8–6. CHD by smoking and age (discrete)—interaction

Variable	Term	Estimate	Std. Error	p-value	$\widehat{or}$
Constant	$\hat{a}$	− 3.319	0.175	—	—
Age 45–54	$\hat{b}_1$	0.735	0.218	<0.001	2.087
Age ≥ 55	$\hat{b}_2$	1.469	0.268	<0.001	4.346
Smoking	$\hat{c}$	0.027	0.003	<0.001	1.029
Interaction	$\hat{d}_1$	− 0.00162	0.009	0.860	0.998
Interaction	$\hat{d}_2$	− 0.0228	0.013	0.080	0.978

−2 Loglikelihood = 1,706.868; number of model parameters = 6.

Comparison of the two likelihood statistics ($L_0 = 1,710.557$ and $L_1 = 1,706.868$ gives $L_0 - L_1 = X^2 = 3.689$ with $6 - 4 = 2$ degrees of freedom, yielding a p-value $= 0.158$) shows no persuasive evidence, but perhaps an indication of an interaction between smoking and age with regard to coronary heart disease when age is treated as an unordered categorical variable.

Categorizing age into three somewhat arbitrary groups causes some loss of statistical efficiency and requires a more complicated model. Additionally, categorizing continuous data influences the analytic results (e.g., $\hat{c}_{\text{discrete}} = 0.027$, Table 8–6 and $\hat{c}_{\text{continuous}} = 0.058$, Table 8–4), emphasizing the importance of the definition and measurement of risk variables in general. Figure 8–3 (bottom) displays the results from the estimated logistic regression equations for both the additive (left) and the interaction (right) models for age (categorized) and smoking risk.

Conceptually the description and display of continuous relationships is not as easy as relationships that involve a small number of discrete classes. To make interpretation simpler, continuous variables are made often discrete (a topic in Chapter 2). For example, low birth weight is defined as an infant weighing less than 2,500 grams, and AIDS is defined as an HIV individual with two tests that show a T-cell count less than 200. Clearly, such categories are useful in many contexts but should not determine the statistical approach. An alternative is to analyze continuous data as measured and then form discrete categories based on the estimated analytic model to describe the results. For example, the logistic regression analysis (Table 8–3) yields the coefficients $\hat{b} = 0.0764$ for age and $\hat{c} = 0.0239$ for smoking exposure estimated from the data as measured. These coefficients relate the likelihood of a coronary event to the risk variables but not in a very intuitive or descriptive way. However, the estimated model makes it a simple task to estimate values for specific levels of the risk variables. The probability of a coronary event is estimated by

$$\text{probability of a CHD event} = \frac{1}{1 + e^{-(-6.360 + 0.0764x + 0.0239y)}}.$$

The estimated additive model [expression (8.4) and Table 8–3] allows a table, such as Table 8–7, to be constructed showing the important properties of the bivariate analysis. The relationship of age and smoking to the risk of CHD is simply expressed in terms of these estimated probabilities. For example, it is easy to see that the probability of a CHD event roughly doubles when a nonsmoker is compared to a person who smokes 30 cigarettes per day or the likelihood of a CHD event more than triples when age 50 is compared to age 70. The analysis as well as the statistical tests are based on the data as reported, so that the issues of cut-points and efficiency do not arise. The description of the analytic results, however, can be displayed in any creative way that helps in understanding the risk/disease relationships.

Interaction

A bivariate logistic regression analysis of the influence of body weight and cholesterol on the risk of coronary disease provides an opportunity to explore the consequences of an interaction. Employing both variables in their natural units [cholesterol (mg per 100 ml) = x and weight

Table 8–7. Probabilities of a coronary event estimated from the logistic bivariate regression model, where age and smoking are risk factors

Cigarettes/Day	$y = 0$	$y = 10$	$y = 20$	$y = 30$
x = age 50	0.073	0.091	0.113	0.139
x = age 60	0.145	0.177	0.215	0.258
x = age 70	0.267	0.316	0.370	0.427

Table 8–8. CHD by weight and cholesterol—interaction model

Variable	Term	Estimate	Std. Error	p-value	$\widehat{or}$
Constant	$\hat{a}$	-13.21	2.58	—	—
Cholesterol	$\hat{b}$	0.0373	0.010	<0.001	1.038
Weight	$\hat{c}$	0.0450	0.015	0.003	1.046
Interaction	$\hat{d}$	-0.000142	0.000058	0.014	0.999

-2 Loglikelihood $= 1,684.702$; number of model parameters $= 4$.

(pounds) $= y$] produces the parameter estimates for a bivariate logistic model [expression (8.5)] given in Table 8–8 where an interaction term is included.

Evaluation of the coefficient $\hat{d}$ ($z = 2.448$ and p-value $= 0.014$) yields no evidence to justify excluding a weight/cholesterol interaction term from the model. A similar result is achieved by comparing the respective likelihood statistics (i.e., $L_{d=0} - L_{d\neq0} = 1,690.221 - 1,684.702 = 5.519$, also note that $z^2 = (2.448)^2 = 5.992$). The estimated log-odds plots (Figure 8–4) and the plot of the estimated logistic functions (Figure 8–5) both show the modeled influence of the interaction effect. The lines representing risk associated with cholesterol for different weights are not parallel on the log-odds scale. If no interaction exists, then the increased risk of disease would be the same regardless of the individual's weight. Since weight and cholesterol interact, the risk from increase in cholesterol depends on weight. A 50% increase for a 190-pound individual increases, via the logistic model, the probability of a CHD event from 0.088 to 0.235, whereas the same cholesterol increase for a person weighing 250 pounds produces a smaller increase in CHD risk, from 0.174 to 0.205. The interaction between cholesterol and weight implies that, in the context of the logistic model, the risk to heavier individuals is less affected by increases in cholesterol levels.

In geometric terms, the slope of the line describing the increase in log-odds of disease with increasing values of cholesterol decreases in magnitude as weight increases (i.e., the slope associated with cholesterol risk is slope $= \hat{b} - \hat{d} \times$ weight $= 0.0373 - 0.000142 \times$ weight, see Figure 8–4). A direct consequence of an interaction is that the risk factor coefficients (linear effects; $\hat{b}$ and $\hat{c}$) in the logistic model no longer directly measure the isolated effects of the risk variables but reflect a more complex combination of influences. The influence of weight cannot be summarized without accounting for the levels of cholesterol and, similarly, cholesterol cannot be summarized without accounting for weight.

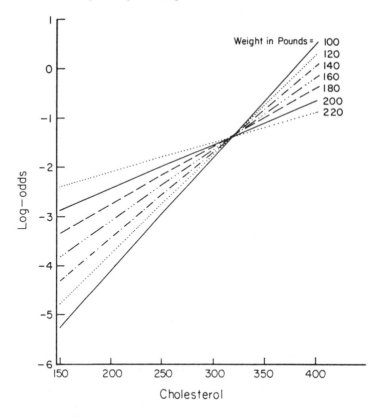

Figure 8–4. Log-odds measure of risk of CHD by levels of cholesterol for a series of selected weights based on estimated logistic parameters

A formal expression derived from the weight/cholesterol logistic model that defines the impact of an interaction on the calculation and interpretation of the odds ratio is

$$\widehat{or} = e^{(\hat{b} + \hat{d} \times \text{weight}) \times (\text{difference in cholesterol levels})}$$

or, specifically,

$$\widehat{or} = e^{(0.0373 - 0.000142 \times \text{weight}) \times (\text{difference in cholesterol levels})}, \tag{8.8}$$

where the odds ratio reflects the risk from differences in cholesterol levels compared for individuals with the same weight. Expression (8.8) shows that the odds ratio is related to the difference in cholesterol, as expected, but the magnitude of the odds ratio is also influenced by the value of *weight*. Therefore, an interpretation of $\widehat{or}$ is conditional on the weight of the individuals being compared. To be specific, $\widehat{or} = 4.950$ for two men weighing 150 pounds and $\widehat{or} = 2.435$ for two men weighing 200 pounds for the same 100 mg per 100 ml difference in their

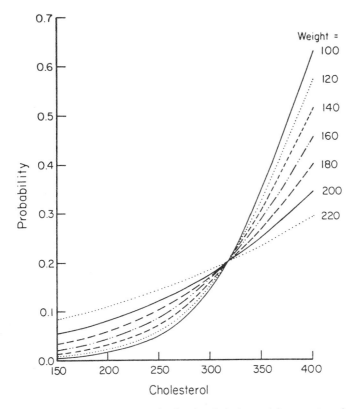

Figure 8–5. Probability of a CHD event by levels of cholesterol for a series of selected weights based on estimated logistic probabilities

cholesterol levels. Only when $d = 0.0$ (no interaction) are inferences concerning cholesterol "free" from influences of weight.

Logistic Regression Coefficients: General Considerations

A general additive multivariate logistic model (i.e., without interaction terms) is

$$\text{log-odds} = a + \sum_{i=1}^{k} b_i x_i \quad \text{and} \quad p_x = \frac{1}{1 + e^{-(\text{log-odds})}} \tag{8.9}$$

and the odds for two sets of x-values $(x_1, x_2, \ldots, x_k$ and $x'_1, x'_2, \ldots, x'_k)$ are

$$\frac{p_x}{1 - p_x} = e^{a + \sum b_i x_i} \quad \text{and} \quad \frac{p_{x'}}{1 - p_{x'}} = e^{a + \sum b_i x'_i}, \tag{8.10}$$

giving the associated odds ratio as

$$\text{odds-ratio} = \frac{p_x/(1-p_x)}{p_{x'}/(1-p_{x'})} = e^{\sum b_i(x_i - x_i')} = e^{b_1(x_1 - x_1')} e^{b_2(x_2 - x_2')} e^{b_3(x_3 - x_3')} \ldots e^{b_k(x_k - x_k')}.$$

(8.11)

If one risk variable in the set is increased by one unit while the other variables are unchanged ($x_i' = x_i + 1$ while for the other $k - 1$ variables $x_1 = x_1'$, $x_2 = x_2'$, ..., $x_k = x_k'$), then

$$\text{odds-ratio} = e^{b_i}.$$

(8.12)

That is, the coefficient b_i or odds ratio e^{b_i} expresses the influence of one unit difference in the variable x_i on the risk of disease while the other $k - 1$ variables are equal or held constant. In effect, the logistic model allows two hypothetical individuals or groups to be compared that differ with respect to one variable and have identical values for the other $k - 1$ risk factors when an additive model is used to represent the relationships among the measured variables. The odds ratio is, in this way, adjusted for the presence of the other risk factors. Like randomized data, the impact measured by the regression coefficient is attributable only to a specific variable since the influence of the other measured variables are "equalized" between the two groups or two individuals compared. Randomized data remain superior in the sense that randomization likely equalizes all confounding variables between compared groups; whereas a logistic model allows adjustment only for confounding influences from measured variables entered in the model and, of course, the adjustment depends on the validity (or, at least, the goodness-of-fit) of the additive model [expression (8.9)]. Nevertheless, the logistic model isolates the influence of a specific variable making it "free" of the confounding influences of the other variables in the analysis. The assessment of these independent effects is a basic objective of a linear logistic regression analysis.

"Centering"

Problems arise when highly correlated risk variables are used in a regression analysis. High correlation means that two variables have essentially indistinguishable influences on an outcome, making it difficult to produce accurate estimates of the regression coefficients associated with each variable. In other words, separation of the individual influences on the outcome by means of a regression coefficient becomes difficult (unreliable) when the two variables are themselves almost identical. This phenomenon is called collinearity, and the topic is discussed in detail in textbooks on regression analysis (e.g., [1]). Collinearity in the context of logistic regression and a method for potentially improving the precision of the estimated coefficients associated with nearly collinear variables is illustrated with the WCGS data.

The size of an individual is reflected by a body-mass index, defined as weight (kilograms) divided by a function of height (meters^2). The body-mass index $(q = kg/m^2)$ calculated from the WCGS data is potentially related to CHD risk. A simple linear regression model is

$$\text{log-odds} = a + bq, \tag{8.13}$$

which gives the parameter estimates in Table 8–9.

Clearly, the body-mass index is associated with CHD risk (p-value < 0.001). However, it is possible that for high values of body-mass index, risk increases more slowly than for low or intermediate values. One way to incorporate this nonlinearity into the analysis is to modify the simple logistic model by adding a quadratic term. The model becomes

$$\text{log-odds} = a + bq + cq^2. \tag{8.14}$$

Parenthetically, a quadratic term in a logistic equation describes a special type of interaction. The risk variable can be viewed as interacting with itself, which means that the level of risk associated with the outcome variable depends on the level of the risk factor itself. The estimated parameters of the quadratic model are given in Table 8–10.

Table 8–9. CHD by body-mass index

Variable	Term	Estimate	Std. Error	p-value	$\widehat{or}$
Constant	$\hat{a}$	−4.509	0.606	—	—
q	$\hat{b}$	0.085	0.0241	<0.001	1.088

−2 Loglikelihood = 1,769.426; number of model parameters = 2.

Table 8–10. CHD by body-mass index—quadratic term included

Variable	Term	Estimate	Std. Error	p-value	$\widehat{or}$
Constant	$\hat{a}$	−8.217	3.58	—	—
q	$\hat{b}$	0.373	0.276	0.177	1.452
q^2	$\hat{c}$	−0.0055	0.0053	0.295	0.995

−2 Loglikelihood = 1,768.227; number of model parameters = 3.

The addition of the quadratic term changes strikingly the results observed from the linear logistic model. The coefficient measuring the effects of the body-mass index on the risk of a CHD event increases from 0.085 to 0.373, and the precision, as reflected by the standard error, increases from 0.0241 to 0.276 (a more than ten-fold increase!). These changes are predominately due to the high correlation between q and q^2. The correlation is $r = 0.995$, and this high degree of correlation (nearly collinear) disrupts the estimation process.

If the body-mass index is simply transformed by subtracting the overall mean value from each observed value ($q_i - \bar{q}$, where $\bar{q} = $ mean $= 24.52$), the logistic analysis becomes considerably more reliable. This centered variable remains useful for estimating the risk/disease association when a quadratic term is added to the model. Two inconsequential changes occur. The constant term in the model is different, and the units of measurement are relative to the mean. The transformed risk values have mean zero, causing extreme individuals to have either positive or negative values. The logistic analysis using centered body-mass index values gives the parameter estimates in Table 8–11.

Note that the estimate of the influence of body mass on the risk of CHD is the same in both logistic analysis ($\hat{b} = 0.085$, with standard error $= 0.241$ for both the transformed and nontransformed risk variable, Tables 8–9 and 8–11). More important, the estimates (particularly the standard errors) are not highly affected when q^2 is added to the model using the centered variable. The estimates of the quadratic model parameters using the centered variable are given in Table 8–12.

Precision improves when the risk factors (body mass and body mass squared) are centered and no longer highly correlated ($r' = 0.359$). The estimated coefficient measuring the influence of body mass is $\hat{b} = 1.101$ with a standard error of 0.029, only slightly increased over the estimates from the additive model [expression (8.14)]. The reduction in correlation between risk factor variables (q and q^2) has the desired effect of producing an analysis hardly affected by highly

Table 8–11. CHD by body-mass index—centered

Variable	Term	Estimate	Std. Error	p-value	$\widehat{or}$
Constant	$\hat{a}$	−2.443	0.066	—	—
$(q - \bar{q})$	$\hat{b}$	0.085	0.0241	<0.001	1.089

−2 Loglikelihood = 1,769.212; number of model parameters = 2.

Table 8–12. CHD by body-mass index—centered with quadratic term included

Variable	Term	Estimate	Std. Error	p-value	$\widehat{or}$
Constant	$\hat{a}$	-2.412	0.072	—	—
$(q - \bar{q})$	$\hat{b}$	0.101	0.0293	<0.001	1.106
$(q - \bar{q})^2$	$\hat{c}$	-0.00545	0.0053	0.302	0.995

-2Loglikelihood $= 1,768.050$; number of model parameters $= 3$.

correlated risk variables. The small price for the improved estimate of b is the use of transformed measurements rather than natural units. Centering a risk variable can, but may not always, increase the precision of a variable used in a regression analysis.

Figure 8–6 shows the curves associated with both the linear (first row) and quadratic (second row) models relating body mass to CHD risk. The log-odds, odds ratio (relative to $\bar{q} = 24.52$), and the probability of a coronary event are shown in each column based on a logistic model. The differences in the shape of the curves associated with these two models shows the critical importance of selecting a model to describe appropriately the risk/disease relationship.

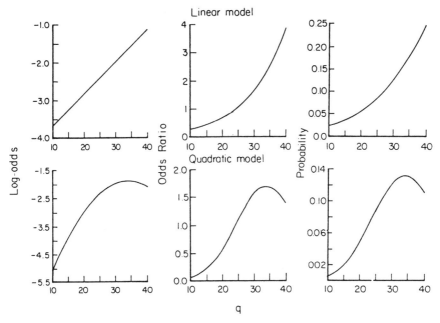

Figure 8–6. Two logistic models (linear and quadratic) showing the relationship of a body-mass index to the risk of CHD for three measures (log-odds, odds ratio, and probability) of association

The WCGS Additive Model

The additive model is the simplest description of the influence of a series of risk factors. All variables are entered into the analysis only as additive influences and the log-odds is expressed, as shown earlier, as

$$\text{log-odds} = a + \sum_{i=1}^{k} b_i x_i. \qquad (8.15)$$

For the WCGS data, eight risk factors ($k = 8$) employed in the additive model produce the nine estimated parameters (eight risk factor coefficients and a constant term) shown in Table 8–13.

Using all eight risk factors in a logistic analysis substantially improves the summary model (reduces the likelihood statistic) over the situation where no risk factors are considered. That is, $L_0 = 1{,}781.244$ when all eight risk factors are ignored, and $L_1 = 1{,}580.738$ when all risk factors are included. The reduction $L_0 - L_1 = 200.506$ (p-value < 0.001) is attributable to the inclusion of these eight risk factors in describing CHD. risk. The overall influence of all risk factors simultaneously entered into an analysis is rarely of interest. More important questions focus on the relative role of each risk factor in determining the probability of disease occurrence.

The relative impact of each variable is related to its corresponding coefficient in the logistic regression equation. However, direct comparison of the coefficients (b_i's) does not account for the fact that the variables are measured in different units. For example, age in the WCGS data is not four times more important than height in determining the risk of CHD, because the age coefficient is about four times larger ($b_1 = 0.0648$ versus $b_2 = 0.016$). Three common ways to measure the relative role of each variable in a logistic regression equation are:

Table 8–13. Full model—no interaction

Variable	Term	Estimate	Std. Error	p-value	$\widehat{or}$
Constant	$\hat{a}$	−13.55	2.32	—	—
Age	$\hat{b}_1$	0.0648	0.012	<0.001	1.067
Height	$\hat{b}_2$	0.0160	0.033	0.629	1.016
Weight	$\hat{b}_3$	0.00782	0.0038	0.044	1.008
Systolic bp	$\hat{b}_4$	0.0177	0.0064	0.005	1.018
Diastolic bp	$\hat{b}_5$	−0.0015	0.011	0.989	1.000
Cholesterol	$\hat{b}_6$	0.0111	0.0015	<0.001	1.011
Smoking	$\hat{b}_7$	0.0209	0.0043	<0.001	1.021
A/B	$\hat{b}_8$	0.653	0.145	<0.001	1.922

−2 Loglikelihood = 1,580.738; number of model parameters = 9.

the use of standardized coefficients (two methods) and the comparison of specific likelihood statistics. These methods allow the influence from variables measured in different units, such as age and height, to be directly compared.

Method 1

To make the regression coefficients commensurate (comparable units), they can be multiplied by the standard deviation of the associated variable (denoted by S_i). For example, a one-year increase in age results in an increase of 0.0648 in the log-odds of disease. Since the estimated standard deviation from the distribution of ages of WCGS participants is 5.524 (Table A–1 in Appendix A), the quantity $(0.0648)(5.524) \doteq 0.358$ is an estimate of the increase in the log-odds for a one standard deviation increase in age. Similarly, all values $\hat{b}_i S_i$ estimate the change in the log-odds of disease for a one standard deviation increase in the ith risk factor. These standardized coefficients have the same units (response in log-odds per standard deviation of the risk factor), producing comparable measures of response directly reflecting the role of each variable in the risk of disease. For example, comparing age and height, the standardized coefficients are 0.358 (age) and 0.040 (height)—age has about nine times more influence than height when measurement units are taken into account.

Method 2

When a specific variable is deleted from the logistic regression analysis (keeping the rest of the variables in the equation), the increase in the likelihood statistic based on $k - 1$ variables is attributable specifically to the influence of the deleted variable. This fact produces another technique to evaluate the role of each variable in a logistic equation. The difference between the likelihood statistic for the k-variable model (L_k) and the likelihood statistic for the model with the variable x_i excluded (L_{k-1}) measures the role of the removed variable. The difference $L_{k-1} - L_k$ directly measures the magnitude of the contribution of the variable x_i that is not reflected by the other variables in the logistic model. The unique contributions of each variable to the regression analysis provide a series of commensurate measures of each risk factor's relative influence on the probability of disease. Again, comparing age and height—28.552 (age) versus 0.234 (height).

Method 3

The third approach consists of dividing the regression coefficient $\hat{b}_i$ by its standard error. The quantity $\hat{b}_i/S_{\hat{b}_i}$ also measures the role of the risk factor x_i in the logistic model. Similar to the likelihood measure, these standardized values are unitless and produce commensurate measures of risk associated with each individual risk factor. One further note: standardizing a coefficient by its standard error and the difference between likelihood statistics are both related to a chi-square distribution (as already discussed). These two measures are not likely to substantially differ in a specific analysis, particularly when large sample sizes are involved. Table 8–14 illustrates the three methods applied to the WCGS data using the eight-variable additive logistic model.

The three approaches give essentially the same results. Cholesterol makes the strongest contribution to CHD risk, followed by roughly equal contributions from age, smoking, and behavior type. Weight and systolic blood pressure play lesser roles in the logistic equation, while the variables diastolic blood pressure and height have almost no independent influence on CHD risk.

Confounder Bias in the WCGS Data

The definition of confounding is essentially the same whether the analysis involves continuous or discrete variables (discussed previously in Chapters 2, 6, and 7). Confounder bias in the context of logistic regression is most naturally measured in terms of the changes in the estimated regression coefficients or the estimated odds ratios. The impact of confounding bias on the relationship between a specific variable (x_i) and the disease outcome is seen by the changes in the coefficient $(\hat{b}_i)$ caused by deleting one or more risk factors to an additive logistic model. This "before-after" comparison yields a

Table 8–14. Comparisons of three commensurate measures of impact on the risk of CHD

Variable	Coefficient	S_i	$\hat{b}_i S_i$	$L_7 - L_8$	$X^2 = (\hat{b}_i/S_{\hat{b}_i})^2$
Age	$\hat{b}_1$	5.524	0.358	28.522	29.160
Height	$\hat{b}_2$	2.529	0.040	0.234	0.235
Weight	$\hat{b}_3$	21.100	0.165	4.015	4.235
Systolic b.p.	$\hat{b}_4$	15.112	0.267	7.512	7.649
Diastolic b.p.	$\hat{b}_5$	9.727	−0.015	0.001	0.019
Cholesterol	$\hat{b}_6$	43.420	0.482	57.727	54.760
Smoking	$\hat{b}_7$	14.518	0.303	23.057	23.624
A/B	$\hat{b}_8$	0.500	0.327	21.226	20.281

measure of confounder bias $\hat{B}_i - \hat{b}_i$, where $\hat{B}_i$ is the estimated logistic coefficient when one or more confounding variables are eliminated from the model and $\hat{b}_i$ is the estimated logistic coefficient when the confounding variable or variables are included in the model. Implicit in assessing a confounding influence is the assumption that no inter-action exists among the variables considered.

The additive model applied to the WCGS data provides a look at the issue of confounder bias. Consider the behavior type variable. The estimate of the logistic regression coefficient associated with behavior type when no other risk factors are considered is 0.864. The confounder bias from the other seven variables (change in the value 0.864) is seen in Table 8–15, where the rows contain the estimated logistic regression coefficients for a series of models that include the variables given by the columns. The confounder bias influencing the A/B behavior type regression coefficient produces a range from 0.864 to 0.653 (column 1 of Table 8–15).

Confounder bias for a specific measure of association is a somewhat arbitrary quantity since its magnitude depends on both the variables included in the model and the order in which they are entered into the logistic equation. For example, if the cholesterol variable is added to the model first rather than sixth, the coefficient associated with behavior type changes from 0.864 to 0.819 (confounder bias = 0.045) rather than the observed change of 0.752 to 0.715 (confounder bias = 0.037).

The same table can be expressed in terms of the estimated adjusted odds ratios and the impact of confounding on this measure of the impact of behavior type on the probability of a CHD event is given in Table 8–16.

The WCGS example data illustrate that confounding bias is generally a function of the combined influences of all the risk factors entered

Table 8–15. Confounding and the A/B association with CHD risk

A/B	Age	Ht	Wt	SBP	DBP	Chol	Cigs
0.864	—	—	—	—	—	—	—
0.799	0.069	—	—	—	—	—	—
0.791	0.071	0.039	—	—	—	—	—
0.780	0.070	−0.013	0.012	—	—	—	—
0.751	0.062	0.008	0.007	0.020	—	—	—
0.752	0.062	0.006	0.007	0.022	−0.005	—	—
0.715	0.030	0.006	0.021	0.021	−0.006	0.012	—
0.653	0.065	0.016	0.008	0.018	−0.001	0.011	0.021

Table 8-16. Odds ratios: confounding and the A/B association with CHD

A/B	Age	Ht	Wt	SBP	DBP	Chol	Cigs
2.373	—	—	—	—	—	—	—
2.223	1.071	—	—	—	—	—	—
2.206	1.074	1.040	—	—	—	—	—
2.181	1.073	1.013	1.012	—	—	—	—
2.119	1.064	1.008	1.007	1.020	—	—	—
2.121	1.064	1.006	1.007	1.022	0.995	—	—
2.044	1.030	1.006	1.021	1.021	0.994	1.012	—
1.921	1.067	1.016	1.008	1.018	0.999	1.011	1.021

into the equation (confounder bias $= 0.653 - 0.864 = -0.211$). Extreme examples can be constructed such that two risk factors do not cause confounding bias when treated individually, but when they are considered together confounding occurs [2]. It is unlikely that this complete dependency on only a joint influence occurs in actual data. However, it is important to keep in mind that confounding bias is a function of all risk factors, and its magnitude cannot be inferred from analyses dealing with each variable separately (sometimes called the marginal analyses).

Goodness-of-Fit: Continuous Case

Assessing the fit of a logistic model when some or all of the risk factors are continuous is not straightforward. In the discrete case, an expected number based on the model is calculated and compared to the observed number for each category of data. In the continuous case, no natural categories exist leading to a variety of proposals for measures of "fit" [3]. A common approach involves forming somewhat arbitrary categories and applying a chi-square statistic much like the previously discussed discrete case (Chapter 7).

One strategy uses categories based on levels of risk estimated from the logistic model under investigation. Traditionally ten groups are formed, each containing approximately one-tenth of the data. The members of the first group are the subjects with the lowest probability of the event estimated by the logistic model, while the second group makes up the next 10% of the subjects with respect to risk and so forth until the tenth group consists of all individuals above the 90th percentile based on their estimated logistic risk probabilities. The percentile groups are sometimes called "deciles of risk." Once the groups are formed the average logistic probability per group is calculated. That is, the logistic probabilities for each one-tenth of the data are summed and divided by the number of members of that group or for the kth decile group the average probability is

$$\bar{p}_k = \frac{1}{n_k} \sum_{j=1}^{n_k} p_j, \tag{8.16}$$

where $n_k \approx n/10$, and n represents the total observed number of individuals. To be perfectly clear, the value p_j is the probability of disease based on the estimated logistic coefficients ($\hat{b}_i's$), the values of an individual's risk factors, and the logistic model, producing one estimate per study subject. The expected number of events in the kth group is then $\hat{e}_k = n_k \bar{p}_k = \sum p_j$. Also for each of the ten groups the observed number of events is recorded, symbolized by o_k. A similar expected number of nonevents can be calculated ($n_k - \hat{e}_k$) and compared to the observed number ($n_k - o_k$) in each decile. The pairs of observed and expected counts generated for each decile of risk are compared (20 pairs) with the usual chi-square statistic or, in symbols,

$$X^2 = \sum \frac{(\text{observed} - \text{expected})^2}{\text{expected}} \tag{8.17}$$

and, specifically,

$$X^2 = \sum_{i=1}^{10} \frac{(o_i - \hat{e}_i)^2}{\hat{e}_i} + \sum_{i=1}^{10} \frac{([n_i - o_i] - [n_i - \hat{e}_i])^2}{n_i - \hat{e}_i} = \sum_{i=1}^{10} \frac{(o_i - \hat{e}_i)^2}{n_i \bar{p}_i (1 - \bar{p}_i)}. \tag{8.18}$$

The test statistic X^2 has an approximate chi-square distribution with eight degrees of freedom when the logistic model is "correct."

Once again the WCGS data serves as an example. The eight-parameter, additive model (Table 8–13) produces the components for assessing the fit shown in Table 8–17.

Table 8–17. Fit of the additive logistic model to the WCGS data

	CHD			No CHD		
k	$\bar{p}_k$	o_k	$\hat{e}_k$	$n_k - o_k$	$n_k - \hat{e}_k$	n_k
1	0.0155	1	4.898	315	311.102	316
2	0.0252	5	7.938	310	307.062	315
3	0.0343	14	10.805	301	304.196	315
4	0.0444	9	13.986	306	301.014	315
5	0.0564	17	17.766	298	297.234	315
6	0.0708	17	22.302	298	292.698	315
7	0.0886	24	27.909	291	287.091	315
8	0.1154	43	36.351	272	278.649	315
9	0.1568	48	49.392	267	265.608	315
10	0.2800	79	89.040	239	228.960	318
Summary	0.0890	257	280.706	2,897	2,873.294	3,154

Each row in the table describes a "decile of risk" for the 3,154 subjects. For example, the observed number of coronary events in the fourth decile is $o_k = 9$ among the 315 individuals in that group, and the expected value based on the additive logistic model is $\hat{e}_4 = n_4 \hat{p}_4 = 315(0.0444) = 13.986$. The corresponding values for the individuals who did not experience a coronary event are $315 - 9 = 306$ and $315 - 13.986 = 301.014$, respectively. The summary chi-square statistic for this percentile-type grouping strategy is $X^2 = 12.090$ (degrees of freedom = 8) producing a p-value of 0.147, showing no strong evidence of a lack of fit of the additive model. The degrees of freedom are derived from rather complicated considerations but remain equal to eight whenever ten categories are used.

When a linear regression analysis is used, the squared multiple correlation coefficient (regression sum of squares divided by the total sum of squares) is a common and useful summary of the goodness-of-fit. A parallel concept for a logistic analysis is called a pseudo R-squared value based in likelihood statistics. The pseudo R-squared value is defined as

$$\text{pseudo } R\text{-squared} = R_L^2 = \frac{L_0 - L_k}{L_0 - L_s},$$

where L represents a specific likelihood statistic. The likelihood statistics L are defined as follows: L_0 is the likelihood statistic from the model containing only a constant term, L_k is the likelihood statistic from the model containing k risk variables, and L_s is the likelihood statistic from the saturated model. The likelihood statistic from the saturated model is not simply calculated except when no two observations have the same value of the risk factors, and the number of parameters in the model equals the number of observations, then $L_s = 0$. For most large samples of continuous data, L_s is usually close to zero (i.e., as a first-order approximation $L_s \approx 0$). For the WCGS data, $L_0 = 1,779.200$, for the model containing eight terms (Table 8–12), $L_8 = 1,580.738$ and $L_s = 0$ giving

$$R_L^2 = \frac{1,779.200 - 1,580.738}{1,779.200} = 0.112.$$

The value R_L^2 appears on computer output from logistic regression analysis programs and is sometimes thought to play the same role as the squared multiple correlation coefficient in a linear regression analysis. However, the quantity R_L^2 is not a measure of goodness-of-fit. It is a combination of likelihood statistics producing a number between 0 and 1 rather than a comparison of values estimated from a specific model to observed values.

Case/Control Sampling

The odds ratio measure of association is central to much of epidemiologic analyses. One reason for the reliance on this measure is its usefulness in describing associations for a variety of sampling patterns (e.g., cohort, cross-sectional, and case/control data).

Cohort sampling produces two groups of a predetermined number of individuals, one exposed and one not exposed to a risk factor. Subsequent numbers of cases of disease are then recorded for each group. Such cohort data is represented in Table 8–18. The odds ratio is estimated by ad/bc. The number of exposed n_1 and the number of unexposed n_2 individuals are determined by the investigator. The ratio a/b estimates the odds of disease associated with the exposed group and c/d estimates the odds of disease associated with the unexposed group. The estimated odds ratio is, then,

$$\widehat{or} = \frac{a/b}{c/d} = \frac{ad}{bc}. \tag{8.19}$$

The ratios a/c and b/d are influenced by the sample sizes n_1 and n_2 and have no importance as measures of association.

Case/control sampling also produces two groups, but the number of cases (diseased individuals) and controls (nondiseased individuals) are determined by the investigator. For example, 100 cases (n_1 cases) of prostatic cancer could be collected in a specific hospital and 200 noncancer cases (n_2 controls) sampled from the same hospital population to make up a case/control sample of 300 individuals. The number of individuals exposed to a risk factor is ascertained for each group. Such case/control data is represented in Table 8–19. The odds ratio is also

Table 8–18. Data collected by exposure

	Disease	No Disease	Total
Exposed	a	b	n_1
Not exposed	c	d	n_2

Table 8–19. Data collected by disease

	Disease	No Disease
Exposed	a	b
Not exposed	c	d
Total	n_1	n_2

estimated by the quantity ad/bc but for different reasons. Here the odds of being exposed to the risk factor among the cases are estimated by a/c, and the odds of being exposed among the controls are estimated by b/d. However, the odds ratio remains

$$\widehat{or} = \frac{a/c}{b/d} = \frac{ad}{bc}. \tag{8.20}$$

The ratios a/b and c/d have relatively little meaning since they are influenced largely by the numbers of cases and controls selected.

The fact that the odds ratio is the same for both cohort and case/control sampling patterns suggests that the coefficients in a simple logistic regression analysis will also be the same for both types of data.

The following demonstrates that, for a simple logistic regression analysis, case/control sampling produces the same assessment of risk as the analysis of cohort or cross-sectional data. Consider the simple logistic equation where p_x represents the probability of the disease for a specific value of a variable represented as x or, as before,

$$p_x = \frac{1}{1 + e^{-(a+bx)}} \quad \text{and, therefore,} \quad \log\left(\frac{p_x}{1 - p_x}\right) = a + bx. \tag{8.21}$$

Let $s_1 = P(\text{sampled}|\text{case})$ and $s_0 = P(\text{sampled}|\text{control})$. Recall that Bayes's theorem (slightly complicated by the presence of event C) applied to arbitrary events denoted A, B, and C states

$$P(A|BC) = \frac{P(B|AC)P(AC)}{P(BC)}, \tag{8.22}$$

then, specifically

$$P(\text{disease}|x \text{ and sampled}) = \frac{s_1 p_x}{s_1 p_x + s_0(1 - p_x)}, \tag{8.23}$$

where $A = $ disease, $B = $ sampled, and $C = $ value of the variable x. The log-odds is

$$\text{log-odds} = \log\left(\frac{P(\text{disease}|x \text{ and sampled})}{P(\text{no disease}|x \text{ and sampled})}\right), \tag{8.24}$$

and it follows that

$$\text{log-odds} = \log\left(\frac{s_1 p_x/[s_1 p_x + s_0(1 - p_x)]}{s_0(1 - p_x)/[s_1 p_x + s_0(1 - p_x)]}\right) = \log\left(\frac{s_1}{s_0}\frac{p_x}{1 - p_x}\right)$$

$$= A + \log\left(\frac{p_x}{1 - p_x}\right) \tag{8.25}$$

giving

$$\text{log-odds} = A + a + bx = a' + bx. \tag{8.26}$$

Expression (8.26) shows that the coefficient b is not influenced by the case/control sampling. The coefficient b, as before, indicates the change in risk of the disease measured in log-odds for a one unit change in x for either cohort or case/control sampling. Only the constant term in the logistic model (a) is affected by the sampling process.

Similarly, regression coefficients from a multiple logistic analysis produce the same results for cohort and case/control sampling of data. Only the constant term is affected by the sampling pattern. The constant term has no useful interpretation since it is made up of an unknown mixture of two elements (the probabilities s_0 and s_1 as well as the frequency of the disease in the sampled population). However, the constant term in the logistic model does not play an important role and can be ignored in the study of a series of risk factors. Therefore, the properties of a logistic regression apply equally to case/control data, adding flexibility to this analytic technique and, more important, providing a powerful tool for investigating rare diseases. Texts are completely devoted to the analysis of case/control data (e.g., [4] and [5]).

9 The Analysis of Matched Data

A statistical model is a principal tool used to adjust the relationship between risk factor and outcome for the influence of confounding variables (e.g., Chapter 2). An alternative strategy to control the influence of a confounding variable is to collect data in a matched pattern. By "matched," it is meant that the observations are collected in sets so that each set is as similar as possible with respect to a confounding variable or several confounding variables. Therefore, any observed differences within the matched set cannot be attributed to confounding since the confounding variable is essentially constant within each set. Another reason to collect data in a matched design is to increase the precision of the analytic methods used to explore the data. These two goals (removing bias and increasing precision) are the essence of a matched pattern of data collection.

Matching strategies bring balance to a data set and thus increase estimation precision. For example, matching primarily increases the precision of a statistical analysis in a controlled trial with randomization, where confounding is not an issue (Chapter 2). Matching is also used in epidemiologic cohort and case-control studies where both confounding and precision are issues. The principle of matching to remove confounding influences, on the surface, appears simple. However, a number of complications arise and the process of drawing inferences from matched sets of observations is often surprisingly complicated. Particularly for case-control data, the analytic approach to eliminate confounding bias is not intuitive and requires specialized analytic methods to produce accurate inferences.

The following definitions describe four types of sampling patterns and serve as a starting point for studying the analysis of matched data:

Frequency matching: Sampling a predetermined proportion of cases at random and selecting controls in such a way as to guarantee the same number of control observations per category of a predetermined variable or variables.

Stratified sample: Sampling a predetermined number of cases and a predetermined number of controls at random within each of a series of categories.

Post-stratification: Classifying the sampled observations into a series of categories based on the values of a variable or variables observed as part of the study—stratification after selecting the sample.

Matching: Selecting a case at random and finding a corresponding control or controls so that the observations within a set are as similar as possible for a predetermined variable or variables—special case of frequency matching.

These definitions applied to a sample collected to study birth defects over an entire state serve as an illustration where the county of birth (a potential confounder) is a consideration in the sampling strategy. A frequency matched sample would consist of selecting 10% of the birth defects (cases) at random and then selecting a matching number of normal births from each county as controls so that each county has the same number of cases and controls. A stratified sample consists of collecting 200 newborn infants with birth defects and 200 normal births from each county. A post-stratification sampling strategy involves collecting a sample of 2,000 births from the entire state, sorting these data into county groups, and comparing infants with and without birth defects within counties. A matched sample is created by selecting 1,000 infants with birth defects at random and then selecting a normal birth corresponding to each case from the same county to form a matched pair.

These definitions are the basis of different matched data collection strategies. The corresponding analytic approaches are described with particular emphasis on matched pairs. The first third of this chapter deals with matched analysis of a continuous outcome variable. The second third of the chapter describes matching in terms of tables and chi-square analyses of categorical variables. The last part describes the logistic model used to analyze both discrete and continuous data collected in a matched pattern. In the simplest situations these two methods (chi-square and logistic regression) do not differ but, as before, a model approach allows large numbers of risk factors as well as continuous risk variables to be efficiently analyzed.

Sampling Example

A frequency matched pattern of collecting case/control data does not completely remove bias from a confounding variable. Confounding from a variable can be reduced by stratification or removed using a statistical model, but confounder bias remains in directly analyzed case/control data. The following hypothetical data illustrate:

Hypothetical Population

C	D	$\bar{D}$	Total		$\bar{C}$	D	$\bar{D}$	Total
F	60	59,940	60,000		F	20	39,980	40,000
$\bar{F}$	20	39,980	40,000		$\bar{F}$	15	59,985	60,000
Total	80	99,920	100,000		Total	35	99,965	100,000

Two-hundred thousand individuals divided into two subpopulations defined by the variable C form a hypothetical population. The probability of disease among those with the risk factor F is $P(\text{disease}\,|\,C \text{ and } F) = 60/60,000 = 0.001$ when the variable C is present and $P(\text{disease}\,|\,\bar{C} \text{ and } F) = 20/40,000 = 0.0005$ when the variable C is absent. Additionally, the proportion with the risk factor among those individuals with variable C is $P(F\,|\,C) = 0.6$ and among those individuals without variable C is $P(F\,|\,\bar{C}) = 0.4$. The odds ratio measuring the association between risk factor F and disease D is 2.0 in both subpopulations (i.e., no noticeable interaction). The odds ratios calculated for each of the subpopulations (C present and C absent) as well as the population ignoring the variable C are:

$$or_{FD|C} = 2.00, \quad or_{FD|\bar{C}} = 2.00, \quad \text{and} \quad or_{FD} = 2.29.$$

The difference in the proportions with the risk factor F in the two subpopulations, as well as the association between variable C and disease, cause confounding associated with the variable C (i.e., $or_{FD} \neq or_{FD|C}$ and $or_{FD} \neq or_{FD|\bar{C}}$).

A frequency matched cohort study created by sampling one person out of ten from this hypothetical population gives the following idealized "data":

Cohort Sample

C	D	$\bar{D}$	Total		$\bar{C}$	D	$\bar{D}$	Total
F	6	5,994	6,000		F	2	3,998	4,000
$\bar{F}$	3	5,997	6,000		$\bar{F}$	1	3,999	4,000
Total	9	11,991	12,000		Total	3	7,997	8,000

A specific proportion (0.1) of individuals is selected from a hypothetical population with the factor (F) for both confounder present (C) and confounder absent $(\bar{C})$, and a matching number without the factor $(\bar{F})$ are also selected. The odds ratios calculated for each of the subtables (C present and C absent) as well as the table ignoring the confounding variable C are:

$$\widehat{or}_{FD|C} = 2.00, \quad \widehat{or}_{FD|\bar{C}} = 2.00, \quad \text{and} \quad \widehat{or}_{FD} = 2.00.$$

A frequency matched pattern of data collection removes the confounding bias present in the population, allowing an unbiased estimate of the odds ratio ignoring the variable C (i.e., the estimation of or_{FD} is unaffected by the variable C). Note that $\widehat{or}_{FC} = 1.0$, which is a property of a frequency matched cohort sample in general. However, cohort studies are frequently expensive, time-consuming, and require the disease to be at least moderately frequent [1].

Construction of a frequency matched case/control study from this hypothetical population gives the following idealized "data":

Case/Control Sample

C	D	$\bar{D}$	Total		$\bar{C}$	D	$\bar{D}$	Total
F	60	48	108		F	20	14	34
$\bar{F}$	20	32	52		$\bar{F}$	15	21	36
Total	80	80	160		Total	35	35	70

Once the cases (D) are selected, then corresponding controls are selected $(\bar{D})$ for both levels of the confounding variable. The risk/disease odds ratios calculated for each of the subtables (C present and C absent) as well as the table ignoring the confounder C are:

$$\widehat{or}_{FD|C} = 2.00, \quad \widehat{or}_{FD|\bar{C}} = 2.00, \quad \text{and} \quad \widehat{or}_{FD} = 1.95.$$

This example shows a slight bias in the odds ratio towards 1.0 associated with collecting the data in a frequency matched case/control pattern. The odds ratio is 1.95 instead of the 2.0 which is the population odds ratio. A bias between a risk factor and an outcome will exist unless the risk factor is equally distributed between the two subtables, $P(F|C) = P(F|\bar{C})$, or the odds ratio measuring the association between risk factor and disease is 1.0. In most cases, the bias associated with case/control sampling is not large. Nevertheless, case/control data is best analyzed with an approach that compensates for this inherent bias.

This example brings up an important question: If frequency matching does not completely control for confounding bias in a case-control design, what is the principal reason for pursuing this sample selection strategy? One answer is statistical precision.

Balancing a set of observations to improve precision is optimal for comparing two samples with a t-test (described in Chapter 2). The variance of the difference between two mean values is smallest (maximizing the power) when the sample sizes selected from each group are equal ($n_1 = n_2$, where $n = n_1 + n_2$ observations are available for study), when the variances for compared populations are the same. This principle applied to the estimate of an odds ratio. For example, when $or = 1$, the variance of an odds ratio is smallest when $n/2$ cases are compared to $n/2$ controls [2]. A general demonstration that balance increases precision is complex, and even special cases are rather complicated. The following example should lead to an intuitive understanding of why balanced data produce more precise estimates.

When an age-stratified series of diseased individuals is compared to a series of controls (nondiseased individuals), groups of older individuals are likely to have a larger number of cases than the controls. The opposite is true of the younger age groups, where larger numbers of controls and fewer cases of disease are likely. Unbalanced groups lead to increased variance of statistical estimates calculated from the combined data. A matched strategy guarantees that the same number of cases and controls occur in each group so that imbalance does not occur. Pair matching is the extreme case. In this instance, every pair constitutes a group containing two individuals regardless of the level of a confounding variable. If age is the matching variable, then a case who is 80 years old is matched to a control who is close to 80 years old, and a case who is 20 years old is matched to a control close to 20 years old, regardless of the scarcity of the case or control individuals. Balance is a basic feature of a matched pattern of data collection and produces an increased precision for summary statistics based on information from a series of groups.

Stratification/Post-Stratification

A common way to control the disruptive influence of confounding is to stratify the data by the confounding variable. Such strata restrict the range of any confounding variable. When the range of a confounding variable is restricted, the impact on the variable being studied is minimized. Estimates can be made within each stratum and combined to give an overall summary that is minimally influenced by the confounding variable. For example, the mean difference in blood pressures might be calculated for each of a series of five-year age intervals for black and white coronary patients. If the data are not classified into a series of age categories, differences in age between white and black samples will affect the observed differences in blood pressure. When the data are stratified by age, the difference between the means within each age category is not highly affected by age, since age only spans five years. The members of each group are about the same age. The estimated mean differences within each age category can then be combined to form an overall estimate of the racial differences in blood pressure essentially "free" from the confounding influence of age.

A simple illustration shows the reduction in bias from stratifying a variable into a series of groups. Consider a variable influenced by a confounding variable in the comparision of two groups (Figure 9–1). Estimates of the mean difference between these two groups, based on stratifying the outcome variable (y) into various numbers of strata (k), are given in the Table 9–1.

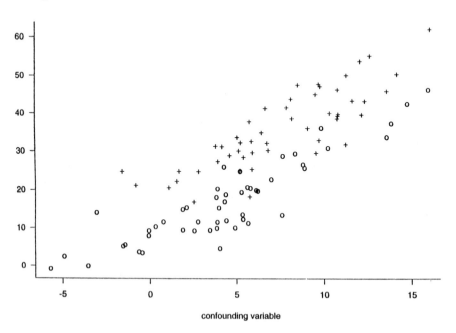

Figure 9–1. Hypothetical data illustrating the influence of a confounding variable on a measured response

Table 9–1. Illustration of the influence of differing numbers of strata (k) in reducing bias from a confounding variable

k = Groups	$\bar{y}_2 - \bar{y}_1$	Reduction	Percentage Decrease*
1	18.2	—	—
2	12.7	5.5	67.0
3	11.6	6.6	80.5
4	11.1	7.1	86.6
5	10.7	7.5	91.5
6	10.6	7.6	92.7

$* = \dfrac{\text{reduction}}{18.2 - 10} \times 100$, where 10 is the actual difference between the two means used to generate the "data."

Under rather general conditions [3], the following is true:

Number of strata = k	2	3	4	5	6
% Bias decrease	62	79	86	89	92

Forming a few strata has an important impact by limiting the influence of a confounding variable. Creating more than five or six categories produces only slight further reductions in bias.

Matching Analysis: A Continuous Variable

One Control for Each Case (1:1 Matching)

Each of a series of malformed infants collected from rural French villages were matched to a control for sex, date of birth, and location (in fact, the sampling design produced two controls, and multiple controls will be discussed next). A continuous variable y representing the distance to the nearest electric power line (distance to the nearest source of electromagnetic radiation measured in meters) was recorded for each observation. The notation for such a 1:1 matched data set is given in Table 9–2.

Table 9–2. Notation for a matched pairs design where the risk variable is continuous

Case	y_{01}	y_{02}	y_{03}	$\cdots$	y_{0N}
Control	y_{11}	y_{12}	y_{13}	$\cdots$	y_{1N}

Table 9–3. Matched pair data consisting of malformation (outcome) and distance to electromagnetic radiation exposure (risk factor) for births in rural France (1988–91)

Case	1,150	100	2,000	350	400	2,700	1,200	1,800	10	250	350
Control	300	100	2,150	1,350	800	1,250	450	400	900	1,950	1,050

A total of N pairs are collected (case $= 0$ and control $= 1$). Data created by matching a newborn infant with a malformation (case) to a nonmalformed infant (control) for the study of electromagnetic radiation are given in Table 9–3. A total of $N = 11$ pairs illustrate (the original study contained over 151 pairs). The mean distances for cases $\bar{y}_{case} = 937.273$ and for controls $\bar{y}_{control} = 972.727$ are natural summary statistics of the differences observed within the matched pairs of observations.

It is strategic to analyze the differences—$d_i = y_{1i} - y_{0i}$. Since pairs of infants were matched for sex, date of birth, and location, these factors do not influence the observed case/control differences in the measured distance. The mean difference is $\bar{y}_{control} - \bar{y}_{case} = \bar{d} = 35.454$ with estimated standard deviation $S_D = 1,033.841$. A t-test yields,

$$T = \frac{\bar{d} - 0}{S_{\bar{d}}} = \frac{\bar{d} - 0}{\sqrt{S_D^2/N}} = \frac{35.454}{311.715} = 0.114.$$

The degrees of freedom are $N - 1 = 10$, giving a p-value of 0.912, showing no evidence that the differences observed within the 11 pairs are due to anything but random variation.

The same analysis can be viewed as a two-way classification, and an analysis of variance yields identical results. The summary statistics are given in Table 9–4. An f-statistic to assess differences within pairs (rows) is

$$F = \frac{6,914.0}{534,413.6} = 0.0129 = (0.114)^2 = T^2.$$

The p-value is again 0.912.

Table 9–4. Analysis of variance summaries of the relationship between case/control status and distance to a source of electromagnetic radiation

Source	Sum of Squares	Degrees of Freedom	Mean Square
Rows (case/control)	6,914.0	1	6,914.0
Columns (pairs)	7,179,500.0	$N - 1 = 10$	717,950.0
Residual	5,344,136.0	$N - 1 = 10$	534,413.6
Total	12,530,550.0	$2N - 1 = 21$	—

Table 9–5. Notation for matched data (two controls per case) where the outcome variable is continuous

Case	y_{01}	y_{02}	y_{03}	$\cdots$	y_{0N}
Control 1	y_{11}	y_{12}	y_{13}	$\cdots$	y_{1N}
Control 2	y_{21}	y_{22}	y_{23}	$\cdots$	y_{2N}

Two Controls for Each Case (1:2 Matching)

The t-test and the f-test will always yield identical results for matched pair data. When more than one control is collected per case, the t-test no longer applies but the f-test (analysis of variance) can be used to evaluate observed case/control differences in mean response. The notation for two controls per case is displayed in Table 9–5 where the studied variable is continuous. A total of N matched sets of data are collected (case $= 0$, first control $= 1$, and second control $= 2$). Data consisting of one case matched to two controls from the study of malformations in France are given in Table 9–6. The illustrative number of matched sets remains $N = 11$.

The differences among the means $\bar{y}_{case} = 937.273, \bar{y}_{control_1} = 972.727$, and $\bar{y}_{control_2} = 1,024.456$ are the focus of the analysis of variance (i.e., differences among the mean values from the rows in the 3×11; Table 9–6). The analysis of variance to evaluate the impact of electromagnetic radiation on the risk of a birth defect follows the same pattern as the comparison for matched pairs data. The summary statistics are given in Table 9–7. An alternative approach would be to combine the two control groups and use a two-sample t-test. A combined sample of controls would have greater power but is only useful if the controls do not systematically differ. An analysis of variance approach allows possible identification of heterogeneity among the samples of control observations. An f-test of the hypothesis that the differences observed among the three observations within each

Table 9–6. Matched data (two controls per case) consisting of malformations (outcome) and distance to electromagnetic radiation exposure (risk factor) for births in rural France (1988–91)

Case	1,150	100	2,000	350	400	2,700	1,200	1,800	10	250	350
Control 1	300	100	2,150	1,350	800	1,250	450	400	900	1,950	1,050
Control 2	750	650	4,050	450	700	2,850	50	2,300	150	300	1,000

Table 9–7. Analysis of variance (two controls per case) summaries of the relationship between case/control status and exposure to electromagnetic radiation

Source	Sum of Squares	Degrees of Freedom	Mean Square
Rows (case/control)	463,581.8	2	231,790.9
Columns (pairs)	18,948,090.9	$N - 1 = 10$	1,894,809.1
Residual	10,222,818.2	$2(N - 1) = 20$	511,140.9
Total	29,634,490.9	$3N - 1 = 32$	—

matched set are due strictly to random variation is

$$F = \frac{231,790.9}{511,140.9} = 0.453,$$

producing an f-statistic with 2 and 20 degrees of freedom, making the p-value 0.642. Again, no evidence is apparent of a systematic effect from electromagnetic radiation.

Matched Pairs Data: Binary Data

Matched pair data where the outcome and the risk factor are both binary variables produce a 2×2 table. This 2×2 table differs in important ways from the 2×2 table generated by unmatched data. If F symbolizes the presence of a risk factor and $\bar{F}$ symbolizes the absence of a risk factor, then matched data are usually displayed in a 2×2 table based on pairs (Table 9–8). The values a, b, c, and d represent counts of pairs and $N = a + b + c + d$ is the total number of pairs sampled. Each pair is constructed so that the level of a confounding variable is the same (or close to the same) for each case and control observation.

Another representation of matched data is possible in terms of a series 2×2 tables where each of N tables displays a specific matched pair. Each pair is a stratum, making the number of strata equal to the

Table 9–8. Notation for matched pairs data with a binary outcome and with a binary risk factor

	Control F	Control $\bar{F}$	Total
Case F	a	b	$a + b$
Case $\bar{F}$	c	d	$c + d$
Total	$a + c$	$b + d$	N

number of matched pairs. Furthermore, each stratum contains a single pair with essentially constant levels of the confounding variable. There are four possible types of matched pairs for two binary factors (Table 9–9). The count of each pair type produces summary Table 9–8 (i.e., a represents number of type 1 pairs, b represents number of type 2 pairs, c represents number of type 3 pairs, and d represents number of type 4 pairs).

The probability that a case possesses the risk factor is estimated by $\hat{p}_1 = (a + b)/N$, where N represents the total number of pairs sampled.

Table 9–9. The four possible types of matched pairs

Type 1

	F	$\bar{F}$	Total
Case	1	0	1
Control	1	0	1
Total	2	0	2

Type 2

	F	$\bar{F}$	Total
Case	1	0	1
Control	0	1	1
Total	1	1	2

Type 3

	F	$\bar{F}$	Total
Case	0	1	1
Control	1	0	1
Total	1	1	2

Type 4

	F	$\bar{F}$	Total
Case	0	1	1
Control	0	1	1
Total	0	2	2

Table 9–10. Matched pairs data where the outcome is low birth weight (<2,500 grams), and the risk factor is the presence or absence of maternal smoking

	Control F	Control $\bar{F}$	Total
Case F	15	40	55
Case $\bar{F}$	22	90	112
Total	37	130	167

Similarly, the probability that a control possesses the risk factor is estimated by $\hat{p}_2 = (a + c)/N$. The quantity $\hat{p}_1 - \hat{p}_2 = (b - c)/N$ measures the difference in the proportions with the risk factor between the case and control individuals.

For example, to study an association between low birth weight and maternal smoking an infant who weighs less than 2,500 grams at birth (case) was matched to an infant whose birth weight is greater than 2,500 grams (control), so that the mother of each infant had the same prepregnancy weight. The risk factor is the mother's smoking exposure (F = smoker and $\bar{F}$ = nonsmoker). These pairs, matched on the mother's prepregnancy weight, produce the $N = 167$ pairs in Table 9–10. The data were tabulated from a larger data set (Table 9–11) and are no more than a count of the four types of matched pairs; (F, F—type 1), (F, $\bar{F}$—type 2), ($\bar{F}$, F—type 3), and ($\bar{F}$, $\bar{F}$—type 4).

Matched pair data do not give information on the influence of the variable used to form the pairs. Since the value of the matching variable maternal prepregnancy weight is the same for each pair (stratum), information derived from comparing differences within each pair is not affected by the matching variable. The pairs are formed for just this reason. A cost of removing confounding bias by matching is the inability to study the influence of the matching variable.

Point Estimates

A natural measure of the impact of the risk factor is $\hat{p}_1 - \hat{p}_2$. If the risk factor is associated with case/control status, then p_1 differs from p_2 and the estimates of these two quantities should reflect this difference. The estimated difference $\hat{p}_1 - \hat{p}_2 = (b - c)/N$ has an estimated variance of

$$v = \text{variance } (\hat{p}_1 - \hat{p}_2) = \frac{([b + c]N - [b - c]^2)}{N^3}. \tag{9.1}$$

Table 9–11. Data from a matched pairs study of $N = 167$ low birth weight infants

Id = matched pairs
Status: case = 1, control = 0
Cigs: smoker = 1, nonsmoker = 0
Parity: first child = 0, one or more children = 1
Ppwt: prepregnancy weight, as reported in kilograms
Gest: gestation < 37 weeks = 0, gestation ≥ 37 = 1
Gain: maternal weight gained during pregnancy, as reported in kilograms

Id	Status	Cigs	Parity	Ppwt	Gest	Gain
1	1	1	1	40.9	1	6.1
1	0	0	1	40.9	0	21.0
2	1	1	0	43.0	1	9.2
2	0	1	1	43.0	1	10.0
3	1	0	0	44.5	1	3.4
3	0	0	0	44.5	0	15.4
4	1	0	1	44.5	1	4.4
4	0	0	1	44.5	0	18.1
5	1	0	1	44.5	1	6.1
5	0	0	0	44.5	0	19.3
6	1	0	0	45.5	0	1.0
6	0	1	0	45.5	0	1.5
7	1	0	0	45.5	0	8.4
7	0	0	1	45.5	0	8.9
8	1	1	0	45.5	1	6.5
8	0	0	0	45.5	1	8.8
9	1	1	1	46.8	0	6.9
9	0	1	0	46.8	0	7.7
10	1	1	0	46.8	0	8.4
10	0	0	0	46.8	0	9.3
═	═	═	═	═	═	═
163	1	1	1	91.0	1	2.7
163	0	1	0	91.0	0	16.2
164	1	0	0	93.2	1	4.5
164	0	0	0	93.1	1	25.8
165	1	1	0	97.7	1	10.6
165	0	1	0	97.7	0	18.7
166	1	0	0	105.0	0	3.6
166	0	1	1	105.0	0	10.7
167	1	1	0	118.0	1	0.0
167	0	1	0	118.0	0	5.5

This estimated variance allows the construction of an approximate $(1 - \alpha)$-level confidence interval, or

$$
\begin{aligned}
\text{lower bound} &= (\hat{\beta}_1 - \hat{\beta}_2) - z_{1-\alpha/2}\sqrt{v} \quad \text{and} \\
\text{upper bound} &= (\hat{\beta}_1 - \hat{\beta}_2) + z_{1-\alpha/2}\sqrt{v}.
\end{aligned}
\tag{9.2}
$$

From the smoking data example (Table 9–10),

$$\hat{p}_1 = \frac{55}{167} = 0.329, \quad \hat{p}_2 = \frac{37}{167} = 0.222, \quad \hat{p}_1 - \hat{p}_2 = 0.108,$$

and the approximate 95% confidence interval is (0.017, 0.199). Note that the estimated variance depends on pairs concordant for the risk factor, a and d. For example, increased numbers of concordant pairs decreases the variance. Therefore, concordant pairs play a role in determining the width of the confidence interval.

Odds Ratio

The Mantel-Haenszel summary odds ratio (repeated from Chapter 7) derived from combining a series of k separate 2×2 tables, is estimated by

$$\text{odds ratio} = \widehat{or}_{MH} = \frac{\displaystyle\sum_{i=1}^{k} \frac{a_i d_i}{n_i}}{\displaystyle\sum_{i=1}^{k} \frac{b_i c_i}{n_i}}. \tag{9.3}$$

Matched pairs data is a series of 2×2 tables each with two observations (Table 9–9). The Mantel-Haenszel estimate can be applied to produce an estimate of the summary odds ratio for a set of matched pairs. To summarize, the values

Type of Pair	$a_i d_i / n_i$	$b_i c_i / n_i$	Number of Pairs
1	0	0	a
2	$\frac{1}{2}$	0	b
3	0	$\frac{1}{2}$	c
4	0	0	d

show the relationship between Table 9–9 and expression (9.3). Since $n_i = 2$ for all tables, combining information from the N pairs (strata) gives

$$\text{odds ratio} = \widehat{or}_m = \frac{\displaystyle\sum_{i=1}^{N} \frac{a_i d_i}{n_i}}{\displaystyle\sum_{i=1}^{N} \frac{b_i c_i}{n_i}} = \frac{0a + \frac{1}{2}b + 0c + 0d}{0a + 0b + \frac{1}{2}c + 0d} = \frac{b}{c}. \tag{9.4}$$

The estimated odds ratio depends only on the discordant pairs.

For the example data (Table 9–10), $\widehat{or}_m = 40/22 = 1.818$. Although the details are not presented, the estimate $\widehat{or}_m$ is also the maximum likelihood estimate of the odds ratio from a matched pairs data set.

Confidence Interval for the Odds Ratio

Two types of pairs do not provide information when an odds ratio is used to assess whether a risk factor has an impact on an outcome. When both the case and control possess the risk factor, the influence on the outcome cannot be determined. If a study is made up only of pairs where both members have the risk factor, no conclusion can be drawn about the influence of the risk factor on the outcome. The same argument holds for the situation where both members of a pair do not possess the risk factor. Again, no inferences about the outcome can be drawn from these pairs. Therefore, pairs concordant for the risk factor are not informative, and the analysis of matched data focuses on only the discordant pairs. The a and d concordant pairs are eliminated from the analysis, and the b and c discordant pairs become the data set (Table 9–8). Under these conditions, the data collected in a matched pairs format represent a sample from a binomial distribution as long as the pairs of observations are sampled independently. If p represents the probability that a case possesses the risk factor (see Appendix B) among the discordant pairs (i.e., $P(\text{case} = F \,|\, \text{all pairs are discordant}) = p$), then the probability of k pairs occurring with the case having the risk factor is

$$\text{binomial probability} = \binom{n}{k} p^k (1 - p)^{n-k} \tag{9.5}$$

and $k = 0, 1, 2, \ldots, n$; where n represents the total number of discordant pairs, $n = b + c$. The term $\binom{n}{k}$ is the number of different ways k discordant pairs with the risk factor associated with the case can occur among n discordant pairs. As usual, the term $\binom{n}{k} = n!/k!(n - k)!$ produces the actual count of these pairs. The term $p^k(1 - p)^{n-k}$ is the probability of a specific configuration of k discordant pairs where the case has the risk factor, and $n - k$ discordant pairs where the control has the risk factor. The product of the two terms is the probability that k discordant pairs occur with the case having the risk factor [expression (9.5)].

Table 9–12. Four approaches to calculating a confidence interval for the odds ratio from matched pairs data (a, b, c, and d are defined in Table 9–8, and $n = b + c$)

Exact Method

$$df_1 = 2c + 2 \qquad df_2 = 2b \qquad f_1 = f_{1-\alpha/2, df_1, df_2} \quad \text{from a } f\text{-distribution}$$

$$t_{\text{lower}} = \frac{b}{b + (c + 1)f_1}$$

$$or_{\text{lower}} = \frac{t_{\text{lower}}}{1 - t_{\text{lower}}}$$

$$df_1 = 2b + 2 \qquad df_2 = 2c \qquad f_2 = f_{1-\alpha/2, df_1, df_2} \quad \text{from a } f\text{-distribution}$$

$$t_{\text{upper}} = \frac{b + 1}{c + (b + 1)f_2}$$

$$or_{\text{upper}} = \frac{t_{\text{upper}}}{1 - t_{\text{upper}}}$$

Approximate Method—*Small Sample Size*

$$A = (c + 0.5)^2$$
$$B = (0.5 - 2bc - b + c - z_{1-\alpha/2}^2)$$
$$C = (b - 0.5)^2$$

$$or_{\text{lower}} = \frac{-B - \sqrt{B^2 + 4AC}}{2A}$$

$$A = (c - 0.5)^2$$
$$B = (0.5 - 2bc + b - c - z_{1-\alpha/2}^2)$$
$$C = (b + 0.5)^2$$

$$or_{\text{upper}} = \frac{-B + \sqrt{B^2 + 4AC}}{2A}$$

Approximate Method—Large Sample Size

$$p_{\text{lower}} = \hat{p} - z_{1-\alpha/2}\sqrt{\frac{\hat{p}(1 - \hat{p})}{n}} - \frac{1}{2n}, \quad \text{where} \quad \hat{p} = \frac{b}{n}$$

$$or_{\text{lower}} = \frac{p_{\text{lower}}}{1 - p_{\text{lower}}}$$

$$p_{\text{upper}} = \hat{p} + z_{1-\alpha/2}\sqrt{\frac{\hat{p}(1 - \hat{p})}{n}} + \frac{1}{2n}$$

$$or_{\text{upper}} = \frac{p_{\text{upper}}}{1 - p_{\text{upper}}}$$

Asymptotic Method

$$\widehat{or}_m = \frac{b}{c}$$

$$v = \text{variance}\ (\log[\widehat{or}_m]) = \frac{1}{b} + \frac{1}{c}$$

$$or_{\text{lower}} = \widehat{or}_m e^{-z_{1-\alpha/2}\sqrt{v}} \quad \text{and} \quad or_{\text{upper}} = \widehat{or}_m e^{+z_{1-\alpha/2}\sqrt{v}}$$

An estimate of p is $\hat{p} = b/(b + c)$. There are a number of ways confidence intervals can be constructed for the parameter p from a binomial distribution based on the estimate $\hat{p}$. This fact leads to a number of ways to construct a confidence interval for the odds ratio from a matched pairs study, since

$$\hat{p} = \frac{\widehat{or}_m}{1 + \widehat{or}_m}, \quad \text{therefore} \quad \widehat{or}_m = \frac{\hat{p}}{1 - \hat{p}}. \tag{9.6}$$

If a confidence bound for p, say p_{bound}, is found, then a bound for the confidence interval for the odds ratio or is $or_{\text{bound}} = p_{\text{bound}}/(1 - p_{\text{bound}})$. Table 9–12 gives four expressions for confidence bounds for the odds ratio from a matched pairs study (three methods based on the binomial distribution [expression (9.5)] and the other based on the variance of $\log[\widehat{or}_m]$).

Using the data (Table 9–10) on low birth weight infants and smoking, $b = 40$ and $c = 22$ gives the following 95% confidence intervals:

	Lower	Upper
Exact*	1.055	3.212
Small sample*	1.052	3.160
Large sample*	1.075	3.392
Asymptotic**	1.081	3.059

*Based on the binomial distribution when $n = 62$.
**Asymptotic variances come from the maximum likelihood estimation process (Appendix E) discussed in advanced mathematical statistic text (e.g., [4]).

Evaluating the Observed Odds Ratio

Again relying on the binomial distribution to describe the data resulting from a matched pairs design, statistical test procedures can be developed to evaluate the observed differences within each matched pair. The null hypothesis states that only random differences exist between cases and controls, which translates into $p = 0.5$, where p is again the probability that a case possesses the risk factor among discordant pairs. If only random differences occur within pairs, then it is equally likely that a risk factor is associated with either a case or a control. That is,

$$H_0: p = 0.5$$

or

$$p = P(\text{case} = F | \text{discordant pair}) = P(\text{control} = F | \text{discordant pair}).$$

Stated either way, a test generated under this null hypothesis based on the normal distribution as an approximation to the binomial distribution is the most common approach to evaluating the association between two binary variables observed in matched pairs data.

Let b represent the number of observed discordant pairs where the case possesses the risk factor, then the expected value of b is $np = n/2$ and the variance of b is $np(1 - p) = n/4$ under the null hypothesis that $p = 0.5$ (from the binomial distribution, see Appendix B), giving the test statistic

$$z = \frac{|b - n/2| - \frac{1}{2}}{\sqrt{n/4}}, \tag{9.7}$$

where z has an approximate standard normal distribution. Equivalently the test statistic X_m^2 is

$$X_m^2 = z^2 = \frac{[|b - c| - 1]^2}{b + c}, \tag{9.8}$$

where X_m^2 has an approximate chi-square distribution with one degree of freedom, called McNemar's test. A correction factor of $\frac{1}{2}$ improves the correspondence between the normal distribution (the approximate distribution) and the binomial distribution (the exact distribution).

Using the smoking and low birth weight data,

$$z = \frac{|40 - 62/2| - \frac{1}{2}}{\sqrt{62/4}} = 2.159$$

or

$$X_m^2 = \frac{[|40 - 22| - 1]^2}{40 + 22} = 4.661 = (2.159)^2.$$

Both test statistics necessarily yield the same p-value of 0.031.

Note that the correction factor used in McNemar's test improves the accuracy, particularly for small sample sizes. For example, if $b = 2$ and $c = 8$, then $X_m^2 = 2.5$ with a p-value of 0.114. The uncorrected chi-square statistic yields a p-value of 0.058 for the same data. The exact value based on the binomial distribution is 0.109. Not surprisingly as the sample size becomes larger, the difference between the corrected and uncorrected chi-square statistics disappears.

The test of the hypothesis $p = 0.5$ does not depend on the concordant pairs; however, the concordant pairs are relevant to other calculations involving matched pairs data. If power calculations are made or sample sizes are predicted for matched pairs analysis, the concordant pairs play a role in these calculations.

The issue of overmatching relates to the proportion of concordant pairs. The term overmatching refers to a matched study where a loss of efficiency occurs because the risk factor distribution is very similar for both cases and controls. For example, in a study of the influence of air pollution (risk factor) on respiratory illness where individuals (case) are matched to selected controls from the household next door, it is likely that the study will suffer from overmatching. In almost all situations both the case and the control will have the same air quality—both will have high levels of pollution or both will have low levels of pollution. These pairs concordant for the risk factor are not used in the statistical test [expressions (9.7) or (9.8)]. A low proportion of discordant pairs makes it hard to study effectively the relationship between risk factor and disease. This illustration of overmatching is an extreme case where the risk factor and the matching variable are almost perfectly correlated, but it demonstrates the increase in concordant pairs due to this correlation (pairs labeled a and d in Table 9–8). The correlation leads to small numbers of discordant pairs, making it less likely that differences associated with the risk factor can be detected (loss of power).

Controlling for an Additional Variable in a Matched Design

To clearly describe an association, data are frequently stratified into groups where the value of a particular confounding variable is constant. This strategy to control for the influence of a confounding variable applies as well to matched pairs data. A 2×2 table of matched pairs data can be constructed so that the pairs are homogeneous for a confounding variable, thereby eliminating its influence. For example, restricting the pairs of smoking/birth weight data to only mothers with parity greater than one (i.e., not having their first child) results in Table 9–13. The stratified data give an odds ratio of $\widehat{or} = 29/19 = 1.526$ with an exact 95% confidence interval of (0.827, 2.881). The influence measured by the odds ratio cannot be from the

Table 9–13. Smoking/birth weight data stratified so that all pairs consist of mothers' parity ≥ 1

	Control F	Control $\bar{F}$	Total
Case F	15	29	44
Case $\bar{F}$	19	27	46
Total	34	56	90

influence of parity greater than one—all pairs have parity greater than one. Furthermore, the observed association is not affected by maternal prepregnancy weight, since all pairs were matched so that both cases and controls have the same prepregnancy weight.

Each stratum formed contains fewer and fewer discordant pairs (e.g., $n = 48$ for parity ≥ 1, where the total sample size is 62), which reduced the power to describe an association. If a large or even moderate number of homogeneous strata are created, the number of observations is reduced to a point where analysis becomes meaningless—the major disadvantage to controlling for confounder bias by stratification.

Disregarding Matching

Data collected in a matched pairs design can be analyzed as if the data were not matched. Matched data ignoring the paired design produce Table 9–14. The symbols a, b, c, and d again represent the counts of the four types of matched pairs. For the maternal smoking data, the counts of low birth weight infants classified by their mother's smoking exposure (F) ignoring the matching are given in Table 9–15. The resulting odds ratio is $\widehat{or} = 55(130)/[37(112)] = 1.723$ with an approximate 95% confidence interval of (1.060, 2.809), showing that the odds of a smoker having a low birth weight infant are about 1.7 times the odds of a nonsmoker. Note that this odds ratio is somewhat lower than $\widehat{or}_m = 1.818$ calculated earlier (Table 9–10 from the same

Table 9–14. Data resulting from ignoring the matched pairs design

	Case	Control	Total
F	$a + b$	$a + c$	$2a + b + c$
$\bar{F}$	$c + d$	$b + d$	$2d + b + c$
Total	N	N	$2N$

Table 9–15. Smoking/birth weight data ignoring the matched design

	Case	Control	Total
F	55	37	92
$\bar{F}$	112	130	242
Total	167	167	334

Table 9–16. Matched data on smoking and mortality stratified into five-year age categories

Age	a_i	b_i	c_i	d_i
40–44	3,355	40	15	0
45–49	10,217	192	59	0
50–54	9,214	246	117	6
55–59	6,089	310	122	13
60–64	3,608	232	128	22
65–69	1,800	185	90	8
70–74	597	86	52	12
75–79	111	31	16	2

Note: a = both men lived
  b = nonsmoker lived and smoker died
  c = nonsmoker died and smoker lived
  d = both men died.

data). Also, the width of the confidence interval is narrower. Although there is a gain in power (shorter confidence interval), disregarding the matched pairs structure produces an estimated odds ratio biased towards one.

In general, ignoring the matching in a data set will produce only a slight bias in the expected odds ratios toward one (i.e., $or_m < or < 1$ or $or_m > or > 1$), but often random variation in the estimated odds ratios obscures this bias (e.g., $\widehat{or}_m > \widehat{or}$, by chance).

Consider a matched pairs data set [5] collected to study mortality and smoking (one member of each pair is a nonsmoker). Men were matched on 17 variables such as age, state of health, exercise, sleep, ... The outcome variable of interest is death. The data are given in Table 9–16.

Table 9–17. Odds ratios and corrected chi-square statistics of the smoking/mortality association for matched and unmatched analysis

Age	$\widehat{or}_m$	$\widehat{or}$	X_m^2	X_c^2
40–44	2.67	2.69	10.47	10.56
45–49	3.25	3.30	69.42	70.26
50–54	2.10	2.08	45.14	44.56
55–59	2.54	2.47	80.95	79.12
60–64	1.81	1.74	29.47	27.66
65–69	2.06	2.07	31.13	32.64
70–74	1.65	1.61	7.89	7.54
75–79	1.94	2.05	4.17	4.57

Table 9–17 compares the chi-square statistic for matched pairs (X_m^2; McNemar's corrected chi-square statistic) with the chi-square statistic from the analysis where the matching is ignored (X_c^2; the usual corrected chi-square statistic). The fundamental property illustrated by the smoking data is that when the sample size is large the difference between the odds ratios ($\widehat{or}$ and $\widehat{or}_m$) is usually not remarkable and ignoring the matching does not consistently increase or decrease the chi-square value (X_c^2 and X_m^2). For an appreciable difference in the chi-square values to occur, the matching must be used to control a strongly confounding variable.

Interaction with the Matching Variable

As mentioned, the direct influence of the variable used to match the observations cannot be studied with paired observations. However, interactions can be estimated and evaluated. In this context, an interaction is the failure of the odds ratios, measuring the association between case/control status and a risk factor, to be the same at differing levels of the matching variable. For example, the maternal smoking data matched for prepregnancy weight produces a simple question: Are the odds ratios measuring the association between low birth weight and maternal cigarette exposure the same for all levels of the mother's prepregnancy weight? To start to answer this question, the data can be divided into those pairs where mother's prepregnancy weight is equal to or above the median value and those pairs below the median value. Table 9–18 shows the smoking/birth weight data divided into two parts based on the mother's median prepregnancy weight.

The estimated odds ratio measuring the association between low birth weight and smoking for mothers whose weight is equal to or greater than the median is $\widehat{or}_m = 23/11 = 2.091$ and for those mothers less the median $\widehat{or}_m = 17/11 = 1.545$. Exact 95% confidence intervals (Table 9–12) are respectively (0.979, 4.751) and (0.683, 3.650), indicating no evidence of a nonrandom difference between these two estimates.

A test of the homogeneity of these two estimated odds ratios comes from applying the usual chi-square test of independence to a table constructed from the discordant pairs (values b and c) from each subtable. A table constructed to test for homogeneity of the odds ratio for the maternal smoking data is shown in Table 9–19.

A chi-square test of independence indicates the likelihood of equality between the two odds ratio as reflected by their estimates. That is, the

Table 9–18. Data on smoking exposure and low birth weight separated into two tables based on mothers' prepregnancy weights

Mother's weight ≥ 56 kilograms (median)

	Control F	Control $\bar{F}$
Case F	10	23
Case $\bar{F}$	11	36

Mother's weight < 56 kilograms (median)

	Control F	Control $\bar{F}$
Case F	5	17
Case $\bar{F}$	11	54

Note: F stands for a smoker and $\bar{F}$ stands for a nonsmoker.

hypothesis of independence is the same as postulating that the ratios within the two columns are the same. The resulting chi-square value $X^2 = 0.321$ with one degree of freedom produces a p-value of 0.570. The analysis gives no reason to believe that an interaction exists between prepregnancy weight and smoking exposure.

Testing homogeneity of a series of odds ratios from a matched design can be applied to any number of subtables. Again, consider the smoking/mortality data (Table 9–20). The usual chi-square test of independence (b_i/c_i odds ratios are constant) applied to a $2 \times K$ table can be used to evaluate the homogeneity of these odds ratios among the eight age categories. For these data, the chi-square value is $X^2 = 15.622$ with degrees of freedom $= k - 1 = 7$ giving a p-value of 0.029, indicating that the odds ratios are likely to vary among at least some of the age categories.

Table 9–19. Numbers of pairs discordant for smoking exposure from data divided into two categories based on mothers' prepregnancy weights

	Below the Median	Above the Median
$F/\bar{F}$	23	17
$\bar{F}/F$	11	11

Table 9–20. Numbers of pairs discordant for smoking/mortality data divided into categories based on age

Age	b_i	c_i	$\widehat{or}_m$
40–44	40	15	2.667
45–49	192	59	3.254
50–54	246	117	2.103
55–59	310	122	2.541
60–64	232	128	1.812
65–69	185	90	2.056
70–74	86	52	1.654
75–79	31	16	1.938

Matching Using More Than One Control

If two controls are used for each case, there are six possible combinations of outcomes when two binary variables are studied. The case can have the risk factor or not; the two controls can both have the risk factor or one control can have the risk factor or neither control can have the risk factor. Since there are two possibilities for the cases and three for the controls, there are a total of six different types of $1:2$ matched data sets. The six possibilities are displayed in Table 9–21. Symbolically, the observed counts of each type of outcome are

Table 9–21. The six possible types of $1:2$ matched sets of data

Type 1

	F	$\bar{F}$	Total
Case	1	0	1
Control	2	0	2
Total	3	0	3

Type 2

	F	$\bar{F}$	Total
Case	1	0	1
Control	1	1	2
Total	2	1	3

Type 3

	F	$\bar{F}$	Total
Case	1	0	1
Control	0	2	2
Total	1	2	3

Type 4

	F	$\bar{F}$	Total
Case	0	1	1
Control	2	0	2
Total	2	1	3

Type 5

	F	$\bar{F}$	Total
Case	0	1	1
Control	1	1	2
Total	1	2	3

Type 6

	F	$\bar{F}$	Total
Case	0	1	1
Control	0	2	2
Total	0	3	3

represented by n_{ij} or:

Table type 1 produces n_{12} matched sets or strata,
Table type 2 produces n_{11} matched sets or strata,
Table type 3 produces n_{10} matched sets or strata,
Table type 4 produces n_{02} matched sets or strata,
Table type 5 produces n_{01} matched sets or strata,
Table type 6 produces n_{00} matched sets or strata,

where case = 0 or 1 and control = 0, 1, or 2. The subscripts indicate the number of cases and controls with the factor. The usual table

Table 9–22. The notation for a $1:2$ matched data set

	Control F and F	Control $\bar{F}$ or F	Control $\bar{F}$ and $\bar{F}$
Case F	n_{12}	n_{11}	n_{10}
Case $\bar{F}$	n_{02}	n_{01}	n_{00}

format summarizing data from a $1:2$ matched design is shown in Table 9–22 and again, the total number of matched sets is N.

Like matched pairs data, each stratum is a 2×2 table, and the Mantel-Haenszel estimate can be applied to produce an estimate of the odds ratio. To summarize, the values

Type of Pair	$a_i d_i / n_i$	$b_i c_i / n_i$	Number of Pairs
1	0	0	n_{12}
2	1/3	0	n_{11}
3	2/3	0	n_{10}
4	0	2/3	n_{02}
5	0	1/3	n_{01}
6	0	0	n_{00}

show the relationship between Table 9–22 and expression (9.3). Since $n_i = 3$ for all matched pairs, an estimate of the odds ratio is

$$\text{odds ratio} = \widehat{or_m} = \frac{\displaystyle\sum_{i=1}^{N} \frac{a_i d_i}{n_i}}{\displaystyle\sum_{i=1}^{N} \frac{b_i c_i}{n_i}} = \frac{0 n_{12} + 1 n_{11} + 2 n_{10}}{2 n_{02} + 1 n_{01} + 0 n_{00}} = \frac{n_{11} + 2 n_{10}}{2 n_{02} + n_{01}}. \quad (9.9)$$

For example, consider the distance data from the French malformation study, where the risk factor is defined as $F = 1 = $ distance < 500 meters and $\bar{F} = 0 = $ distance ≥ 500 meters. The binary response data are ($N = 11$ sets) given in Table 9–23. The $1:2$ matched sample produces an estimated odds ratio of

$$\widehat{or_m} = \frac{0(0) + 1(4) + 2(2)}{2(1) + 1(2) + 0(2)} = \frac{8}{4} = 2.0.$$

Table 9–23. The study of malformations in rural France where distance is defined as a binary variable—distance < 500 meters $= 1$ and distance ≥ 500 meters $= 0$

	Control F and F	Control $\bar{F}$ or F	Control $\bar{F}$ and $\bar{F}$
Case (F)	$n_{12} = 0$	$n_{11} = 4$	$n_{10} = 2$
Case ($\bar{F}$)	$n_{02} = 1$	$n_{01} = 2$	$n_{00} = 2$

Also, a chi-square evaluation of the hypothesis that the risk factor has no relationship to case/control status employs the test statistic

$$X^2_{MH} = \frac{[(n_{11} + 2n_{10}) - (n_{01} + 2n_{02})]^2}{2(n_{11} + n_{10} + n_{02} + n_{01})}, \tag{9.10}$$

where X^2_{MH} has an approximate chi-square distribution with one degree of freedom when the risk factor is unrelated to case/control status. For the example data (Table 9–23), the chi-square statistic $X^2_{MH} = (8 - 4)^2/18 = 0.889$ yields a p-value of 0.346. The test statistic X^2_{MH} is a special application of the Mantel-Haenszel chi-square statistic [6]. Notice again that when all members of a set possess or do not possess the risk factor (n_{12} and n_{00}), these two types of concordant observations do not play a role in the estimate of the odds ratio or the test of association.

An approximate $(1 - \alpha)$-confidence interval can be constructed from the estimated variance

$$v = \text{variance } (\log[\widehat{or}_m]) = \left[2\widehat{or} \left(\frac{n_{10} + n_{01}}{(2 + \widehat{or}_m)^2} + \frac{n_{11} + n_{02}}{(1 + 2\widehat{or}_m)^2} \right) \right]^{-1} \tag{9.11}$$

giving an approximate $(1 - \alpha)$-confidence interval for the odds ratio of

$$or_{\text{lower}} = \widehat{or}_m e^{-z_{1-\alpha/2}\sqrt{v}} \quad \text{and} \quad or_{\text{upper}} = \widehat{or}_m^{+z_{1-\alpha/2}\sqrt{v}}.$$

Again from the example data, $n_{11} + n_{02} = 5$, $n_{10} + n_{01} = 4$ and using $\widehat{or}_m = 2.0$ produces an approximate 95% confidence interval of $(0.481, 8.321)$.

Similar tests and confidence intervals can be developed for any number of controls per case. Even when the data consist of matched sets with different numbers of controls per case, estimates of the odds ratio and confidence intervals can be found with specialized expressions

[7] or with a logistic regression approach, to be described in the next sections.

CONDITIONAL LOGISTIC ANALYSIS

A standard logistic regression analysis requires close to one parameter for each stratum (actually k strata require $k - 1$ estimated parameters), which in the case of matched pairs data almost equals the number of sampled pairs. For matched data or any data with a large number of strata, the estimates resulting from the application of a standard logistic regression model are biased, sometimes seriously [7]. An approach that produces estimates of the important parameters for the logistic model but does not incur the bias associated with estimating a large number of parameters provides a solution to this problem. Such a technique is called conditional logistic regression analysis. A conditional logistic regression analysis is designed to produce unbiased estimates of the parameters that describe the relationship between risk factors and out-come but does not produce estimates of the large number of parameters necessary to identify differences among strata. Typically, the differences among strata are not an issue when the data are matched, making a conditional logistic analysis an ideal technique for analyzing matched data. The technical details describing the differences between a standard (unconditional) logistic analysis and conditional logistic analysis are explored elsewhere [7]. In practical terms, there are basically two choices: If the number of strata is small, then an unconditional logistic analysis is appropriate and gives estimates of the impact of the strata classification on the outcome. If the number of strata is large relative to the number of observations, the conditional logistic analysis is appropriate and gives unbiased estimates of the regression coefficients but no assessment of the impact of the stratum variable on the outcome.

For matched data, the relationships between risk factors and case/control status can be studied with a conditional logistic analysis, but nothing can be learned about the relationship between the variable used to match the observations and the case/control variable. This property was already discussed for the analysis of matched pairs data using tables evaluated with chi-square statistics. The statistical assessment of matched pairs data is conditional on using only the discordant pairs (eliminating the concordant pairs) to describe the relationship of the risk factor to the outcome variable. As will be seen, the conditional logistic regression analysis applied to the case of two binary variables is not different from restricting the data to discordant pairs (condition) and using a binomial distribution to evaluate the impact of a risk factor.

Conditional Logistic Regression Model for the Two × Two Case

Consider once again the case where both the outcome and the risk factor are measured by binary variables. A logistic regression model describing a series of 2×2 tables (one for each matched set) is

$$\text{log-odds} = a_i + fF, \tag{9.12}$$

where F is a binary variable (e.g., $F = 1$ for smokers and $F = 0$ for nonsmokers) and a_i reflects the overall level of the log-odds within each matched set (stratum), and as usual, the log-odds measures the risk associated with a binary outcome. Using the maternal smoking/birth weight data, the log-odds is a function of the probability of a low birth weight infant ($1 = \text{case} = \text{infant} < 2,500$ grams and $0 = \text{control} = \text{infant} \geq 2,500$ grams). A conditional logistic analysis yields an estimate of the model parameter f of $\hat{f} = 0.598$ with a standard error of $S_{\hat{f}} = 0.265$, relating the binary risk factor smoking to the likelihood of a low birth weight infant. The approximate 95% confidence interval is $(0.079, 1.117)$. An estimate of the odds ratio is $\widehat{or}_m = e^{\hat{f}} = 1.818$. The conditional logistic approach allows an unbiased estimate of the parameter f despite the fact that the model contains one parameter associated with each matched pair (a_i). The cost of an unbiased estimate of f is that the direct influences of the matching variable cannot be studied (no estimates of the a_i-parameters are possible).

Testing whether the estimate $\hat{f}$ indicates an association between smoking and low birth weight presents nothing new. The null hypothesis is $H_0: f = 0$, generating a test statistic

$$z = \frac{\hat{f}}{S_{\hat{f}}} = \frac{0.598}{0.265} = 2.257$$

where, as usual, z has an approximate normal distribution when $f = 0$. The variance is, as before (Table 9–12), estimated by variance $(\log[\widehat{or}_m]) = \text{variance} (\hat{f}) = 1/b + 1/c$.

This same issue can also be addressed by comparing log-likelihood statistics from two nested models. If $f \neq 0$, then the log-likelihood statistic is $L_1 = 226.209$. For the nested hypothesis $f = 0$, the log-likelihood statistic is $L_0 = 231.511$. The difference $L_0 - L_1 = 231.511 - 226.209 = 5.302$ has an approximate chi-square distribution with one degree of freedom yielding a p-value of 0.021. This result is essentially the same as using the z-statistic since $z^2 = (2.257)^2 = 5.094$, which also has an approximate chi-square distribution with one degree of freedom when $f = 0$, yielding a p-value of 0.024. Additionally, McNemar's chi-square statistic also gives a similar result ($X^2 = 4.661$ with a p-value $= 0.031$).

An estimate of the influence of smoking on the probability of a low birth weight infant is reflected by the estimated odds ratio $\widehat{or}_m = e^f = e^{0.598} = 1.818$, which is identical to the estimate from the previous 2×2 table analysis (i.e., Table 9–10; $\widehat{or}_m = b/c = 40/22 = 1.818$). For the 2×2 case, the conditional logistic model generated odds ratio is always identical to b/c—the basic difference is that a logistic model approach generalizes to a wide variety of situations.

Multiple Controls per Case

The logistic model [expression (9.12)] can be applied to data where more than one control is used. All that is needed are three variables, one identifying which observations are matched (strata), one which indicates case/control status (case $= 1$ or control $= 0$), and one which indicates the presence or absence of the risk factor ($F = 1$ or 0). The data are once again simply a series of individual 2×2 tables (strata) each containing the counts from matched sets of observations. These tables can contain different numbers of observations since a logistic approach does not require the same number of controls per case in each stratum. Application of the logistic model [expression (9.12)] produces the estimated coefficient $\hat{f}$, reflecting the influence of the risk factor and its estimated standard error. An estimate of the odds ratio and an assessment of its impact easily follow.

Consider the $1:2$ matched set of observations from the distance data for the malformation study carried out in rural France. The data from Table 9–23 displayed by strata (11 matched sets) are given in Table 9–24.

Each strata constitutes a 2×2 table. For example, stratum 4 is (type 2)

	F	$\bar{F}$	Total
Case	1	0	1
Control	1	1	2
Total	2	1	3

The conditional analysis of these data (Table 9–24) using a logistic model yields $\hat{f} = 0.693$ with estimated standard error $S_{\hat{f}} = 0.745$ (from

Table 9–24. Binary data from the French malformation study

Strata	Status	F	Strata	Status	F
1	1	0	7	1	0
1	0	1	7	0	1
1	0	0	7	0	1
2	1	1	8	1	0
2	0	1	8	0	1
2	0	0	8	0	0
3	1	0	9	1	1
3	0	0	9	0	0
3	0	0	9	0	1
4	1	1	10	1	1
4	0	0	10	0	0
4	0	1	10	0	1
5	1	1	11	1	1
5	0	0	11	0	0
5	0	0	11	0	0
6	1	0	—	—	—
6	0	0	—	—	—
6	0	0	—	—	—

the computer algorithm) where F represents the presence of a risk factor (distance < 500 meters) and $F = 0$ represents the absence of the risk factor (distance ≥ 500 meters). The estimated odds ratio is, therefore, $\widehat{or}_m = e^{0.693} = 2.000$, which is the same as the Mantel–Haenszel estimate of 2.0 [expression (9.9)]. In most situations, these odds ratio estimates will be similar. An evaluation of the hypothesis H_0: $b = 0$ with the test statistic $z = 0.693/0.745 = 0.930$ yields a p-value of 0.352, which is expectedly similar to the Mantel–Haenszel, the chi-square test based on $\widehat{or}_m = 2.0$ where the p-value is 0.346.

A sophisticated mathematical argument shows that the relative efficiency of employing multiple controls increases as the number of controls used per matched set increases. Approximately, the gain relative to McNemar's chi-square test is $2R/(R+1)$, where R is the number of controls—$1:R$ matched sets. For example, if five controls $(R = 5)$ are used per case $(1:5)$, the analysis is 1.7 times more effective than the $1:1$ matched pairs analysis, but for an additional three controls per case $(1:8)$, the efficiency only increases slightly.

A small note: As R increases, the likelihood decreases of observing a matched set where the cases and controls are concordant for the risk factor. Therefore, overmatching can become less of a problem when R is large, making it more likely that every collected matched set plays a role in the statistical testing procedure (i.e., using multiple controls increases power).

Bivariate Conditional Logistic Analysis of Matched Pairs Data

A bivariate logistic model is

$$\text{log-odds} = a_i + fF + gG + hFG. \tag{9.13}$$

A bivariate model allows estimates of the association between case/control status and the risk factor F while including the possibility of an interaction between the risk factor and a second variable G. Using a conditional logistic analysis [expression (9.13)] yields the summary statistics given in Table 9–25 where $F = 0$ or 1 represents whether a mother is a nonsmoker or a smoker and $G = 0$ or 1 represents whether she is having her first child or not. The outcome, matched for prepregnancy weight, is again the presence and absence of a low birth weight infant (Table 9–11).

This bivariate model (9.13) can be used to produce estimated odds ratios for the four combination of the two binary risk factors where

$$\widehat{or}_m = e^{\hat{f}F + \hat{g}G + \hat{h}FG} \tag{9.14}$$

and the four estimates are shown in Table 9–26.

Table 9–25. Estimated coefficients from the conditional logistic analysis describing the relationship of smoking exposure and parity to the risk of a low birth weight infant

Parameter	Estimate	Std. Error	p-value	$\widehat{or}_m$
f	0.232	0.333	0.486	1.261
g	−0.204	0.260	0.432	0.815
h	0.945	0.536	0.078	2.573

−2 Log Likelihood(L) = 222.971; number of parameters = 3.

Table 9–26. Odds ratio estimates from the conditional logistic analysis of the birth weight data using the binary risk factors maternal smoking exposure and parity

	Smoker, $F = 1$	Nonsmoker, $F = 0$
Parity ≥ 1, $G = 1$	2.646	0.815
Parity $= 0$, $G = 0$	1.261	1.0

To evaluate the interaction term $(h = 0?)$ either a z-statistic or a comparison of log-likelihoods can be used. The z-statistic is $z = \hat{h}/S_{\hat{h}} = 1.763$ producing a p-value of 0.078. The likelihood approach gives $L_0 = 226.198$ when $h = 0$ (Table 9–27) and $L_1 = 222.971$ when $h \neq 0$ (Table 9–25), yielding $L_1 - L_0 = 226.198 - 222.971 = 3.227$ with a p-value of 0.072 which is, as expected, not very different from the z-statistic evaluation.

If no interaction term is included $(h = 0)$, the bivariate model reduces to

$$\text{log-odds} = a_i + fF + gG \tag{9.15}$$

giving the estimates in Table 9–27 based on a conditional analysis.

The influence of smoking on the risk of a low birth weight infant is measured by $\widehat{or}_m = e^{0.595} = 1.813$ which is adjusted for the influence of parity. An approximate 95% confidence interval is $(1.074, 3.060)$. The length of the confidence interval is slightly shorter than the similar interval calculated from Table 9–13 where the data are stratified to estimate the effects of smoking "free" from the confounding influence of parity. The model-based approach is more powerful and, therefore, less affected by small numbers of observations. The cost, however, is the assumption that the effects of smoking and parity are additive on the log-odds scale.

The confounding influence of a variable can always be assessed by comparing two models—one without the variable to one including the variable. Specifically, the matched pairs analysis ignoring the issue of parity [expression (9.12)] yields an estimated odds ratio of $\widehat{or}_m = 1.818$ measuring the association between smoking and low birth weight. From the additive logistic model including the influence of parity, the analogous odds ratio is $\widehat{or}_m = e^{0.595} = 1.813$ (Table 9–27). The similarity of these two estimates shows little confounding influence on the relationship between smoking and birth weight from the binary parity variable.

Table 9–27. Estimated coefficients for the additive logistic model relating smoking exposure and parity to low birth weight

Parameter	Estimate	Std. Error	p-value	$\widehat{or}_m$
f	0.595	0.267	0.026	1.813
g	0.024	0.224	0.914	1.024

-2 Log Likelihood$(L) = 226.198$; number of parameters $= 2$.

Logistic Model—Interactions with the Matching Variable

To repeat once again, it is not possible to study the variable or variables used to form matched sets of data. For example, the conditional logistic analysis of low birth weight (Table 9–10) does not produce information on the direct effect of maternal prepregnancy weight. However, questions concerning interactions with the matching variable can be addressed with a logistic model. For example, does the odds ratio measuring the association between smoking exposure and low birth weight vary among different levels of maternal prepregnancy weight? This same question was addressed with two individual 2×2 tables, where the matched pairs were divided into groups depending on whether paired mothers were above or below the median prepregnancy weight. A logistic model using conditional estimation produces the same results. That is, the model

$$\text{log-odds} = a_i + fF + hFH \qquad (9.16)$$

is used, where F is the binary variable indicating smoking or not, while H indicates below the median prepregnancy weight ($H = 0$; represents less than 56 kilograms) or above the median weight ($H = 1$; represents greater than or equal to 56 kilograms). For matched data, no estimate is possible of the coefficient g in the previous bivariate model [expression (9.13)] when the pairs are matched on values of H, so the term gH is not included in the model but an estimate of the coefficient h indicates the degree of interaction. As usual, conditional logistic regression does not allow the estimation of the a_i-terms in the model. Using the smoking and low birth weight data, the two estimated parameters of the model are given in Table 9–28.

Odds ratio estimates from the logistic model [expression (9.16)] are the same odds ratios that arise from analyzing two individual 2×2 tables. For mothers with prepregnancy weight less than 56 kilograms the odds ratio is $\widehat{or}_m = e^{\hat{f}} = 1.545$, and for mothers who weigh more than 56 kilograms the odds ratio is $\widehat{or}_m = e^{\hat{f} + \hat{h}} = e^{0.737} = 2.091$, as before.

Table 9–28. Estimated coefficients from a conditional logistic analysis of smoking and low birth weight, including a possible interaction with prepregnancy weight

Parameter	Estimate	Std. Error	p-value	$\widehat{or}_m$
f	0.435	0.387	0.261	1.545
h	0.302	0.533	0.571	1.353

-2 Log Likelihood$(L) = 225.888$; number of parameters $= 2$.

Comparing log-likelihood statistics from nested models once again produces results similar to the chi-square analysis. For the interaction model, $L_1 = 225.888$ $(h \neq 0$; Table 9–28) and when the interaction term is removed from the model, $L_0 = 226.209$ $(h = 0)$. The difference $L_0 - L_1 = 0.322$ has an approximate chi-square distribution with one degree of freedom when $h = 0$, giving a p-value of 0.571 (the chi-square analysis yields $X^2 = 0.322$ generating a p-value of 0.570). Also, the direct assessment of the estimated parameter $\hat{h}$ yields almost identical results, or $z = \hat{h}/S_{\hat{h}} = 0.302/0.533 = 0.567$ and $z^2 = (0.567)^2 = 0.321 \approx L_0 - L_1$.

Logistic Models with Continuous Variables

A clear advantage of a model approach over analyzing tabular data is that continuous variables are easily made part of a logistic model. To illustrate, consider the interaction between prepregnancy weight, measured directly as reported, and the relationship between smoking (binary variable) and low birth weight. The logistic model is

$$\text{log-odds} = a_i + fF + gxF, \tag{9.17}$$

where x represents the reported prepregnancy weight in kilograms. Again, the direct effect of prepregnancy weight is not part of the logistic model since this variable was used to form the matched pairs. To assess the possibility of an interaction, the two important parameters for this model are estimated and displayed in Table 9–29.

The odds ratios can be estimated from the model parameters for a given value of x. For example, the impact of prepregnancy weight on the relationship between low birth weight and smoking $(F = 1)$ is reflected by the estimated odds ratio

$$\widehat{or}_m = e^{1.045 - 0.0075x} = (2.843)(0.993)^x.$$

The odds ratio reflecting the association between smoking and low birth weight depends on the level of prepregnancy weight (i.e., multiplied by $(0.993)^x$). Some examples are given in Table 9–30.

Table 9–29. Estimates of the influence of an interaction between prepregnancy weight and smoking exposure

Parameter	Estimate	Std. Error	p-value	$\widehat{or}_m$
f	1.045	1.290	0.419	2.843
g	−0.00749	0.0211	0.723	0.993

-2 Log Likelihood$(L) = 226.084$; number of parameters $= 2$.

Table 9–30. Estimates of the influence of smoking exposure on the risk of a low birth weight infant for selected prepregnancy weights (kilograms)

x	$\widehat{or}_m$
40	2.11
50	1.95
60	1.81
70	1.68
80	1.56

The evaluation of the influence of the interaction effect follows the usual lines. The z-statistic to assess the estimate $\hat{g}$ is $z = -0.0075/0.021 = -0.357$, giving a p-value of 0.723. The parallel comparison of log-likelihoods is $L_0 - L_1 = 0.125$, where $L_1 = 226.084$ (interaction model, Table 9–29) and $L_0 = 226.209$ (g set to zero). This chi-square statistic has one degree of freedom producing a p-value of 0.724 (note; $z^2 = (0.355)^2 = 0.127$).

The assessment of a continuous variable need not be restricted to the variable used in matching the study individuals. In the matched data set displayed in Table 9–11, maternal weight gain is recorded (actually the basic purpose of the data set is to study the influence of maternal weight gain on the risk of a low birth weight infant). An additive logistic model applied to the matched low birth weight data including both the influences of smoking (binary variable) and weight gain (in kilograms, as reported) is

$$\text{log-odds} = a_i + fF + gw, \tag{9.18}$$

where w represents the maternal weight gain in kilograms abstracted from physician records. This model [expression (9.18)] postulates additive influences of smoking and weight gain producing the two estimated parameters in Table 9–31. The magnitude of the coefficient g is influenced by the measurement units and indicates the change in the log-odds for a one-unit increase in the risk factor, namely one kilogram of maternal weight gain. The impact of maternal weight gain can be assessed by comparing log-likelihood statistics where a chi-square statistic with one degree of freedom is $L_{g=0} - L_{g\neq0} = 226.209 - 160.541 = 65.668$ with an associated p-value < 0.001. The impact of weight gain is not in doubt but the question arises: Is the influence adequately summarized by a linear relationship?

Table 9–31. Estimates of the influence of smoking and weight gain on the risk of a low birth weight infant

Parameter	Estimate	Std. Error	p-value	$\widehat{or}_m$
f	0.649	0.321	0.044	1.314
g	−0.257	0.050	<0.001	0.774

−2 Log Likehood(L) = 160.541; number of parameters = 2.

The relationship between the risk variable and the outcome in the additive model [expression (9.18)] is constrained to be linear on a log-odds scale. To study the relationship between a continuous variable and the log-odds, a continuous variable can be temporarily treated as a categorical variable. A series of categories is generated by a set of design variables which allows the estimation of an unconstrained relationship. For maternal weight gain, four useful categories are: less than 5 kilograms, between 5 and 10 kilograms, between 10 and 14 kilograms, and greater than 14 kilograms. These four categories are represented by the three design variables shown in Table 9–32. The logistic model accounting for weight gain in an unconstrained fashion (no assumption about the relationship between risk factor and the log-odds outcome variable) is

$$\text{log-odds} = a_i + fF + g_2G_2 + g_3G_3 + g_4G_4. \tag{9.19}$$

A conditional logistic analysis using expression (9.19) addresses the relationship between weight gain and low birth weight for the $N = 167$ matched pairs without an assumption about the relationship between weight gain and the risk of a low birth weight infant. The binary variable F reflecting smoking exposure is left in the model. Table 9–33 shows the estimated coefficients resulting from this unconstrained model using the four weight gain categories rather than the actual measured weight gain. Since G_1 is set to zero, the estimated odds ratios are relative to the first category (<5 kilograms) where $or = 1.0$.

Table 9–32. Design variables representing four maternal weight gain categories

	G_2	G_3	G_4
<5 Kilograms	0	0	0
5–10 Kilograms	1	0	0
10–14 Kilograms	0	1	0
>14 Kilograms	0	0	1

Table 9–33. Estimated coefficients from a conditional logistic analysis treating weight gain measured as an unordered categorical variable (unconstrained)

Parameter	Estimate	Std. Error	p-value	$\widehat{or}_m$
f	0.677	0.309	0.028	1.968
g_2	−1.116	0.491	0.023	0.327
g_3	−1.953	0.565	0.001	0.141
g_4	−3.666	0.746	<0.001	0.0255

−2 Log Likelihood(L) = 160.541; number of parameters = 4.

The estimated g-coefficients indicate a more or less linear relationship, since the coefficients $g_1 = 0$, $\hat{g}_2 = -1.1$, $\hat{g}_3 = -2.0$, and $\hat{g}_4 = -3.7$ roughly differ by about 1.2 between each of the estimates (a constant difference implies a linear response). Therefore, the use of weight gain as linear contributor to the log-odds [expression (9.18)] has some justification.

Additive Logistic Model

In general, the additive logistic model for a series of matched pairs is

$$\text{log-odds} = a_i + \sum b_j x_j. \tag{9.20}$$

For example, a logistic model employing four risk variables (three binary and one continuous) to study the risk of a low birth weight infant is represented by

$$\text{log-odds} = a_i + b_1 x_1 + b_2 x_2 + b_3 x_3 + b_4 x_4, \tag{9.21}$$

where x_1 is binary (smoker or nonsmokers), x_2 is binary (parity $= 0$ or parity ≥ 1), x_3 is continuous (weight gain, as reported), x_4 is binary (gestation <37 weeks or gestation ≥ 37 weeks). Estimates of the four coefficients based on conditional logistic estimation are given in Table 9–34, using the data represented in Table 9–11.

Table 9–34. Estimates from a four-variable conditional logistic analysis—coefficients associated with smoking, parity, weight gain, and gestation

Parameter	Estimate	Std. Error	p-value	$\widehat{or}_m$
b_1	0.629	0.325	0.053	1.876
b_2	−0.092	0.278	0.738	0.912
b_3	−0.244	0.052	<0.001	0.783
b_4	0.795	0.776	0.305	2.214

−2 Log Likelihood(L) = 159.317; number of parameters = 4.

Before making inferences about the four risk variables from the additive model, it is critical to show that interaction effects are negligible. Postulating a model with a series of terms allowing possible interactions between the matching variable (prepregnancy weight) and the four risk factors yields a log-likelihood statistic of $L_1 = 151.342$ (not shown). The additive model produces a log-likelihood statistic of $L_0 = 159.317$. The difference $L_0 - L_1 = 7.975$ has an approximate chi-square distribution with four degrees of freedom when no interaction exists, producing p-value $= 0.092$. Similarly, assessing all six possible interactions among the four risk factor variables produces a chi-square statistic of 9.364 with six degrees of freedom and a p-value of 0.154. These two chi-square values indicate no strong evidence of any important interactions with the variable used to form the matched sets or among the risk variables. Therefore, the additive model [expression (9.21)] is likely an acceptable representation of the relationships of the four risk factors to the outcome of low birth weight.

The four-variable logistic model shows that weight gain has an important influence on the risk of a low birth weight infant. The coefficient $\hat{b}_4$ is adjusted to be "free" from any confounding influence from maternal prepregnancy weight (due to the matching structure), and any confounding influence from the three other variables is removed by using a logistic model.

If the matching variable is not a strong confounder, a matched and unmatched analysis produce similar results. The impact of a matching variable can be assessed by comparing the conditional and unconditional logistic regression analyses. The $N = 167$ pairs of matched data analyzed with an unconditional logistic regression approach give the estimated coefficients in Table 9–35 using the model

$$\text{log-odds} = a + b_1 x_1 + b_2 x_2 + b_3 x_3 + b_4 x_4 + b_5 x_5, \qquad (9.22)$$

Table 9–35. Estimates from the five-variable unconditional logistic analysis— smoking, parity, weight gain, gestation, and prepregnancy weight

Parameter	Estimate	Std. Error	p-value	$\widehat{or}_m$
a	0.309	0.269	—	—
b_1	0.549	0.268	0.042	1.731
b_2	−0.051	0.242	0.834	0.951
b_3	−0.105	0.021	<0.001	0.900
b_4	0.588	0.257	0.023	1.800
b_5	0.004	0.010	0.712	1.004

$-2 \log \text{Likehood}(L) = 408.086$; number of parameters $= 6$.

which employs the same variables as the matched pairs model [expression (9.21)] but directly includes the measured prepregnancy weight (x_5) and a single constant term (a—the stratified structure of the data is ignored).

The odds ratios from the unconditional analysis (Table 9–35) are closer to 1.0 when compared to the conditional analysis (Table 9–34), but are potentially biased. The standard error associated with each coefficient is smaller in the unconditional analysis. This trade-off— biased estimates with increased precision—is typical in choosing between conditional and unconditional approaches using logistic regression models.

10 Life Tables:
An Introduction

The first formal life tables were developed independently by Edmund Halley (1693) and John Graunt (1662). By the end of the nineteenth century, life tables were routinely computed as part of an emerging awareness of the importance of mortality statistics. The first official U.S. life table published in 1900 showed the expected length of life for white males as 46.6 years and for white females as 48.7 years.

A life table is a systematic record of the mortality experience of a group. A cohort life table is constructed from the mortality records of individuals followed from the birth of the first to the death of the last member of a group. Such life tables are constructed from animal and insect data. For human populations, it is obviously not practical to construct a life table by following a cohort of individuals from birth until all have died. Instead, a life table is constructed from current mortality rates. These rates do not apply to past populations and undoubtedly will not apply to future populations. Nevertheless, mortality patterns can be clearly displayed in a current life table, and the comparison of life tables calculated for different groups is a basic strategy for analyzing survival data.

Aside: It is useful to look at a simple structure which is the basis for the following general, but more complex, development of life tables and other survival curve estimates. Consider a series of consecutive time intervals, where a failure can occur in any one of these intervals with probabilities q_1, q_2, q_3, and so forth. Therefore,

Interval	P(failure interval i)	P(survive interval i)	P(survive beyond interval i)
1	q_1	$p_1 = 1 - q_1$	p_1
2	q_2	$p_2 = 1 - q_2$	$p_1 \times p_2$
3	q_2	$p_3 = 1 - q_3$	$p_1 \times p_2 \times p_3$

where the conditional probability $p_i = P(\text{surviving to interval } i + 1 \mid \text{sur-}$ vived through the interval i). The probability of surviving beyond a given interval is the product of a series of these conditional probabilities. For example, the probability of surviving beyond interval 3 is $p_1 \times p_2 \times p_3$. This product-rule can be used for any number of intervals and is a fundamental part of the description of survival data.

Complete, Current Life Table: Construction

The word *complete* when applied to a life table means that ages are not grouped but recorded in one-year intervals. The actual construction of a complete life table is rather mechanical and consists of seven basic elements:

Age interval (x to $x + 1$): Each age interval consists of one year (age denoted by x) except the last age interval, which is left open ended (e.g., 90^+ years).

Number alive (l_x): The symbol l_x represents the number of individuals alive at exactly age x. The number l_x is the life table population at risk for the interval x to $x + 1$. The number alive at age 0 (l_0) is set at some arbitrary value, such as 100,000, and called the radix.

Deaths (d_x): The symbol d_x represents the number of individuals who died between the ages of x and $x + 1$.

Probability of death (q_x): The symbol q_x represents the conditional probability that an individual who is alive at age x dies before age $x + 1$. That is, $P(\text{death before age } x + 1 \mid \text{alive at age } x) = q_x$, and $q_x = d_x/l_x$. The probability of death within a specific age interval is related to a hazard rate and is distinct from a survival probability. Hazard rates and survival probabilities are topics in the next two sections.

Years lived (L_x): The symbol L_x represents the cumulative time lived by the entire cohort between the ages of x and $x + 1$. Each individual alive at age x contributes to the total time lived, either one year if an individual lives the entire year or the proportion of the year lived if the person died in the interval. The value of L_x is the life table person-years of risk for the interval x to $x + 1$.

Total time lived (T_x): The symbol T_x represents the total time lived beyond age x by all individuals alive at age x. The total time lived is $T_x = L_x + L_{x+1} + L_{x+2} + \cdots$. The value T_x is primarily a computational step in the life table construction.

Expectation of life (e_x): The symbol e_x represents the average number of additional years expected to be lived by those individuals alive at age x, computationally $e_x = T_x/l_x$.

The following relationships are direct consequences of these seven definitions:

1. Number dying in the interval x to $x + 1 = d_x = q_x l_x = l_x - l_{x+1}$;
2. Number surviving at age $x + 1 = l_{x+1} = p_x l_x = l_x - d_x$;
3. Probability of dying in the interval x to $x + 1 = q_x = (l_x - l_{x+1})/l_x = d_x/l_x$; and
4. Probability of surviving from x to $x + 1 = p_x = 1 - q_x = (l_x - d_x)/l_x = l_{x+1}/l_x$.

These definitions apply to a complete life table, using age intervals of one year.

The total person-years at risk for the interval x to $x + 1$ includes one year of survival for each person who did not die during the interval. Individuals who die contribute the proportion of the year they were alive to the total time lived. The average time contributed by those who died in the interval x to $x + 1$ is represented by $\bar{a}_x$. The value $\bar{a}_x$ is close to 0.5 for all ages except the first few years of life. For years 0 to 4 the values of $\bar{a}$·are: $\bar{a}_0 = 0.09$, $\bar{a}_1 = 0.43$, $\bar{a}_2 = 0.45$, $\bar{a}_3 = 0.47$, and $\bar{a}_4 = 0.49$ (determined empirically by Chiang [1]). These values make logical sense. The distribution of survival times in the first year of life is skewed toward the beginning of the interval, because most deaths in the interval 0 to 1 year occur within the first month. Therefore, the average contribution of time lived by those who died to the total years lived is low for the first age interval. For ages 2 to 4 years the mean $\bar{a}_x$ shows slightly earlier deaths within the interval, but these $\bar{a}_x$ values are close to 0.50. For all other age intervals the average value of $\bar{a}_x$ is essentially 0.5 years in most human populations. A value of $\bar{a}_x = 0.5$ means that individuals die randomly throughout the interval producing an average contribution for each person of 0.5 years.

The value $\bar{a}_x$ takes on importance in calculating the person-years of life for a life table because

$$L_x = (l_x - d_x) + \bar{a}_x d_x \tag{10.1}$$

is the life table person-years of risk for the age interval x to $x + 1$. Using L_x, the life table age-specific mortality rate becomes d_x/L_x and provides a link to observed age-specific mortality rates. The life table person-years calculation does not differ from the person-years calculation discussed in Chapter 1 [expression (1.5)].

The starting point for construction of a life table is a set of age-specific probabilities of death (q_x). These probabilities are derived by equating the life table age-specific mortality rates to the age-specific mortality rates from the population of interest, or

$$\text{life table mortality rate} = \frac{d_x}{L_x} = R_x = \text{observed mortality rate,} \quad (10.2)$$

where R_x is the age-specific rate for age x calculated from observed mortality data for a specific year (calendar time). A value for q_x follows from R_x because

$$\text{life table mortality rate} = \frac{d_x}{(l_x - d_x) + \bar{a}_x d_x} = \frac{q_x}{1 - (1 - \bar{a}_x) q_x} = R_x \quad (10.3)$$

and solving for q_x gives

$$q_x = \frac{R_x}{1 + (1 - \bar{a}_x) R_x}. \quad (10.4)$$

A set of observed mortality rates (R_x) produce a set of life table probabilities (q_x). The probabilities q_x generate the rest of the life table functions $(l_x, d_x, L_x, T_x, \text{and } e_x)$ with one exception.

The person-years of life (L_x) for the last interval cannot be calculated directly, because a value for $\bar{a}_x$ is not generally available. The individuals who are present at the start of the last interval all die $(q_{x'} = 1.0)$ so that $l_{x'} = d_{x'}$, where x' symbolizes the final age interval (e.g., if the last interval is 90^+, then $x' = 90$), but $\bar{a}_{x'}$ is certainly greater than 0.5. The calculation of $L_{x'}$ is slightly complicated, because it depends on both the population at risk and the choice of x'. Again equating the observed mortality rate with the life table mortality rate for this last age interval gives a value of $L_{x'}$ because

$$\frac{d_{x'}}{L_{x'}} = \frac{l_{x'}}{L_{x'}} = R_{x'} \quad (10.5)$$

and solving for $L_{x'}$ yields

$$L_{x'} = \frac{l_{x'}}{R_{x'}}, \quad (10.6)$$

where, to repeat, $R_{x'}$ comes from the observed mortality data. For example, if $d_{90+} = 8,366$ (from Table 10–1) and $R_{90+} = 3,487/17,346 = 0.201$ (from 1980 male, California mortality rates), then $L_{90+} = 8,368/0.201 = 41,616.5$ person-years of total additional life lived by those who reached age 90. Therefore, an observed set of age-specific mortality rates is all that is needed to calculate a complete life table.

Table 10–1. California 1980 population of white males

x to $x + 1$	Population	Deaths	R_x^*	q_x	d_x	l_x	L_x	T_x	e_x
0–1	129,602	2,166	1,671.3	0.01647	1,647	100,000	98,518	6,960,692	69.61
1–2	117,753	123	104.5	0.00104	103	98,355	98,295	6,862,175	69.77
2–3	115,003	73	63.5	0.00063	62	98,250	98,217	6,763,880	68.84
3–4	113,314	60	53.0	0.00053	52	98,188	98,161	6,665,663	67.89
4–5	110,822	41	37.0	0.00037	36	98,137	98,118	6,567,502	66.92
5–6	110,548	55	49.8	0.00050	49	98,100	98,076	6,469,384	65.95
6–7	106,857	42	39.3	0.00039	39	98,051	99,032	6,371,308	64.98
7–8	112,184	58	51.7	0.00052	51	98,013	97,988	6,271,276	64.00
8–9	116,423	44	37.8	0.00038	37	97,962	91,944	6,175,288	63.04
9–10	132,952	52	39.1	0.00039	38	97,925	97,906	6,077,344	62.06
10–11	134,266	48	35.7	0.00036	35	97,887	97,869	5,979,438	61.09
11–12	128,938	60	46.5	0.00047	46	91,852	97,829	5,881,569	60.11
12–13	125,502	52	41.4	0.00041	41	97,806	97,786	5,783,740	59.13
13–14	128,212	82	64.0	0.00064	63	97,766	97,735	5,685,954	58.16
14–15	131,775	129	97.2	0.00097	95	97,703	91,656	5,588,219	57.20
15–16	143,600	233	162.3	0.00162	158	97,608	97,529	5,490,563	56.25
16–17	151,840	290	191.0	0.00191	186	91,450	97,357	5,393,034	55.34
17–18	157,365	400	254.2	0.00254	247	97,264	97,141	5,295,677	54.45
18–19	159,476	415	260.2	0.00260	252	97,017	96,891	5,198,535	53.58
19–20	171,235	416	242.9	0.00243	235	96,765	96,648	5,101,644	52.72
20–21	173,682	418	240.7	0.00240	232	96,530	96,414	5,004,996	51.85
21–22	172,656	436	252.5	0.00252	243	96,298	96,177	4,908,582	50.97
22–23	176,544	400	226.6	0.00226	217	96,056	95,947	4,812,405	50.10
23–24	175,732	410	233.3	0.00233	223	95,838	95,726	4,716,458	49.21
24–25	174,780	409	234.0	0.00234	223	95,615	95,503	4,620,731	48.33

(*Continued*)

Table 10–1. California 1980 population of white males—Continued

x to x + 1	Population	Deaths	R_x^*	q_x	d_x	l_x	L_x	T_x	e_x
25–26	173,214	393	226.9	0.00227	216	91,391	95,283	4,525,228	47.44
26–27	169,980	400	235.3	0.00235	224	95,175	95,063	4,429,944	46.55
27–28	168,369	366	217.4	0.00217	206	94,951	94,848	4,334,881	45.65
28–29	157,189	330	209.9	0.00210	199	94,547	94,646	4,240,033	44.75
29–30	162,394	346	213.1	0.00213	201	94,547	94,446	4,145,387	43.84
30–31	161,191	329	204.1	0.00204	192	94,345	94,249	4,050,941	42.94
31–32	154,874	355	229.2	0.00229	216	94,153	94,045	3,956,692	42.02
32–33	162,136	338	208.5	0.00208	196	93,937	93,840	3,862,647	41.12
33–34	163,665	305	187.0	0.00187	175	93,742	93,654	3,768,807	40.20
34–35	127,624	267	209.2	0.00209	196	93,567	93,469	3,675,153	39.28
35–36	128,890	296	229.7	0.00229	214	93,371	93,264	3,581,684	38.36
36–37	127,933	302	236.1	0.00236	220	93,157	93,047	3,488,420	37.45
37–38	127,923	334	261.1	0.00261	242	92,937	92,816	3,395,373	36.53
38–39	109,718	281	256.1	0.00256	237	92,695	92,576	3,302,557	35.63
39–40	108,168	325	300.5	0.00300	277	92,458	92,319	3,209,981	34.72
40–41	104,314	338	324.0	0.00324	298	92,181	92,031	3,117,662	33.82
41–42	100,059	342	341.8	0.00341	314	91,882	91,725	3,025,630	32.93
42–43	97,330	344	353.4	0.00353	323	91,569	91,407	2,933,905	32.04
43–44	92,394	356	385.3	0.00385	351	91,246	91,070	2,842,497	31.15
44–45	91,741	431	469.8	0.00469	426	90,895	90,682	2,751,427	30.27
45–46	92,331	438	474.4	0.00473	428	90,469	90,255	2,660,745	29.41
46–47	88,150	522	592.2	0.00590	532	90,041	89,775	2,576,491	28.55
47–48	90,475	559	617.9	0.00616	551	89,509	89,233	2,480,716	27.71
48–49	90,095	650	721.5	0.00719	639	88,958	88,638	2,391,483	26.88
49–50	97,275	696	715.5	0.00713	630	88,318	88,003	2,302,845	26.07
50–51	98,008	734	748.9	0.00746	654	87,688	87,361	2,214,841	25.26

51–52	93,134	825	885.8	0.00882	768	87,034	86,650	2,127,480	24.44
52–53	94,496	875	926.0	0.00922	795	86,267	85,869	2,040,830	23.66
53–54	93,239	1,010	1083.2	0.01077	921	85,472	85,011	1,954,960	22.87
54–55	96,443	1,126	1167.5	0.01161	981	84,551	84,060	1,869,949	22.12
55–56	97,763	1,197	1224.4	0.01217	1,017	83,569	83,061	1,785,889	21.37
56–57	96,823	1,272	1313.7	0.01305	1,077	82,552	82,014	1,702,829	20.63
57–58	96,189	1,334	1386.9	0.01377	1,122	81,475	80,914	1,620,815	19.89
58–59	98,518	1,553	1576.4	0.01564	1,257	80,353	79,724	1,539,901	19.16
59–60	96,154	1,564	1626.6	0.01613	1,276	79,096	78,458	1,460,177	18.46
60–61	88,552	1,472	1662.3	0.01649	1,283	77,820	77,179	1,381719	17.76
61–62	83,814	1,684	2009.2	0.01989	1,522	76,537	75,776	1,304,541	17.04
62–63	81,464	1,763	2164.1	0.02141	1,606	75,014	74,211	1,228,766	16.38
63–64	76,317	1,871	2451.6	0.02422	1,778	73,408	72,519	1,154,554	15.73
64–65	75,505	2,032	2691.2	0.02656	1,902	71,630	70,679	1,082,035	15.11
65–66	73,832	2,097	2840.2	0.02801	1,953	69,728	68,752	1,011,356	14.50
66–67	69,480	2,121	3052.7	0.03007	2,038	67,776	66,757	942,604	13.91
67–68	65,690	2,130	3242.5	0.03191	2,098	65,738	64,689	875,847	13.32
68–69	62,557	2,256	3606.3	0.03542	2,254	63,640	62,513	811,159	12.75
69–70	57,412	2,327	4053.2	0.03973	2,439	61,386	60,166	748,646	12.20
70–71	53,926	2,205	4088.9	0.04007	2,362	58,947	57,766	688,479	11.68
71–72	50,402	2,376	4714.1	0.04606	2,606	56,585	55,282	630,713	11.15
72–73	47,213	2,342	4960.5	0.04840	2,613	53,979	52,673	575,431	10.66
73–74	42,931	2,233	5201.4	0.05070	2,604	51,366	50,064	522,759	10.18
74–75	39,611	2,300	5806.5	0.05643	2,751	48,762	47,386	472,694	9.69
75–76	36,306	2,408	6632.5	0.06420	2,954	46,011	44,534	425,308	9.24
76–77	33,386	2,251	6742.3	0.06523	2,808	43,057	41,653	380,774	8.84
77–78	30,141	2,102	6973.9	0.06739	2,712	40,249	38,892	339,121	8.43
78–79	26,432	2,272	8595.6	0.08241	3,094	37,536	35,990	300,229	8.00
79–80	26,264	2,093	7969.1	0.07664	2,640	34,443	33,123	264,239	7.67

(Continued)

Table 10–1. California 1980 population of white males—Continued

x to $x+1$	Population	Deaths	R_x^*	q_x	d_x	l_x	L_x	T_x	e_x
80–81	21,846	1,958	8962.7	0.08578	2,728	31,803	30,439	231,117	7.27
81–82	18,868	1,947	10319.1	0.09813	2,853	29,075	27,648	200,677	6.90
82–83	16,653	1,802	10820.9	0.10265	2,692	26,222	24,876	173,029	6.60
83–84	14,825	1,751	11811.1	0.11153	2,624	23,530	22,218	148,153	6.30
84–85	13,137	1,689	12856.8	0.12080	2,525	20,906	19,643	125,935	6.02
85–86	11,350	1,622	14290.7	0.13338	2,452	18,380	17,155	106,292	5.78
86–87	9,442	1,426	15102.7	0.14042	2,237	15,929	14,811	89,137	5.60
87–88	8,047	1,198	14887.5	0.13856	1,897	13,692	12,744	74,327	5.43
88–89	6,091	1,072	17599.7	0.16176	1,908	11,795	10,841	61,583	5.22
89–90	5,382	897	16666.7	0.15385	1,521	9,887	9,126	50,742	5.13
90+	17,346	3,487	20102.6	1.00000	8,366	8,366	41,616	41,616	4.97

* = Rate per 100,000 person-years of risk.

Table 10–2. California 1980 population of white males

x to $x + 1$	Population	Deaths	R_x^*	q_x	d_x	l_x	L_x	T_x	e_x
0–1	123,342	1,635	1325.6	0.01310	1,310	100,000	98,821	7,693,461	76.93
1–2	111,520	64	57.4	0.00057	57	98,690	98,658	7,594,641	76.95
2–3	109,120	41	37.5	0.00038	37	98,633	98,613	7,495,983	76.00
3–4	108,749	22	20.2	0.00020	20	98,596	98,586	7,397,370	75.03
4–5	105,698	41	38.8	0.00039	38	98,576	98,557	7,298,784	74.04
5–6	105,801	37	35.0	0.00035	34	98,538	98,521	7,200,227	73.07
6–7	101,630	37	36.4	0.00036	36	98,504	98,486	7,101,706	72.10
7–8	106,850	32	29.9	0.00030	29	98,468	98,453	7,003,220	71.12
8–9	110,410	32	29.0	0.00029	29	98,438	98,424	6,904,767	70.14
9–10	127,237	33	25.9	0.00026	26	98,410	98,397	6,806,342	69.16
10–11	128,916	33	25.6	0.00026	25	98,384	98,372	6,707,945	68.18
11–12	124,123	32	25.8	0.00026	25	98,359	98,347	6,609,573	67.20
12–13	119,672	28	23.4	0.00023	23	98,334	98,322	6,511,227	66.22
13–14	123,652	48	38.8	0.00039	38	98,311	98,292	6,412,905	65.23
14–15	127,869	68	53.2	0.00053	52	98,273	98,247	6,314,613	64.26
15–16	139,122	98	70.4	0.00070	69	98,220	98,186	6,216,366	63.29
16–17	146,318	93	63.6	0.00064	62	98,151	98,120	6,118,180	62.33
17–18	150,163	132	87.9	0.00088	86	98,089	98,046	6,020,059	61.37
18–19	152,382	121	79.4	0.00079	78	98,003	97,964	5,922,014	60.43
19–20	162,203	138	85.1	0.00085	83	97,925	97,883	5,924,050	59.47
20–21	162,313	118	72.7	0.00073	71	97,842	97,806	5,726,167	58.52
21–22	162,709	104	63.9	0.00064	62	97,771	97,739	5,628,360	57.57
22–23	167,087	96	57.5	0.00057	56	97,708	97,680	5,530,621	56.60
23–24	168,874	121	71.7	0.00072	70	97,652	97,617	5,432,940	55.64
24–25	168,959	119	70.4	0.00070	69	97,582	97,548	5,335,324	54.68

(*Continued*)

Table 10-2. California 1980 population of white males—Continued

x to $x+1$	Population	Deaths	R_x^*	q_x	d_x	l_x	L_x	T_x	e_x
25–26	168,414	110	65.3	0.00065	64	97,513	97,481	5,237,776	53.71
26–27	165,167	141	85.4	0.00085	83	97,450	97,408	5,140,295	52.75
27–28	164,403	123	74.8	0.00075	73	97,366	97,330	5,042,887	51.79
28–29	154,062	137	88.9	0.00089	86	97,294	97,250	4,945,557	50.83
29–30	158,102	135	85.4	0.00085	83	97,207	97,166	4,848,307	49.88
30–31	157,975	134	84.8	0.00085	82	97,124	97,083	4,751,141	48.92
31–32	153,534	134	87.3	0.00087	85	97,042	97,000	4,654,058	47.96
32–33	160,016	157	98.1	0.00098	95	96,957	96,910	4,557,058	47.00
33–34	160,299	127	79.2	0.00079	77	96,862	96,824	4,460,149	46.05
34–35	125,826	144	114.4	0.00114	111	96,785	96,730	4,363,324	45.08
35–36	126,747	158	124.7	0.00125	120	96,675	96,614	4,266,594	44.13
36–37	125,960	155	123.1	0.00123	119	96,554	96,495	4,169,980	43.19
37–38	127,942	161	125.8	0.00126	121	96,436	96,375	4,073,485	42.24
38–39	109,358	169	154.5	0.00154	149	96,314	96,240	3,977,110	41.29
39–40	106,481	196	184.1	0.00184	177	96,166	96,077	3,880,870	40.36
40–41	103,828	171	164.7	0.00165	158	95,989	95,910	3,784,793	39.43
41–42	99,325	205	206.4	0.00206	198	95,831	95,732	3,688,883	38.49
42–43	96,380	228	236.6	0.00236	226	95,633	95,520	3,593,151	37.57
43–44	93,276	256	274.5	0.00274	261	95,407	95,276	3,497,631	36.66
44–45	92,873	258	277.8	0.00277	264	95,146	95,014	3,402,355	35.76
45–46	92,183	246	266.9	0.00267	253	94,882	94,755	3,307,341	34.86
46–47	88,595	274	309.3	0.00309	292	94,629	94,483	3,212,586	33.95
47–48	91,046	323	354.8	0.00354	334	94,337	94,170	3,118,103	33.05
48–49	89,588	384	428.6	0.00428	402	94,003	93,802	3,023,934	32.17
49–50	97,274	398	409.2	0.00408	382	93,601	93,409	2,930,132	31.30

50–51	98,371	449	456.4	0.00455	425	93,218	93,006	2,836,722	30.43
51–52	95,717	474	495.2	0.00494	458	92,794	92,565	2,743,716	29.57
52–53	99,570	557	559.4	0.00558	515	92,335	92,078	2,651,152	28.71
53–54	101,653	687	675.8	0.00674	618	91,820	91,511	2,559,074	27.87
54–55	105,815	675	637.9	0.00636	580	91,202	90,912	2,467,563	27.06
55–56	108,657	737	678.3	0.00676	613	90,622	90,316	2,376,651	26.23
56–57	106,689	784	734.8	0.00732	659	90,009	89,680	2,286,336	25.40
57–58	106,142	842	793.3	0.00790	706	89,350	88,997	2,196,656	24.58
58–59	107,384	929	865.1	0.00861	764	88,644	88,263	2,107,659	23.78
59–60	103,981	1,007	968.4	0.00964	847	87,881	87,457	2,019,396	22.98
60–61	97,063	964	993.2	0.00988	860	87,034	86,604	1,931,939	22.20
61–62	93,115	1,033	1109.4	0.01103	951	86,174	85,698	1,845,335	21.41
62–63	90,046	1,070	1188.3	0.01181	1,007	85,223	84,720	1,759,637	20.65
63–64	86,916	1,141	1312.8	0.01304	1,098	84,216	83,667	1,674,917	19.89
64–65	85,726	1,282	1495.5	0.01484	1,234	83,118	82,501	1,591,250	19.14
65–66	86,996	1,387	1594.3	0.01582	1,295	81,884	81,237	1,508,749	18.43
66–67	83,258	1,400	1681.5	0.01668	1,344	80,589	79,917	1,427,513	17.71
67–68	79,961	1,428	1785.9	0.01770	1,403	79,245	78,544	1,347,595	17.01
68–69	78,039	1,485	1902.9	0.01885	1,467	77,842	77,109	1,269,052	16.30
69–70	74,389	1,617	2173.7	0.02150	1,642	76,375	75,554	1,191,943	15.61
70–71	70,163	1,614	2300.4	0.02274	1,700	74,733	73,883	1,116,389	14.94
71–72	67,599	1,816	2686.4	0.02651	1,936	73,033	72,065	1,042,506	14.27
72–73	65,045	1,813	2787.3	0.02749	1,954	71,097	70,120	970,441	13.65
73–74	60,676	1,905	3139.6	0.03091	2,137	69,143	68,074	900,320	13.02
74–75	57,975	1,889	3258.3	0.03206	2,148	67,006	65,931	832,246	12.42
75–76	54,912	1,995	3633.1	0.03568	2,314	64,857	63,700	766,315	11.82
76–77	51,217	2,089	4078.7	0.03997	2,500	62,543	61,293	702,615	11.23
77–78	48,251	1,993	4130.5	0.04047	2,430	60,043	58,828	641,322	10.68
78–79	43,234	2,344	5421.7	0.05279	3,041	57,613	56,093	582,494	10.11

(Continued)

Table 10–2. California 1980 population of white males—Continued

x to x + 1	Population	Deaths	R_x^*	q_x	d_x	l_x	L_x	T_x	e_x
79–80	47,158	2,399	5087.2	0.04961	2,707	54,572	53,218	526,401	9.65
80–81	39,462	2,318	5874.0	0.05706	2,960	51,865	50,385	473,183	9.12
81–82	36,295	2,416	6656.6	0.06442	3,151	48,905	47,330	422,798	8.65
82–83	31,875	2,360	7403.9	0.07140	3,267	45,755	44,121	375,468	8.21
83–84	30,470	2,535	8319.7	0.07987	3,394	42,488	40,791	331,347	7.80
84–85	27,904	2,540	9102.6	0.08706	3,404	39,094	37,392	290,556	7.43
85–86	24,712	2,458	9946.6	0.09475	3,382	35,690	34,000	253,163	7.09
86–87	21,302	2,383	11186.7	0.10594	3,423	32,309	30,597	219,164	6.78
87–88	19,402	2,120	10926.7	0.10361	2,993	28,886	27,389	188,567	6.53
88–89	14,905	1,993	13371.4	0.12533	3,245	25,193	24,270	161,177	6.22
89–90	13,873	1,900	13695.7	0.12818	2,903	22,648	21,196	136,907	6.05
90$^+$	47,650	8,131	17064.0	1.00000	19,745	19,745	115,710	115,710	5.86

* = Rate per 100,000 person-years of risk.

Specifically, consider the age interval 65 to 66 for white males from the 1980 California data:

1. $q_{65} = \dfrac{R_{65}}{1 + 0.5R_{65}} = \dfrac{0.0284}{1 + 0.5(0.0284)} = 0.0280,$ since $R_{65} = \dfrac{2{,}097}{73{,}832} =$ 0.0284 (note: $\bar{a}_{65} = 0.5$),

2. $d_{65} = l_{65}q_{65} = 69{,}728(0.0280) = 1.953,$

3. $L_{65} = (l_{65} - d_{65}) + 0.5d_{65} = (69{,}728 - 1{,}953) + 0.5(1{,}953) = 68{,}752,$

4. $T_{65} = L_{65} + L_{66} + \cdots + L_{90+} = 68{,}752 + 66{,}757 + \cdots + 9{,}126$ $+ 41{,}616 = 1{,}011{,}356,$ and

5. $e_{65} = \dfrac{T_{65}}{l_{65}} = \dfrac{1{,}011{,}356}{69{,}728} = 14.504.$

These five steps are sequentially applied to each age interval, starting at age 0, resulting in the entire current life table from a set of mortality rates (R_x) and an arbitrary starting value (l_0).

Two complete life tables are given in Tables 10–1 and 10–2 for male and female residents of California based on mortality rates from the year 1980. The expected number of years of life remaining after age x is an effective summary of the entire mortality pattern described by a life table (e_x; last column in Tables 10–1 and 10–2). The expectation of life is no more than a special mean value and is calculated in the same way as most mean values, where

$$\text{mean years remaining} = e_x = \frac{\text{total years lived beyond age } x}{\text{number of individuals age } x} = \frac{T_x}{l_x}. \quad (10.7)$$

Perhaps the most common single summary value calculated from a life table is the expectation of life at birth (e_0). For the California data, $e_0 = 69.61$ years for males and $e_0 = 76.93$ years for females, based on 1980 mortality patterns.

Expectations of life at birth are compared among countries and among groups within a country. The U.S. life expectancy e_0 has steadily increased over the last 80 years and the difference between males and females has also increased, as Table 10–3 shows.

Table 10–3. U.S. expectation of life for white males and females (1900–80)

Year	1900	1910	1920	1930	1940	1950	1960	1970	1980
Male	46.6	48.6	54.5	59.7	62.1	66.5	67.4	68.0	70.7
Female	48.7	52.0	55.6	63.5	66.6	72.2	74.1	75.6	78.1

Source: Vital Statistics of the United States, 1983, U.S. Department of Health and Human Services.

The expectation of life has a geometric interpretation related to a survival curve. The expectation of life (e_0) is approximately equal to the area under the survival curve. In Chapter 11 this property is discussed further [expressions (11.29) and (11.30)].

Another single summary value that indicates the overall mortality pattern found in a life table is the median age at death. The median age at death is that age where half the life table population is still alive and half have died. More simply, it is that age where exactly $\frac{1}{2}l_0$ individuals are alive (dead). It is a relatively simple matter to find this median age in a life table. The l_x column is searched to find the age interval that contains $\frac{1}{2}l_0$ individuals. This interval is denoted $\tilde{x}$ to $\tilde{x} + 1$. Then, using linear interpolation (other more elegant interpolation schemes are certainly possible) gives an approximate median value of

$$\text{median} = \hat{x}_{0.5} = \tilde{x} + \frac{l_{\tilde{x}} - \frac{1}{2}l_0}{l_{\tilde{x}} - l_{\tilde{x}+1}}.$$

From the California life table (Table 10–1) for male residents in 1980, the age interval containing $\frac{1}{2}l_0 = 50{,}000$ individuals is age 73 to 74 and

$$\hat{x}_{0.5} = 73 + \frac{51{,}366 - 50{,}000}{51{,}366 - 48{,}762} = 73.525$$

is the median remaining age at death. For the females, the age interval containing the median is 80 to 81 (Table 10–2) giving

$$\hat{x}_{0.5} = 80 + \frac{51{,}865 - 50{,}000}{51{,}865 - 48{,}905} = 80.630.$$

That is, half the women experiencing the 1980 pattern of mortality will live beyond the age of 80.6 years old. Another estimate of the median is the end point of the interval containing the value $\frac{1}{2}l_0$ or, for the California data, 74 years (males) and 81 years (females).

The crude mortality rate associated with a life table is the total persons who died divided by the total number of person-years lived by the entire life table population or

$$\text{crude mortality rate} = \frac{\sum d_x}{T_0} = \frac{l_0}{T_0}. \tag{10.8}$$

The life table crude mortality rate is the reciprocal of the expectation of life at birth or

$$\text{crude mortality rate} = \frac{l_0}{T_0} = \frac{1}{e_0} \quad \text{or} \quad e_0 = \frac{1}{l_0/T_0} = \frac{1}{\text{crude mortality rate}}. \tag{10.9}$$

Referring to the life table for males (Table 10–1), the crude mortality rate is $100,000/6,960,692 = 0.0144$ or $1,437$ deaths per 100,000 person-years and $1/0.0144 = 69.607$ years of life are expected to be lived by a newborn male infant who experiences the exact 1980 age-specific mortality rates. A life table formally shows the expected relationship that survival time (average remaining lifetime) is inversely related to risk (rate of death).

Three assumptions are implicit in constructing and interpreting a life table. The life table structure assumes that the same number of births occur each year (l_0 constant). The deaths are also assumed to be randomly distributed within each interval for ages greater than four (thus resulting in $\bar{a}_x = 0.5$), and population size does not change (the number of births is equal to the number of deaths each year, and no immigration or emigration occurs). When a population conforms to these three properties, it is called a stationary population. Although stationary human populations do not exist, in many cases changes are sufficiently small so that postulating that the mortality pattern of a group has an approximately stationary structure is not unreasonable, making a life table a useful tool to describe human mortality experience.

Life Table Survival Curve

A fundamental summary statistic derived from a life table is an estimate of a survival curve (introduced in Chapter 1); that is, the probability of surviving beyond a specific point in time. In symbols, $S(x)$ represents the probability of surviving beyond age x. Two identical ways of computing $S(x)$ from a life table are:

$$S(x) = \frac{l_x}{l_0} \qquad (10.10)$$

or

$$S(x) = \sum_{i=0}^{x-1} p_i. \qquad (10.11)$$

The equivalence of these two calculations comes from the fact that

$$S(x) = \sum_{i=1}^{x-1} p_i = \frac{l_1}{l_0} \frac{l_2}{l_1} \frac{l_3}{l_2} \frac{l_4}{l_3} \cdots \cdots \frac{l_{x-1}}{l_{x-2}} \frac{l_x}{l_{x-1}} = \frac{l_x}{l_0}, \qquad (10.12)$$

because $p_i = l_{i+1}/l_i$ is the probability of surviving from age i to age $i + 1$ given that the individual is alive at the beginning of the interval. Also note that $S(0) = 1$, which is a property of survival curves in general.

The survival curves for the male (solid line) and female (dotted line)

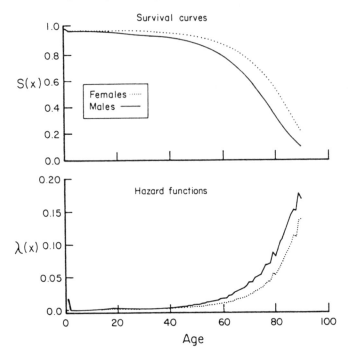

Figure 10–1. Survival curve and hazard function from the life table for white males and females, California 1980

1980 California populations are displayed in Figure 10–1 (top). A small but sharp decrease in $S(x)$ caused by high rates of infant mortality in the first year of life is followed by a slight and gradual decrease in the probability of survival until about ages 60 or 70, where the $S(x)$ curve begins to fall rapidly. This pattern is frequently observed in modern human populations. The probability of living more than 90 years is given by the values $S(90) = 0.084$ for males and $S(90) = 0.197$ for females (females are 2.4 times more likely than males to live beyond the age of 90).

Life Table Hazard Function

The slope of the survival curve or the derivative of $S(x)$ at the point x ($dS(x)/dx$) measures the impact of mortality on a population at a specific age x. The slope indicates the rate of change of the curve representing the probability of surviving beyond a particular point (intensity of mortality). To measure risk, this slope is divided by the probability of surviving beyond age x. Analogous to the definition of a mortality rate [expression (1.2)], if the instantaneous slope of the survival curve is measured relative to the proportion surviving beyond age x, then the previous definition of a hazard rate emerges, given as

$$\lambda(x) = -\frac{dS(x)/dx}{S(x)}, \tag{10.13}$$

where $\lambda(x)$ represents the hazard rate and the negative sign makes it a positive quantity. A hazard rate applied to mortality or disease data is the instantaneous rate of death, which sensitively reflects risk. Because a hazard rate is an instantaneous quantity, it must be approximated when the survival curve $S(x)$ comes from a life table.

To calculate the hazard rate from a complete life table, it is necessary to make a series of approximations to calculate this theoretical quantity. The slope of the survival curve at the midpoint of the interval x to $x + 1$ is approximately $S(x + 1) - S(x)$, and the value of the survival curve at the midpoint $x + 1/2$ is approximately $[S(x + 1) + S(x)]/2$. These two approximations are exact if the survival curve is a straight line. Combining these two quantities gives an approximate expression for the hazard rate at age $x + 1/2$ of

$$\lambda(x + 1/2) = -\frac{dS(x + 1/2)/dx}{S(x + 1/2)} \approx -\frac{S(x + 1) - S(x)}{[S(x + 1) + S(x)]/2}. \tag{10.14}$$

This expression in terms of the number of persons alive at age x (l_x) is

$$\lambda(x + 1/2) \approx -\frac{l_{x+1} - l_x}{(l_{x+1} + l_x)/2} = -2\frac{p_x - 1}{p_x + 1} = \frac{2q_x}{p_x + 1}, \tag{10.15}$$

because $S(x) = l_x/l_0$ [expression (10.10)] and $p_x = l_{x+1}/l_x$.
Since $\log(p) \approx 2(p - 1)/(p + 1)$ for $p > 0.7$, then

$$\lambda(x + 1/2) \approx -\log(p_x), \tag{10.16}$$

which provides a useful approximation of the hazard rate for life tables based on human mortality. An expression for the hazard rate at age x is the average of the hazard rates at age $x - 1/2$ and $x + 1/2$ or

$$\lambda(x) \approx \frac{-[\log(p_{x+1}) + \log(p_x)]}{2}. \tag{10.17}$$

A further simplification is achieved by using yet another approximation, because $\log(p) \approx p - 1$ for $p > 0.9$, then

$$\lambda(x + 1/2) \approx -\log(p_x) \approx q_x \tag{10.18}$$

and, as before, an approximation for the hazard rate at age x is

$$\mu(x) \approx \frac{q_{x-1} + q_x}{2} \tag{10.19}$$

for age intervals with low probabilities of death ($q_x < 0.10$). Expression (10.18) shows that a hazard rate is not very different from the conditional probability of death in a specific life table age interval when p_x is close to 1.

Another view of the hazard rate $\lambda(x + 1/2)$ comes from utilizing the fact that a hazard rate is an instantaneous age-specific rate. An average age-specific rate from a life table is

$$\text{life table mortality rate} = \frac{d_x}{l_x - 0.5d_x}. \tag{10.20}$$

For a small interval (say, one year), the age-specific life table mortality rate is approximately equal to the hazard rate at the middle of an age interval or

$$\lambda(x + 1/2) \approx \text{life table mortality rate} = \frac{d_x}{l_x - 0.5d_x}. \tag{10.21}$$

Two other versions of this expression are used. They are

$$\lambda(x + 1/2) \approx \frac{q_x}{1 - 0.5q_x} = \frac{2q_x}{p_x + 1}. \tag{10.22}$$

The last expression is the same as the previous expression for the hazard rate [expression (10.15)] derived from different considerations. Again, if d_x is small relative to l_x ($p_x \approx 1$), then $\lambda(x + 1/2) \approx q_x$. In general, an approximate life table hazard rate is

$$\lambda(x + (\tfrac{1}{2})\delta_x) = \frac{d_x}{\delta_x(l_x - 0.5d_x)}, \tag{10.23}$$

where δ_x represents the age interval length. The accuracy of this approximate expression for a hazard rate decreases as the age interval length δ_x increases.

The hazard functions (a series of hazard rates) are plotted in Figure 10–1 (bottom) for the California 1980 life tables for males and females. Detail of the mortality pattern is clearly seen from these hazard functions. For example, an inconsistency in the rise of the hazard function for the older age groups is obvious and undoubtedly due to the lack of reliability in reporting of age for older individuals (about 80 years or so).

The shape of the hazard curve observed for the 1980 California life table populations is typical of most human populations over the entire age span. After the first year of life, the next 60 years are characterized by slightly increasing hazard function followed by a sharp increase. However, hazard functions in other contexts take on a variety of shapes. A population subject to only accidental (random) deaths, for example, would have a mortality pattern with a constant hazard function (a horizontal line). A hazard function and a survival curve are related—higher rates of mortality imply lower probabilities of survival. The exact mathematical relationship is described in Chapter 12, and complete discussions are found in more technical texts on survival analysis (e.g., [2]).

Life tables can be constructed from small sets of data where q_x is estimated directly from the observed data. The principles are the same as those described, but the issue of sampling variation should not be ignored. The values q_x, l_x, etc. are estimated quantities subject to sampling variation which usually requires reporting their associated standard errors. Huge numbers of individuals make up the California life table data sets, so the precision of the estimates is not much of an issue. For a life table based on a small number of individuals, however, the variability of the estimated quantities should be taken into account. Expressions for the variances of life table estimates are based on assuming that the probabilities of death can be modeled by binomial distributions (these expressions are presented in detail elsewhere [11]).

A life table based on small numbers of observations illustrates. Eleven individuals received a special chemotherapy program for the treatment of leukemia, where the time to failure to respond is considered the "survival" time [2]. The times to remission (in weeks) are: 5, 5, 8, 8, 12, 23, 27, 30, 33, 43, 45. A life table, based on 10 week intervals, summarizing these 11 observations is given in Table 10–4.

The size of the sample used to construct this life table is small making the variability of the estimates an issue and, once again, categorizing a continuous variable (survival time) is not an ideal way to proceed. Small sets of survival data are better analyzed by other approaches (presented in Chapters 11 and 12)

Proportional Hazard Rates—An Example

An instructive application of life table properties involves an actuarial-like calculation showing the consequences of lowered hazard rates on a specific population. Suppose a hazard rate is reduced uniformly by

Table 10–4. Life table for small set of data

Interval	Midpoint	"Deaths"	Population	q_x	p_x	l_x	$S(x)$	$\lambda(x+5)$
0–10	5	4	11	0.364	0.636	1,000	1.000	0.044
10–20	15	1	7	0.143	0.857	636	0.636	0.015
20–30	25	2	6	0.333	0.667	545	0.545	0.040
30–40	35	2	4	0.500	0.500	364	0.364	0.067
40–50	45	2	2	1.000	0.000	182	0.182	0.200

a set proportion c (i.e., $\lambda(x) = c\lambda_0(x)$ where $\lambda_0(x)$ is a known or estimated hazard function). Construction of a life table based on such a hazard function describes the resulting mortality experience. Figure 10–2 (top) shows three hypothetical hazard functions based on the 1980 California, white male population mortality rates ($\lambda_0(x)$, top line), where c is set at 0.75, 0.50, and 0.25 (the next three lines). The logarithms of the hazard rates clearly show the detail of these curves (Figure 10–2, bottom). Note that the logarithms of a set of proportional hazard rates produce parallel lines. The associated life table constructed from the $c\lambda(x)$-values describes the impact of the lower hazard rates.

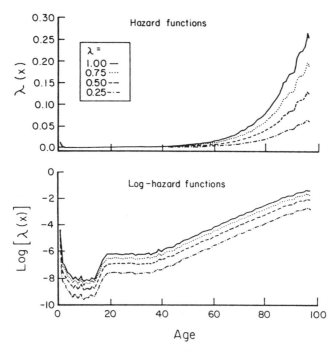

Figure 10–2. Hazard functions and the logarithm of the hazard functions for three hypothetical patterns of mortality based on the white, male mortality rate, California 1980

Table 10–5. Influence of three hypothetical hazard rates on the 1980 California male population

Hazard	$\% \geq 65$ Years*	$\% \geq 75$ Years*	$\% \geq 85$ Years*	Expectation (e_0)
$1.00*\lambda$	69.7	46.0	18.3	69.6
$0.75*\lambda$	78.8	58.7	30.0	74.7
$0.50*\lambda$	85.3	70.2	45.1	79.8
$0.25*\lambda$	92.3	83.8	67.4	87.4

* $= \% \geq x$ Years is $100 \times S(x)$.

That is, $c\lambda(x)$ produces a series of q_x-values which in turn produce the rest of the life table functions allowing a complete description of the three hypothetical populations.

To summarize the life tables constructed from the three reduced hazard functions, the proportion of individuals alive at ages 65, 75, and 85 years $(S(x) = $ survival probabilities) along with the expected length of life at birth $(e_0$-values) for the "proportional populations" are shown in Table 10–5.

It is unlikely that a decrease in mortality would be exactly proportional throughout the life span (i.e., proportional hazards rates); nevertheless some idea of the impact of decreasing mortality risk is gained by life table summary values. The percentage of older individuals increases strikingly as age-specific mortality decreases. For example, about 46% of the 1980 California males are older than 75 years, but, when the mortality is reduced by a factor of 4 $(c = 0.25)$, this value increases to an estimated 84%. The expected length of life at birth is correspondingly increased about 18 years from 69.6 to 87.4 years.

The effects on a population from changes in a hazard rate are not always clear. As the illustration shows, a hazard rate is frequently related to more easily interpreted measures of risk using life table summaries. A decrease in a hazard rate becomes a less abstract expression of risk when translated, for example, into an increase in the number of individuals exceeding a specific age or into an increase in the expected years of remaining life.

LIFE TABLES: THREE APPLICATIONS OF LIFE TABLE TECHNIQUES

Life Table Method for Calculating a Survival Probability from Follow-Up Data

The evaluation of a treatment for a chronic disease usually involves the assessment of survival times or, perhaps, remission times. The probability of surviving five years after receiving treatment is a frequent measure of the efficacy of a drug or surgical procedure. Survival data are often collected and recorded over a period of time, forming a series of cohorts (one for each year of follow-up, for example). This follow-up pattern of data collection allows an efficient estimate of the five-year survival probability or, in general, an estimate of the survival curve associated with the sampled population. A set of follow-up data [3] concerning the survival of six cohorts of kidney cancer patients illustrates (Table 10–6).

A complete display of the data set is presented to show the cohorts formed as each year new patients are added to the sample. The symbol x denotes the years survived after the kidney cancer is diagnosed. The column labeled l_x, contains the count of the individuals alive at the beginning of the time interval x to $x + 1$. The number of deaths in each interval is represented by d_x. The possibility exists that patients are "lost to follow-up" during the time period covered by the study. The count of patients lost during an interval is symbolized by u_x. The last column in the table contains the counts of the patients withdrawn from study (denoted w_x). Individuals are said to be withdrawn when they are no longer relevant to further calculations. For example,

Table 10–6. Calculation of a survival probability: data

Year	x to $x + 1$	l_x	d_x	u_x	w_x
1946	0–1	9	4	1	—
	1–2	4	0	0	—
	2–3	4	0	0	—
	3–4	4	0	0	—
	4–5	4	0	0	—
	5–6	4	0	0	4
1947	0–1	18	7	0	—
	1–2	11	0	0	—
	2–3	11	1	0	—
	3–4	10	2	2	—
	4–5	6	0	0	6
1948	0–1	21	11	0	—
	1–2	10	1	2	—
	2–3	7	0	0	—
	3–4	7	0	0	7
1949	0–1	34	12	0	—
	1–2	22	3	3	—
	2–3	16	1	0	15
1950	0–1	19	5	1	—
	1–2	13	1	1	11
1951	0–1	25	8	2	15

consider the 1950 cohort of 19 patients. Five patients died the first year and one the second year; two were lost (one each year), and the remaining 11 individuals produced information about the first and second year of survival but no information about the third year or beyond, because they were only observed for a maximum of two years. The 11 ($w_2 = 11$) remaining members of this cohort alive at the end of the second year are said to be withdrawn after two years, because they do not contribute to subsequent calculations. They either survived or died after 1951, but this information is not part of the collected data. All that is known about individuals withdrawn is that they were alive at the closing date of the study. The times of these four possible events (l_x, d_x, u_x, and w_x) are tabulated by year for the kidney cancer follow-up data (Table 10–6). A summary table that combines the survival experience of all kidney cancer patients for the six cohorts is given in Table 10–7. The number of individuals who are at risk at the beginning of the interval l_{x+1} result from what has occurred in the previous interval (d_x, u_x, and w_x) or

$$l_{x+1} = l_x - d_x - u_x - w_x. \tag{10.24}$$

If the entire cohort was entered into the study on the first day and followed for at least five years and no one was lost, then the estimated five-year kidney cancer survival probability would be the number who lived more than five years divided by the number who started the study. For most survival data, however, individuals enter the study at different times during the study period. The fact that the data are collected sequentially makes it necessary to piece together the follow-up information.

It is also likely that during the course of collecting a set of follow-up data, individuals will die from causes other than the one being investigated. Somewhat pragmatically, these individuals are usually classified as lost (i.e., u_x is increased) which introduces no bias if these deaths are completely unrelated to the disease under study.

Table 10–7. Calculation of a survival probability from tabled data: summary data

x to $x + 1$	l_x	d_x	u_x	w_x
0–1	126	47	4	15
1–2	60	5	6	11
2–3	38	2	0	15
3–4	21	2	2	7
4–5	10	0	0	6
5–6	4	0	0	4

Notice that 15 individuals in the 1951 cohort were withdrawn after one year. If the exact time these patients were observed was known, then the total person-years of risk would be the sum of their observed individual survival times. When this information is not available, estimates of survival time should be adjusted to compensate for the incomplete nature of the data on withdrawn individuals. One approach is to assume that each person withdrawn during an interval, on the average, contributes one-half an interval of time $(\bar{a}_x = 0.5)$ to the total survival time. That is, it is postulated that individuals come into the study randomly throughout the follow-up period, implying they are withdrawn randomly from observation. If this is the case, then attributing one-half an interval's time to each person withdrawn is "on the average" correct. A similar assumption is usually made about individuals lost from follow-up. That is, individuals are lost at random from follow-up and contribute an average of 0.5 years of observation during the year they were lost. An estimate of the probability of death (q_x) that accounts for the two sources of incomplete information is made by reducing the number of persons beginning the interval (l_x) to compensate for those individuals lost (u_x) and withdrawn (w_x) during the interval. Specifically,

$$l'_x = l_x - 0.5u_x - 0.5w_x, \tag{10.25}$$

where l'_x is called the "effective" number of persons at risk in the interval, and the probability of death within an interval is then estimated by

$$q_x = \frac{d_x}{l'_x}. \tag{10.26}$$

The adjusted persons at risk (l'_x) better reflects the underlying situation.

An alternate view of this adjustment comes from noting that the observed number of deaths is understated since lost and withdrawn individuals are not followed for, on the average, half an interval. Deaths occurring among these individuals during that time will not be recorded. An estimate of the additional number of "missing deaths" is $0.5(u_x + w_x)q_x$. Adding these "deaths" to the number of observed deaths gives an estimate of the probability of death as

$$q_x = \frac{d_x + 0.5(u_x + w_x)q_x}{l_x}, \tag{10.27}$$

and solving for q_x produces the same result as before (i.e., $q_x = d_x/l'_x$). Employing the value q_x to estimate the proportion of deaths among those who were lost or withdrawn implies that these individuals do not differ in their mortality experience from those who continued to be followed. This assumption may not be tenable in some situations. For example, it might be that lost individuals are more likely to have survived or, perhaps, more likely to have died; a suitable q_x should be used under these conditions. A more subtle implication of employing l'_x is the implicit assumption that mortality experience is unrelated to the probability that an individual is withdrawn from follow-up.

Analogous to the life table calculation of a survival curve, the survival probabilities are

$$\hat{P}_x = \prod_{x=0}^{k-1} p_x, \tag{10.28}$$

where, as before, $p_x = 1 - q_x$. The value $\hat{P}_k$ is the probability of surviving beyond the kth time interval. Applying these estimates to the kidney cancer data gives Table 10–8. The estimated five-year survival probability is $\hat{P}_5 = (0.597) \times (0.903) \times (0.934) \times (0.879) \times (1.000) = 0.442$ (standard error $= 0.060$). The variance of these estimates comes from the expression

$$\text{variance}(\hat{P}_k) = \hat{P}_k^2 \sum_{x=0}^{k-1} \frac{q_x}{l'_x p_x}. \tag{10.29}$$

This variance estimate is often referred to as "Greenwood's formula" after Major M. Greenwood, an early contributor to biostatistics. As usual, an estimate of the variance is necessary to test hypotheses or construct confidence intervals for specific estimated survival probabilities.

Another estimate of the five-year survival probability is the number of individuals who survived more than five years divided by those who began the study at least five years previously. Only the 1946 cohort can be used to estimate this five-year survival probability, because the other cohorts contain individuals with less than five years of follow-up time. The five-year survival probability is $4/9 = 0.444$ with a standard

Table 10–8. Calculation of a five-year survival rate from tabled data: calculations

Interval	d_x	l'_x	q_x	p_x	$\hat{P}_x$	$\prod p_x$	Std. Error
0–1	47	116.5	0.403	0.597	$\hat{P}_0$	1.000	—
1–2	5	51.5	0.097	0.903	$\hat{P}_1$	0.597	0.045
2–3	2	30.5	0.066	0.934	$\hat{P}_2$	0.539	0.048
3–4	2	16.5	0.121	0.879	$\hat{P}_3$	0.503	0.051
4–5	0	7.0	0.000	1.000	$\hat{P}_4$	0.442	0.060
5–6	0	2.0	0.000	1.000	$\hat{P}_5$	0.442	0.060

error of 0.166 (assuming the lost individual survived). Using all available data rather than a single cohort produces a more precise estimate of the five-year survival probability (ratio of standard errors = $0.166/0.060 = 2.7$ in the kidney cancer example). However, the cost of this increased precision is possible bias from the assumption that the mortality experience over time is similar enough among cohorts that combining data for all years reflects the overall mortality experience of the sampled population.

Another important summary of survival data is an estimate of the mean survival time. This calculation is complicated by the fact that the time of death is not known for all participating individuals. For the data recorded on the 126 kidney cancer patients, the mean survival time is 3.523 years. Mean survival-time calculations are discussed in Chapter 11.

Survival patterns experienced by different groups can be summarized and compared using specific survival probabilities. Two such groups from the WCGS data are those with high values of the body-mass index (greater than the 75th percentile) and those with smaller body-mass values (less than the 75th percentile). The data and the calculated "survival" probabilities (here "survival" means time free from a coronary event) are given in Tables 10–9 and 10–10.

The comparison of these probabilities shows a lower probability (higher risk) of "survival" for those individuals with a high body-mass index. For example, the five-year survival probability of $\hat{P}_5 = 0.940$ for high values of body-mass index is less than the $\hat{P}'_5 = 0.961$ observed for individuals with "normal" values of the body-mass index. The standard errors for these estimates indicate that this difference is not likely to have occurred by chance variation (i.e., the confidence intervals only slightly overlap). For the greater than 75th percentile

Table 10–9. WCGS data: the body-mass greater than the 75th percentile

x to $x+1$	l_x	d_x	w_x	q_x	$\hat{P}_x$	Std. Error
0–1	871	6	0	0.0069	1.000	—
1–2	865	8	21	0.0094	0.993	0.0028
2–3	836	16	19	0.0194	0.984	0.0043
3–4	801	9	23	0.0114	0.965	0.0063
4–5	769	11	14	0.0144	0.954	0.0072
5–6	744	12	19	0.0163	0.940	0.0082
6–7	713	18	46	0.0261	0.925	0.0092
7–8	649	9	195	0.0163	0.901	0.0106
8–9	445	5	431	0.0218	0.886	0.0115
9–10	9	0	9	0.0000	0.867	0.0141

Table 10–10. WCGS data: the body-mass less than the 75th percentile

x to x + 1	l_x	d_x	w_x	q_x	$\hat{P}_x$	Std. Error
0–1	2,283	9	4	0.0039	1.000	—
1–2	2,270	20	24	0.0089	0.996	0.0013
2–3	2,226	23	50	0.0104	0.987	0.0024
3–4	2,153	18	41	0.0084	0.977	0.0032
4–5	2,094	18	37	0.0087	0.967	0.0037
5–6	2,039	27	61	0.0134	0.961	0.0042
6–7	1,951	14	99	0.0074	0.947	0.0048
7–8	1,838	22	502	0.0139	0.940	0.0051
8–9	1,314	12	1,271	0.0177	0.927	0.0057
9–10	31	0	31	0.0000	0.911	0.0073

group the approximate 95% confidence interval based on $\hat{P}_5 = 0.940$ is (0.924, 0.956), and for the less than 75th percentile group the confidence interval based on $\hat{P}_5 = 0.961$ is (0.953, 0.969). Figure 10–3 is a plot of these two sets of survival probabilities.

The WCGS follow-up times are recorded exactly (to the nearest day) so the probability that a coronary event does not occur ("survival") can be calculated without assumptions about the individuals lost or withdrawn during the follow-up period. Instead of using 0.5 years of

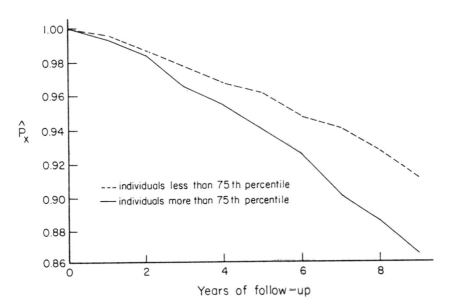

Figure 10–3. Survival probabilities for individuals with a body-mass index less than and greater than the 75th percentile (WCGS data)

risk, the exact total time contributed by individuals lost or withdrawn can be calculated and directly produces the exact "effective" number of persons at risk. The difference between the exact and approximate approaches is inconsequential. The nine-year probability using the exact follow-up times is 0.869 for individuals with body-mass indexes in the upper quartile and 0.913 for the "normal" body-mass individuals, compared to the approximate $(\bar{a}_x = 0.5)$ values 0.867 and 0.911, respectively. In other study settings, however, individuals lost or withdrawn from follow-up may have different experiences, necessitating careful selection of an adjustment method when exact values are not available.

Three assumptions about the structure of the sampled population are made to calculate a survival curve using life table techniques. First, all lost and withdrawn subjects are assumed to contribute, on the average, half the survival information of an individual followed for a complete year (or complete time interval). Second, the data collected for a number of cohorts are combined to maximize the number of observations available in each time interval to calculate the probability of death. To give an unbiased estimate of survival probabilities, all cohorts must experience the same pattern of mortality during the follow-up period (again, the absence of interaction permits the data to be summarized). In terms of the kidney cancer data, the individuals who entered the study in 1947, for example, are assumed to have the same pattern of mortality as the patients who entered in 1951, which allows the data from both groups to be used in the calculation of the probability of surviving the first year after diagnosis. The third assumption is that the lost and withdrawn individuals have the same probability of death as the individuals remaining in the follow-up data set. This conjecture is probably the most tenuous when applied to individuals lost from observation. Situations certainly arise where other assumptions make sense. For example, if it is assumed that all individuals classified as lost actually survived, then

$$q'_x = \frac{d_x + 0.5 w_x q'_x}{l'_x} \quad \text{or} \quad q'_x = \frac{d_x}{l_x - 0.5 w_x} \tag{10.30}$$

or, if all individuals lost in fact died, then

$$q''_x = \frac{d_x + 0.5(u_x + w_x q''_x)}{l_x} \quad \text{or} \quad q''_x = \frac{d_x + 0.5 u_x}{l_x - 0.5 w_x}. \tag{10.31}$$

The probabilities q'_x and q''_x represent the extremes in terms of the impact of the lost individuals on the calculation of the probability of death. These two extremes applied to the kidney cancer data yield five-year survival probabilities of $\hat{P}'_5 = 0.454$ if all lost patients survive and $\hat{P}''_5 = 0.387$ if all lost patients die, where $\hat{P}_5 = 0.442$ when individuals are assumed to be lost at random from follow-up. The range 0.387 to 0.454 provides limits to the potential bias caused by differences in survival between individuals lost and individuals not lost to follow-up.

Life Table Measures of Specific Causes of Death

Hundreds of causes of death act simultaneously within human populations. Two approaches based on life table methods provide an opportunity to isolate the individual impact of specific causes on the pattern of human mortality. These methods help resolve two questions:

1. What is the age structure throughout the life span associated with a specific cause of death, taking into account other causes?
2. How does the probability of death from a specific cause change when other causes are "eliminated" from the population?

The first question is answered by applying a multiple-cause life table (also called a multiple-decrement life table). The second question is addressed by a competing risk analysis.

Multiple-Cause Life Table

A multiple-cause life table is similar to the single cause life table but describes simultaneously the mortality patterns of a number of diseases in a population. The goal of such a table is to organize and display the age structure of individuals dying of specific causes. The mechanics of constructing these age distributions are defined and illustrated by a set of data consisting of California resident males who died during 1980. The causes of death come from death certificates, classified according to the ninth revision of the International Classification of Diseases (ICD9) [4]. These deaths are classified into four categories: death from lung cancer (ICD9, code 162), deaths from ischemic heart disease (ICD9, codes 410 to 414), deaths from motor vehicle accidents (ICD9, codes E810 to E819), and deaths from all other causes. Also necessary is a series of age-specific population counts—the 1980 U.S. Census counts of California male residents are used. The following life table construction is abridged, which means that the lengths of the age intervals are not consistently one year. Most age intervals are five-year lengths (represented as δ_x; for example, $\delta_{60} = 5$ years). Although the example uses five-year age intervals, a life table can be organized into intervals of any lengths, even varying lengths. Regardless of the choice of the interval length, the principles of constructing a life table remain unchanged—clearly some technical details differ.

The basic components required to construct a multiple-cause life table are the age-specific midyear populations and the age-, cause-specific numbers of deaths. That is,

D_x = total number of deaths in the age interval x to $x + \delta_x$,

$D_x^{(i)}$ = number of deaths from i^{th} cause in the age interval x to $x + \delta_x$, and

P_x = total number of individuals at risk ages x to $x + \delta_x$ at midyear.

These quantities for male residents of California (1980) are given in Table 10–11.

Average age-specific mortality rates calculated from Table 10–11 are $R_x = D_x/P_x$ for the age interval x to $x + \delta_x$ and, similar to the single-cause, complete life table,

$$q_x = \frac{\delta_x R_x}{1 + 0.5\delta_x R_x} \tag{10.32}$$

Table 10–11. Deaths from four causes: California, males, 1980

	P_x	$D_x^{(1)}$	$D_x^{(2)}$	$D_x^{(3)}$	$D_x^{(4)}$	D_x
Age	Population	Lung Cancer	IHD*	Motor*	All Other	Total
0–1	193,310	1	2	3	2,507	2,513
1–4	515,150	1	3	58	375	437
5–9	843,750	0	2	90	195	287
10–14	915,240	0	1	80	248	329
15–19	1,091,684	3	1	523	1,162	1,689
20–24	1,213,068	4	6	965	1,507	2,482
25–29	1,132,811	3	13	627	1,665	2,308
30–34	1,008,606	12	63	437	1,547	2,059
35–39	776,545	36	136	277	1,371	1,820
40–44	629,452	85	306	201	1,510	2,102
45–49	578,420	225	567	197	2,115	3,104
50–54	578,795	445	1,050.	150	3,163	4,808
55–59	573,119	786	1,807	147	4,663	7,403
60–64	467,607	1,059	2,528	129	5,603	9,319
65–69	378,259	1,297	3,328	97	7,014	11,736
70–74	269,849	1,266	3,815	89	7,423	12,593
75–79	175,580	941	3,793	99	7,508	12,341
80–84	95,767	557	3,452	44	6,202	10,255
85+	78,832	430	5,249	61	8,222	13,962
Total	11,515,844	7,151	26,122	4,274	64,000	101,547

*IDH = Ischemic heart disease; Motor = Motor vehicle accidents.

is the conditional probability of death within the interval x to $x + \delta_x$, where δ_x is the length of the interval starting at age x. These probabilities are an extension of those calculated in the single-cause life table [expression (10.4)] applied to age intervals with length of δ_x years. For example, the probability of death for individuals age 60 before age 65 is

$$q_{60} = \frac{5(0.0199)}{1 + 0.5(5)0.0199} = 0.0949, \quad \text{where} \quad R_{60} = \frac{9.319}{467,607} = 0.0199.$$

$$(10.33)$$

To "fine tune" these calculations, the 0.5 in the denominator is sometimes replaced by better values of the average time lived by those who died. Values other than 0.5, generally, have little impact on the final calculations for data covering the entire life span.

To compute the cause-specific conditional probabilities of death, the q_x values are distributed proportionally (prorated) by the observed numbers of death. Since

$$q_x^{(i)} = \frac{\delta_x D_x^{(i)}}{P_x + 0.5\delta_x D_x} \quad \text{and} \quad q_x = \frac{\delta_x D_x}{P_x + 0.5\delta_x D_x}, \quad (10.34)$$

then

$$q_x^{(i)} = \frac{D_x^{(i)}}{D_x} q_x. \quad (10.35)$$

The values $q_x^{(i)}$ is the age-, cause-specific conditional probability of death for cause i before age $x + \delta_x$ for those individuals alive at age x. Continuing the illustration for the age interval 60 to 65, the probability of dying from lung cancer before age 65 for individuals age 60 is

$$q_{60}^{(\text{lung})} = \frac{1,059}{9,319} 0.0949 = 0.0108. \quad (10.36)$$

These conditional probabilities for the illustrative data are given in Table 10–12.

Since all causes of death are included, $q_x = \sum q_x^{(i)}$. The $q_x^{(i)}$ probabilities calculated from the California mortality data indicate that the cause-specific conditional probabilities for lung cancer $(q_x^{(1)})$ increase rapidly after age 40 until about age 70 and then increase less rapidly in the older ages. The probabilities for ischemic heart disease $(q_x^{(2)})$ also increase sharply at about age 70 but are generally associated with older individuals (shifted to the right). The conditional probabilities describing deaths from motor vehicle accidents $(q_x^{(3)})$, however, increase until ages 20 to 25, decrease and remain fairly constant until age 70, where they again sharply increase. The cause-specific probability

Table 10–12. Conditional probabilities: California, males, 1980

Age	q_x Total	$q_x^{(1)}$ Lung Cancer	$q_x^{(2)}$ IDH	$q_x^{(3)}$ Motor	$q_x^{(4)}$ All Others
0–1	0.01292	0.00001	0.00001	0.00002	0.01289
1–4	0.00339	0.00001	0.00002	0.00045	0.00291
5–9	0.00170	0.00000	0.00001	0.00053	0.00115
10–14	0.00180	0.00000	0.00001	0.00044	0.00135
15–19	0.00771	0.00001	0.00000	0.00239	0.00530
20–24	0.01018	0.00002	0.00002	0.00396	0.00618
25–29	0.01014	0.00001	0.00006	0.00275	0.00731
30–34	0.01016	0.00006	0.00031	0.00216	0.00763
35–39	0.01165	0.00023	0.00087	0.00177	0.00878
40–44	0.01656	0.00067	0.00241	0.00158	0.01190
45–49	0.02648	0.00192	0.00484	0.00168	0.01804
50–54	0.04069	0.00377	0.00889	0.00127	0.02677
55–59	0.06256	0.00664	0.01527	0.00124	0.03941
60–64	0.09492	0.01079	0.02575	0.00131	0.05707
65–69	0.14397	0.01591	0.04082	0.00119	0.08604
70–74	0.20896	0.02101	0.06330	0.00148	0.12317
75–79	0.29891	0.02279	0.09187	0.00240	0.18185
80–84	0.42235	0.02294	0.14217	0.00181	0.25543
85+	1.00000	0.03080	0.37595	0.00437	0.58888

curves for these three causes of death are shown in Figure 10–4 (smoothed). As before, these curves are estimates of the hazard function associated with each specific cause of death.

Again parallel to the single-cause life table, an arbitrary number of individuals (l_0) can be distributed according to the conditional probabilities of death to produce the distribution of the number of life table "deaths" for a population with a pattern of age-specific mortality described by the $q_x^{(i)}$-values. The cohort constructed from the California data is shown in Table 10–13.

The life table deaths (Table 10–13) result from applying the relationship

$$d_x^{(i)} = l_x q_x^{(i)} \tag{10.37}$$

where, as before, l_x represents the number of persons alive at the beginning of age interval x. For example, the number of persons age 60 who die from lung cancer between age 60 to 65 is

$$d_{60}^{(\text{lung})} = 802{,}800(0.0108) = 8{,}659.$$

An additional table calculated by accumulating the deaths in each cause-specific category is also a useful description of the life table

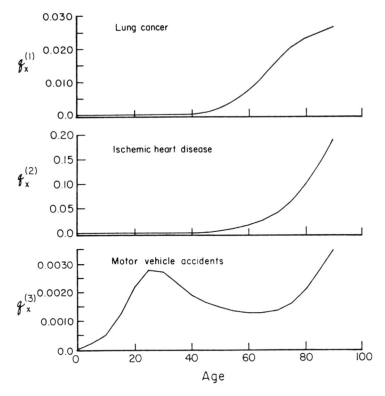

Figure 10–4. Cause-specific probabilities of death for three specific diseases (lung cancer, ischemic heart disease and motor vehicle accidents) for California, males, 1980

population. These sums represent the number of individuals who reach age x and will ultimately die of a specific cause. In symbols,

$$W_x^{(i)} = d_x^{(i)} + d_{x+\delta_x}^{(i)} + \cdots + d_{x'}^{(i)}. \qquad (10.38)$$

To illustrate,

$$W_{60}^{(\text{lung})} = 8,659 + 11,560 + \cdots + 7,913 + 6,137 = 58,550$$

is the number of individuals who reach age 60 and eventually die of lung cancer. Again from the California data, these accumulated life table deaths are given in Table 10–14.

The cumulative numbers of deaths provide the values necessary to calculate the probability of death before age x for each cause. That is, for the ith cause

$$F_x^{(i)} = 1 - \frac{W_x^{(i)}}{W_0^{(i)}} \qquad (10.39)$$

Table 10–13. Life table "deaths" from four causes: California, males, 1980

Age	l_x Total	$d_x^{(1)}$ Lung Cancer	$d_x^{(2)}$ IHD	$d_x^{(3)}$ Motor	$d_x^{(4)}$ All Other
0–1	1,000,000	5	10	15	12,885
1–4	987,084	8	23	444	2,869
5–9	983,740	0	12	524	1,136
10–14	982,069	0	5	429	1,329
15–19	980,305	13	4	2,339	5,197
20–24	972,751	16	24	3,849	6,012
25–29	962,850	13	55	2,651	7,040
30–34	953,091	56	296	2,054	7,272
35–39	943,412	217	821	1,673	8,280
40–44	932,421	624	2,248	1,476	11,091
45–49	916,982	1,760	4,435	1,541	16,543
50–54	892,703	3,362	7,933	1,133	23,896
55–59	856,379	5,689	13,078	1,064	33,748
60–64	802,800	8,659	20,671	1,055	45,814
65–60	726,601	11,560	29,663	865	62,517
70–74	621,996	13,066	39,374	919	76,611
75–79	492,026	11,214	45,203	1,180	89,476
80–84	344,954	7,913	49,042	625	88,111
85+	199,263	6,137	74,913	871	117,343

Table 10–14. Expected number of life table deaths after age x: California, males, 1980

Age	$W_x^{(1)}$ Lung Cancer	$W_x^{(2)}$ IHD	$W_x^{(3)}$ Motor	$W_x^{(4)}$ All Other
0–1	70,313	287,809	24,707	617,171
1–4	70,308	287,799	24,691	604,285
5–9	70,301	287,776	24,238	601,416
10–14	70,301	287,765	23,723	600,280
15–19	70,301	287,759	23,295	598,951
20–24	70,287	287,755	20,955	593,754
25–29	70,271	287,731	17,106	587,742
30–34	70,259	287,676	14,455	580,702
35–39	70,202	287,380	12,401	573,430
40–44	69,985	286,558	10,728	565,151
45–49	69,360	284,311	9,251	554,059
50–54	67,601	279,876	7,711	537,516
55–59	64,239	271,943	6,577	513,620
60–64	58,550	258,865	5,513	479,872
65–69	49,891	238,194	4,459	434,058
70–74	38,330	208,531	3,594	371,540
75–79	25,264	169,157	2,676	294,929
80–84	14,050	123,955	1,496	205,454
85+	6,137	74,913	871	117,343

is the probability of dying before age x. Among individuals dying of lung cancer, the probability of dying before age 60 is

$$F_{60}^{(\text{lung})} = 1 - \frac{58{,}550}{70{,}313} = 0.1673, \tag{10.40}$$

or about 17% of the lung cancer deaths occur before age 60. Table 10–15 shows the cumulative probabilities of death ($F_x^{(i)}$ probabilities) for the California 1980 data.

The age structure for each cause of death throughout the life span is apparent from the F_x probabilities, and the patterns for separate causes of death can be contrasted. For example, 78% of all motor vehicle accident deaths occur by age 60, while 17% of lung cancer deaths occur before age 60. These cumulative distributions are shown in Figure 10–5, and a few representative summary values are given in Table 10–16.

The cumulative distributions reveal distinct patterns of mortality associated with three specific causes. Motor vehicle accidents, expectedly, have the greatest impact at the younger ages (median age of death = 36.40) while, perhaps less expectedly, the ischemic heart

Table 10–15. Cumulative distributions for four causes of death: California, males, 1980

Age	$F_x^{(1)}$ Lung Cancer	$F_x^{(2)}$ IHD	$F_x^{(3)}$ Motor	$F_x^{(4)}$ All Other
0–1	0.00000	0.00000	0.00000	0.00000
1–4	0.00007	0.00004	0.00062	0.02088
5–9	0.00018	0.00012	0.01859	0.02553
10–14	0.00018	0.00016	0.03980	0.02737
15–19	0.00018	0.00017	0.05716	0.02952
20–24	0.00037	0.00019	0.15184	0.03794
25–29	0.00060	0.00027	0.30764	0.04768
30–34	0.00078	0.00046	0.41494	0.05909
35–39	0.00158	0.00149	0.49809	0.07087
40–44	0.00467	0.00435	0.56580	0.08429
45–49	0.01355	0.01216	0.62555	0.10226
50–54	0.03858	0.02757	0.68792	0.12906
55–59	0.08640	0.00513	0.73379	0.16778
60–64	0.16730	0.10057	0.77685	0.22246
65–69	0.29045	0.17239	0.81954	0.29670
70–74	0.45486	0.27545	0.85453	0.39799
75–79	0.64069	0.41226	0.89181	0.52213
80–84	0.80018	0.56932	0.93946	0.66710
85+	0.91272	0.73971	0.96476	0.80987

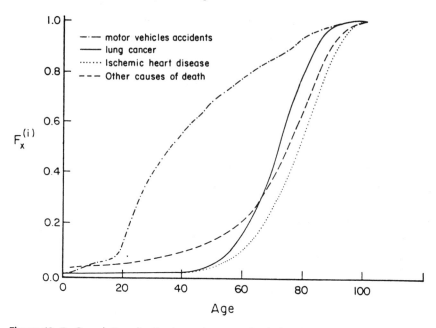

Figure 10–5. Cumulative distributions of age at death for three specific diseases (lung cancer, ischemic heart disease and motor vehicle accidents) for California, males, 1980

disease is associated with older ages, producing a median age at death of 78.8 years.

Lifetime Probability of Death

A multiple-cause life table allows a direct calculation of the lifetime probability of death from a specific cause, which is occasionally a useful summary of risk. The probability of dying of a specific cause is calculated by the number of people who died of that cause divided by the number of persons who could have died (those at risk). The table of the expected numbers of deaths after a specific age contains this information (Table 10–14). The first row in the table contains the

Table 10–16. Median age (as well as 25th and 75th percentiles) at death

	25th Percentile	Median	75th Percentile
Lung cancer	64.45	71.98	78.77
Ischemic heart disease	69.34	78.82	86.40
Motor vehicle accidents	24.20	36.40	58.09
Other causes	63.16	75.03	83.79
All causes	63.37	74.64	83.86

total number of individuals ultimately dying from each cause over the entire life span. Since 1,000,000 males make up the 1980 California life table "population at risk" (sum of the first row of Table 10–14), then

P(dying from lung cancer) = 70,313/1,000,000 = 0.070

P(dying from ischemic heart disease) = 287,809/1,000,000 = 0.288

P(dying from motor vehicle accident) = 24,707/1,000,000 = 0.025

P(dying from other causes) = 617,170/1,000,000 = 0.617

are the lifetime probabilities of dying from any one of the three specific causes.

Each row in the table allows the calculation of the lifetime probability associated with individuals of a specific age. For example, for males age 60, the lifetime probability of dying of lung cancer is 58,550/ 802,800 = 0.073, where 802,800 individuals are alive at the beginning of the age interval 60–65 (the sum of the row age 60–65 of Table 10–14) and 58,550 is the number who died of lung cancer after age 60. Three cause-specific conditional probabilities for the 1980 California data are:

P(dying from lung cancer after age 60) = 58,550/802,800 = 0.073

P(dying from ischemic heart disease after age 60) = 258,865/802,800 = 0.322

P(dying from motor vehicle accident after age 60) = 5,513/802,800 = 0.007

P(dying from other causes after age 60) = 479,872/802,800 = 0.598.

The cumulative probability of death from a multiple-cause life table is related to the lifetime probability of death from a specific cause. The probability $1 - F_x^{(i)}$ is the conditional probability of death after age x among those who ultimately die of cause i. The lifetime probability of death from a specific cause i is the conditional probability of death from cause i for all individuals who reach age x. That is, the first probability is P(death after age x|death from cause i), and the second is P(death from cause i|death after age x). Specifically, $1 - F_{60}^{(\text{lung})} = P$(death after 60|death from lung cancer) = 58,550/70,313 = 0.833 and P(death from lung cancer|death after 60) = 58,550/802,800 = 0.073.

Competing Risks

British statistician William Farr (1875) was among the first to discuss the impact on the risk of one disease from other risks operating in the studied population. This problem was also explored by the early French mathematicians Bernoulli and D'Alembert and later by a British actuary Makeham. The issues are neatly summarized by the following simple example given by J. Berkson and L. Elveback [5]:

> Two marksmen shoot at a range of targets under conditions in which, if a target is struck, it instantly drops from view so that it cannot be struck again. Represent the striking rate of marksman 1, that is the probability of a hit when he is firing alone, as Q_1 and similarly the rate of marksman 2 when he is firing alone as Q_2. The probability when one risk operates alone is called the net risk or rate and is represented by upper case Q; when it operates together with another risk it is called the crude risk or rate and is represented by lower case q.
>
> Suppose N targets are exposed and marksman 1 shoots first, followed by marksman 2:
> Rate for 1 is $q_1 = Q_1$
> Rate for 2 is $q_2 = (1 - Q_1)Q_2$
> Total rate is $q = q_1 + q_2 = Q_1 + Q_2 - Q_1 Q_2$
> Suppose marksman 2 shoots first, followed by marksman 1, then:
> Rate for 2 is $q_2 = Q_2$
> Rate for 1 is $q_1 = (1 - Q_2)Q_1$
> Total rate is $q = q_1 + q_2 = Q_1 + Q_2 - Q_1 Q_2$.

It is seen that the total crude rate with both marksmen shooting is the same, whichever marksman shoots first and assuming independence of the net probabilities Q_1 and Q_2, this will be true in general. Regardless of the ordering of the shooting or whether the two marksmen shoot together, the total crude rate is given by the "total rate," which, of course, can be derived as the complement of the product of the probabilities, $P_1 = 1 - Q_1$ and $P_2 = 1 - Q_2$, of not being struck (survival rate).

If, from independent trials, we know Q_1, the net rate of marksman 1, and have a record of q, the crude rate when both shot together, we can derive the net rate Q_2 from "total rate":

$$Q_2 = \frac{q - Q_1}{1 - Q_1}. \tag{10.41}$$

Rarely are the net probabilities Q_1 or Q_2 known, but rather, the crude probabilities q_1, q_2, and q can be estimated from collected data. Manipulation of these crude probabilities, under specific conditions, allows estimation of the net probabilities from observed data.

The following discussion of competing risks is focused on only two causes of death and only a single age interval is considered. These two assumptions do not affect the principles underlying the competing risk argument (mathematicians say, "there is no loss of generality") and simplify the notation.

The formal definitions of the two central probabilities are:

Crude probability: q_i = the probability an individual who is alive at the start of the interval dies from cause i in the presence of cause j, sometimes called the mixed probability of death.

Net probability: Q_i = the probability an individual who is alive at the start of the interval dies from cause i when cause j is not present, sometimes called the pure probability of death

The marksman example shows a relationship between the net and crude probabilities [expression (10.41)], but it is not much use unless one of the net probabilities is known. To estimate the net probabilities, further statistical structure is needed. First, assume that the net probabilities are described by two exponential functions, where λ_1 and λ_2 are hazard rates associated with causes 1 and 2, respectively. The exponential model applied to survival analysis is explored in more detail in the next chapter. Under these conditions the net probabilities of death are assumed to be described by

$$Q_1 = 1 - e^{-\lambda_1} \quad \text{and} \quad Q_2 = 1 - e^{-\lambda_2}. \tag{10.42}$$

Cause 2 can be thought of as a specific cause of death and cause 1 as all the other causes combined. For example, cause 2 could be death from coronary heart disease and cause 1 could be death from any other cause. The net probability Q_1 describes the likelihood of death uninfluenced by death from cause 2. Specifically, Q_1 could be the probability of death with the influence from coronary heart disease "removed." Second, assume that the probability of surviving the interval is

$$P(\text{surviving}) = P_1 P_2 = (1 - Q_1)(1 - Q_2) = (e^{-\lambda_1})(e^{-\lambda_2}) = e^{-\lambda_1 + -\lambda_2} = e^{-\lambda},$$

$$\tag{10.43}$$

where $\lambda = \lambda_1 + \lambda_2$. That is, cause 1 and cause 2 are statistically independent.

Expression (10.43) for the probability of surviving the interval is valid only when cause 1 and cause 2 are statistically independent. Although death from cause 1 is mutually exclusive of death from cause 2, it is still important that the mechanisms underlying these two events act independently. In terms of the marksman example, independence means that the hits and misses of one marksman do not influence the accuracy of the other marksman and vice versa. Equivalently, cause of death 1 is assumed not to be related in any way to cause of death 2. Independence of causes of death is certainly not a realistic assumption for some diseases, particularly chronic diseases. The influence of the dependency among causes of death on the estimate of the net probabilities has not been extensively studied.

These two assumptions (exponential probabilities and independence) make it possible to estimate the probability of death from one cause while the other cause is "eliminated" from consideration (net probability). To estimate the net probability of death, a bit of algebra relates the crude and net probabilities. Consider q = crude probability of death in the interval, death from either cause 1 or 2, then

$$P(\text{death}) = q = 1 - P_1 P_2 = 1 - e^{-\lambda}. \tag{10.44}$$

Note that the crude probability has the same form as both net probabilities. Furthermore,

$$(1 - q)^{\lambda_i/\lambda} = e^{-\lambda_i} = P_i \quad \text{giving} \quad Q_i = 1 - P_i = 1 - (1 - q)^{\lambda_i/\lambda}. \tag{10.45}$$

This basic relationship [expression (10.45)] allows the estimation of the net probabilities, because the ratio of the two hazard rates λ_i/λ is estimated by d_i/d, where d_i represents the number of deaths from cause i and $d = d_1 + d_2$ represents the total number of deaths from both causes in the time interval being considered. The estimated net probability of death from cause i with cause j eliminated is then

$$\hat{Q}_i = 1 - \left(1 - \frac{d}{l}\right)^{d_i/d}, \tag{10.46}$$

where l individuals are at risk from both causes of death at the beginning of the interval.

The assumption that the net probabilities are described by a simple exponential function may not be appealing in some situations [expression (10.42)]. An alternative estimate of the net probability can be derived from intuitive considerations that do not involve an exponential risk model. Individuals can be classified into three categories: (1) died of cause 1, (2) died of cause 2, or (3) lived through the interval. A death from cause 2 can be considered as a person "lost to follow-up" with respect to calculations for cause 1. When cause 2 is "removed," deaths from cause 1 are undercounted because the former "lost to follow-up" are now at risk. That is, the direct estimate of the net probability is too small because a proportion of the individuals who would have died of cause 2 and "lost," can now die of cause 1. Those who would have died of cause 2 are exposed to risk, on the average, for half the interval so that $0.5d_2$ represents an additional "effective" number of individuals at risk when cause 2 is "removed." The value $0.5d_2 Q_1$ estimates the number of additional deaths from cause 1 among the individuals who would have died from cause 2 (if it were present). Therefore, "correcting" the number of deaths d_1 gives

$$\hat{Q}'_1 = \frac{d_1 + 0.5d_2\hat{Q}'_1}{l} \tag{10.47}$$

and solving for the net probability Q'_1 yields

$$\hat{Q}'_1 = \frac{d_1}{l - 0.5d_2}. \tag{10.48}$$

The probability $\hat{Q}'_1$ is another estimate of the net probability of death from cause 1 based on l individuals at risk, where again d_1 represents the number of deaths from cause 1 and d_2 represents the number of deaths from cause 2. The estimated net probability $\hat{Q}'_1$ is greater than crude probability q_1, because additional individuals are at risk and die of cause 1 when cause 2 is "eliminated." In general,

$$\text{net probability} = \hat{Q}'_i = \frac{d_i}{l - 0.5d_j} \geq \frac{d_i}{l} = \hat{q}_i = \text{crude probability.} \tag{10.49}$$

For most applications of competing risk calculations, the crude probability and the net probability hardly differ. Expression (10.49) indicates why. For $\hat{Q}'_i$ and $\hat{q}_i$ to differ substantially, the competing cause of death must be a large proportion of the individuals at risk (d_j has to be large relative to l), which is not usually the case for human mortality data. In fact, it is usually quite the opposite—d_j is almost always much less than l ($d_j \ll l$).

Two small points: Although the exponential and intuitive estimates come from different considerations, they differ little in value ($\hat{Q}_i \approx \hat{Q}'_i$) for most situations. The net probability of death from a specific cause, if other causes of death act independently, can also be estimated by considering deaths from other causes as censored observations. The topic of censored data is developed in the next two chapters. It should simply be noted at this point that methods applicable to censored data apply in the context of competing risks.

Applications

The estimation of the net probabilities (exponential and intuitive) are illustrated by a subset of data from a large study of the effects of smoking on coronary heart disease (CHD) mortality (Hammond and Horn [6] and reported in [5]). A small part of these smoking and CHD data are given in Table 10–17.

Table 10–17. Competing risks: deaths after 44 months of follow-up for ages 60–65

	Nonsmokers	Smokers
CHD = d_1	552	921
Other = d_2	714	1,095
Population	20,278	21,594
Crude	0.0272	0.0427
Exponential	0.0277	0.0438
Intuitive	0.0277	0.0438

Difference—Crude: 0.0427 − 0.0272 = 0.0155
Net: 0.0438 − 0.0277 = 0.0161
Ratio—Crude: 0.0427/0.0272 = 1.567
Net: 0.0438/0.0277 = 1.581.

As expected, the net probabilities of death from CHD for smokers and nonsmokers increase, but slightly, when competing causes of death are "removed." The increase in net risk for CHD among smokers and nonsmokers can be expressed as a difference or as a ratio (Table 10–17), providing an estimate of the "pure" impact of smoking on CHD risk. Some controversy exists over which is the "best" expression of the increased risk from smoking. The issues surrounding the choice of a ratio versus a difference as an expression of risk are basically semantic and are discussed elsewhere (see [5] or [7]).

Occasionally, the argument is put forth that increases in cancer incidence in the last three or four decades, at least in part, are due to the decrease in mortality from infectious diseases. This thought is based on the idea that deaths from infectious diseases operate early in life, thereby eliminating a proportion of individuals who would die of cancer later in life. Data for the years 1900 to 1950 that reflect on this question are given in Table 10–18.

Using competing risk estimates, the net probabilities (infectious disease removed) show no reason to believe that the decreasing mortality from infectious disease plays an appreciable role in the observed increase in cancer mortality. Comparison of the crude and net probabilities (multiplied by 100,000) for cancer deaths shows essentially identical values for all six decades. That is, under the conditions for a competing risk calculation, removing infectious disease as a cause of death competing with cancer mortality does not change the national mortality pattern of cancer deaths over the years 1900 to 1950.

Net probabilities [expression (10.46)] can be calculated from specific causes of death and summarized with life table functions. The

Table 10–18. Competing risks: total cancer and infectious disease deaths by year for the United States 1900–50

Year	1900	1910	1920	1930	1940	1950
Infection	240,077	225,565	191,958	137,971	90,239	60,370
Cancer	48,700	70,414	88,793	119,985	158,943	208,109
Total deaths	1,308,056	1,356,535	1,382,887	1,394,611	1,422,161	1,472,842
Population	76,094	92,407	106,466	123,188	132,122	151,683
Crude*	64.00	76.20	83.40	97.40	120.30	137.20
Intuitive*	64.10	76.29	83.48	97.45	120.34	137.23

*Crude and net probabilities multiplied by 100,000.

The crude cancer mortality rate is $\dfrac{d_{cancer}}{\text{population}} \times 100{,}000$, and population is given in thousands.

exponential-based expression for a net probability of death from cause i at age x using life table deaths is

$$Q_{x.i} = 1 - (1 - q_x)^{d_x^{(i)}/(d_x)}, \tag{10.50}$$

where $d_x^{(i)}$ represents life table deaths from i^{th} cause in the interval x to $x + 1$ and $d_x = d_x^{(i)} + d_x^{(j)}$ represents the total life table deaths. The net probabilities $Q_{x.i}$ reflect the impact of mortality at age x from cause i with the cause j "removed" and can be used to calculate other life table functions, particularly the expectation of life. For example, if all deaths from cardiovascular disease (CVD deaths = cause j) are "eliminated" and a life table based on the remaining causes of death (all non-CVD deaths = cause i) is computed, then an estimate of the years of life lost attributable to cardiovascular disease is found by comparing the "net" expectation of life with the expectation calculated when all causes of death are operating (70.9 years versus 80.6 years—Table 10–19). That is, the life table functions are based on the net probabilities $Q_{x.i}$ rather than the crude probabilities q_x.

Table 10–19 gives the expectation of life for 1980 California males for five selected ages (the third column contains estimates based on the crude probabilities of death q_x—"no causes" removed). Included in Table 10–19 are the expectations of life when four causes of death (cardiovascular disease (CVD), ischemic heart disease (IHD), lung cancer, and motor vehicle accidents) are each "eliminated." Life tables are constructed (not shown) based on $Q_{x.i}$ eliminating each cause of death and producing in the usual fashion the average years of life remaining at age x (e_x). The impact of cardiovascular disease on the total mortality picture is clear. The life table competing risk calculations indicate that the expectation of life would be increased about 10

Table 10–19. Expectation of life with specific competing causes of death "eliminated": California, males, 1980

Age (yrs.)	Expected	No Causes	CVD*	IHD*	Lung Cancer*	Motor*
0	e_0	70.92	80.63	73.79	71.80	71.81
20	e_{20}	52.41	62.61	55.33	53.31	53.19
40	e_{40}	34.49	44.71	37.49	35.41	34.68
60	e_{60}	18.16	28.01	20.08	18.96	18.22
80	e_{80}	7.07	16.56	8.07	7.18	7.07

* = Cause of death eliminated (cause j).

years if cardiovascular disease was "eliminated" as a risk of death. A three-year increase would result if ischemic heart disease was "eliminated." Less of an impact on the expectation of life is observed (about a one-year increase) when lung cancer or motor vehicle accidents are "eliminated" as causes of death.

11 Estimates of Risk from Follow-Up Data

A therapeutic trial, for example, usually involves individuals observed over time where the outcome might be death or occurrence of a specific disease. Such follow-up data typically consist of recording the time elapsed between the beginning of the therapy and a well-defined endpoint such as death. A basic characteristic that separates follow-up data from other types of data is that the outcome is often not observed for all subjects. When death is the endpoint of a follow-up study, for example, a number of the sampled individuals typically are alive at the end of the study period. This lack of knowledge about the exact time of the endpoint biases direct measurement based on the observed survival experience. Special statistical methods, exist, however, to compensate for the incomplete nature of the follow-up data. These techniques allow differing follow-up times to be combined to usefully measure risk regardless of whether the endpoint is observed or not. The theory and application of these methods constitute the major element of the topic usually referred to as survival analysis. Two general approaches are described: one parametric and the other nonparametric. For simplicity, the terminology used in the following, by and large, pertains to mortality and disease outcomes but the methods apply to failure times in general.

Parametric Model

A simple and often useful parametric model postulates that survival probabilities are characterized by an exponential function. More specifically, the probability that an individual will be alive after a time t is

$$P \text{ (surviving beyond time } t) = S(t) = e^{-\lambda t}$$

or equivalently

$$P \text{ (surviving from time } = 0 \text{ until time } = t) = S(t) = e^{-\lambda t}. \quad (11.1)$$

The survival curve $S(t) = e^{-\lambda t}$ is a parametric model of the relationship between time and risk with the potential of providing a compact description of survival data. This model was briefly introduced earlier in the context of the competing risk calculations [expression (10.45)].

An exponential pattern of survival derives from the proposition that the number of deaths in a specific population at risk is proportional only to the number of members of that population. That is, deaths occur at random among the individuals at risk. Proportionality translates into the mathematical expression that

$$\text{decrease in population size} = \frac{dl_t}{dt} = -\lambda l_t, \tag{11.2}$$

which implies that the rate of decrease at a time t is governed only by a constant failure rate λ and the population size l_t. This expression was used earlier in the deviation of the nearest-neighbor distribution [expression (5.8)]. It directly follows that

$$l_t = l_0 e^{-\lambda t}, \tag{11.3}$$

where l_0 is the size of the population at risk when time $t = 0$, or expressed in terms of a survival curve,

$$S(t) = P \text{ (surviving beyond time } t) = \frac{l_t}{l_0} = e^{-\lambda t}. \tag{11.4}$$

The parameter λ does not depend on the time t. Exponential survival implies, for example, that the age of a person is unrelated to a mortality or disease rate. The survival of an individual is a function of time but the failure rate is the same regardless of the age considered. Clearly, this is an unrealistic description for the full spectrum of ages in human population (e.g., 0 to 100 years). In human populations, mortality rates certainly depend on age (mortality rates are usually higher in individuals 80 years old compared to individuals 20 years old, for example). But over short periods of time or under specific conditions, rates can be essentially constant, and an exponential survival model adequately reflects the mortality or disease experience of a human population.

The fact that the probability of living beyond a fixed point in time does not depend on "age" can be seen from the following:

$$P \text{ (surviving 0 to } t_1) = e^{-\lambda t_1} \quad \text{and} \quad P \text{ (surviving 0 to } t_2) = e^{-\lambda t_2}, \tag{11.5}$$

where $t_1 < t_2$. The probability that an individual survives beyond time t_2 given the individual has survived to t_1 is then

$$P \text{ (surviving to } t_2 | \text{surviving to } t_1) = \frac{e^{-\lambda t_2}}{e^{-\lambda t_1}} = e^{-\lambda(t_2 - t_1)}, \tag{11.6}$$

showing that the difference $t_2 - t_1$ is the sole determinant of the probability of surviving to at least t_2, given that the person is alive at t_1. The probability of survival is not influenced by the actual values of t_2 and t_1. For example, the probability of surviving an additional 10 weeks for a person followed 65 weeks is the same as the probability of surviving 10 weeks for an individual followed 5 weeks; the probability of survival depends directly only on the difference $t_2 - t_1 = 10$ weeks. Furthermore, since the probability of survival is not related to the previous amount of follow-up time, then all individuals alive for a specific time are expected to survive the same amount of additional time. A patient followed 65 weeks, for example, has the same expected time of continued survival as a person followed 5 weeks when the distribution of survival times is exponential (i.e., constant hazard rate).

Another view of the "lack of memory" property of the exponential distribution comes from noting that P (*surviving beyond time t* | *survived to time t_1*) $= e^{-\lambda(t - t_1)}$ is also an exponential distribution measured relative to t_1. The distribution of additional survival time is unaffected by knowing that survival has surpassed time t_1—the distribution remains exponential.

To demonstrate that an "exponential" population has a constant average mortality rate, recall the definition of an average rate:

$$\text{average mortality rate} = \frac{\text{number who died}}{\text{total time at risk}}. \tag{11.7}$$

The number of deaths among N individuals between times t_1 and t_2, when survival is described by expression (11.1), is

$$\text{deaths} = N(e^{-\lambda t_1} - e^{-\lambda t_2}) \tag{11.8}$$

and the total time at risk is

$$\text{total time at risk} = N \int_{t_1}^{t_2} e^{-\lambda x} \, dx = N \frac{e^{-\lambda t_1} - e^{-\lambda t_2}}{\lambda}. \tag{11.9}$$

The average mortality rate for the time interval $[t_1, t_2]$ is then given by

$$\text{average mortality rate} = \frac{N(e^{-\lambda t_1} - e^{-\lambda t_2})}{N \dfrac{e^{-\lambda t_1} - e^{-\lambda t_2}}{\lambda}} = \lambda. \tag{11.10}$$

That is, when the average mortality rate is constant, not surprisingly, the average mortality rate and the hazard rate are identical or

$$\text{hazard rate} = -\frac{dS(t)/dt}{S(t)} = \lambda = \text{average mortality rate.} \tag{11.11}$$

The exponential parametric survival time model yields a simple relationship between the average mortality rate and the probability of death. Since

$$P \text{ (death in the interval } [t_1, t_2]) = e^{-\lambda t_1} - e^{-\lambda t_2} \tag{11.12}$$

and when the mortality rate λ is small, $e^{-\lambda t_i} \approx 1 - \lambda t_i$, giving

$$P \text{ (death in the interval } [t_1, t_2]) \approx \lambda(t_2 - t_1). \tag{11.13}$$

The probability of death in an interval is approximately equal to the mortality rate multiplied by the time at risk (e.g., if $t_2 - t_1 = 1$ year, then $rate \approx P$ (death during one year) $\approx \lambda$). A parallel result was noted in Chapter 1 derived without a parametric model [expression (1.12)].

Age Adjustment of Rates

Two traditional procedures for age adjustment of rates were discussed in Chapter 1 [expressions (1.42) and (1.43)]. A less common method, with advantages over the two more usual approaches, is based on modeling the survival experience of individuals within an interval by an exponential survival function. That is, it is assumed that the probability of surviving a specific interval (x_{i-1} to x_i) for all individuals alive at the beginning of the interval is

$$P \text{ (surviving to } x_i | \text{alive at } x_{i-1}) = p_i = e^{-\lambda_i(x_i - x_{i-1})}. \tag{11.14}$$

The value λ_i is the mortality rate associated with the ith age interval which is assumed, at least approximately, constant within a specific interval. However, these constant mortality rates can vary from interval to interval. The probability of surviving over a series of k age intervals, x_0 to x_1, x_1 to $x_2, \ldots, x_{k-1}$ to x_k, is then

$$P = p_1 p_2 \cdots p_k = \prod_{i=1}^{k} p_i = \prod_{i=1}^{k} e^{-\lambda_i(x_i - x_{i-1})} = e^{-\sum_{i=1}^{k} \lambda_i(x_i - x_{i-1})}. \tag{11.15}$$

The cumulative probability symbolized by P summarizes the combined influences of the age-specific rates (λ_i's). This summary value is "age-adjusted" in the sense that comparisons of cumulative probabilities P among different populations are not influenced by differences in age distributions. For most diseases the mortality or incidence rates λ_i are small so that the survival probability for a period x_0 to x_k is approximately $P \approx 1 = \sum \lambda_i(x_i - x_{i-1})$.

A simple illustration comes from the hypothetical data given in Chapter 1 (Table 1–16) where

$$\lambda_1 = 0.001, \ \lambda_2 = 0.002, \ \lambda_3 = 0.004, \quad \text{and} \quad \lambda_4 = 0.008$$

represent four age-specific rates that are identical for two populations (I and II). The probability of surviving from age 40 to 80 (P) is based exclusively on the four age-specific rates. That is,

$$\hat{P} = e^{-10(0.001 + 0.002 + 0.004 + 0.008)} = e^{-0.150} = 0.861 \qquad (11.16)$$

gives the probability of living from age 40 to 80 in the two hypothetical populations. This value is the same for both groups because the age-specific rates are the same for both groups. The estimated probability $\hat{P}$ is unaffected by the differing age distributions in the populations at risk.

Consider again (Table 1–19) the data describing the incidence of breast cancer among women residents of the San Francisco Bay Area (1977–83), where breast cancer rates are to be compared between whites and blacks. The race-, age- and stage-specific incidence rates from these data are shown in Table 11–1.

The probability of being diagnosed with a specific stage of breast cancer $(1 - \hat{P})$ reflects the risk for individuals throughout a specific age range from a series of age-specific rates. Unlike the direct and indirect methods of rate adjustment, the comparison of groups on the basis of $\hat{P}$ or $1 - \hat{P}$ does not require the choice of a standard population. The addition of the estimated age-specific rates each multiplied by the length of the age intervals produces an "age-adjusted" value with a probabilistic interpretation. For the race/cancer example, the value $1 - \hat{P}$ is an estimate of the probability of breast cancer among women for the specified age range. The probability that a white female age 40 will be diagnosed with breast cancer (local stage) before age 80 in the San Francisco Bay Area is estimated by $1 - \hat{P} = 0.059$. The corresponding value for blacks is 0.038. The difference between these two

Table 11–1. Breast cancer by race, age, and stage: incidence rates/100,000 (1977–83)

Age	White		Black	
	Local	Regional	Local	Regional
40–49	87.89	66.55	56.90	56.60
50–59	126.96	96.97	81.18	91.62
60–69	185.46	118.04	109.58	90.04
79–79	211.17	119.11	143.06	94.57
79+	207.80	102.72	138.41	119.54
Crude rate	125.87	88.86	73.74	72.56
$\hat{P}$	0.941	0.961	0.962	0.967
$1 - \hat{P}$	0.059	0.039	0.038	0.033

probabilities is not affected by differences in age distributions (Table 1–18).

Although it is not much of an issue when the estimated cumulative probability $\hat{P}$ is calculated from large numbers of observations such as the breast cancer example, when $\hat{P}$ is estimated from smaller sets of data the variance of this quantity is important. If the mortality or disease rates are small (λ_i less than 0.10 or so), then an estimate of the variance of $\hat{P}$ is

$$\text{variance } (\hat{P}) = \text{variance } (1 - \hat{P}) \approx \sum_{i=1}^{k} \frac{(x_i - x_{i-1})^2 d_i}{l_i^2}, \qquad (11.17)$$

where d_i is the number of deaths among l_i individuals at risk at the beginning of the ith interval of length $(x_i - x_{i-1})$ and k is the number of age-specific rates combined to estimate the "age-adjusted" probability P. Applying the variance expression to the estimated value from the hypothetical data for population I (Table 1–16) gives $\hat{P}_I = 0.861$ with variance $(\hat{P}_I) = 0.00075$, producing an approximate 95% confidence interval of $(0.807, 0.914)$. The same calculation applied to population II rates gives a different result because the variance, unlike $\hat{P}$, depends on the distribution of ages in population at risk. That is, $\hat{P}_{II} = 0.861$ but the estimated variance is 0.00022, producing a smaller approximate confidence interval, $(0.832, 0.890)$.

Censored and Truncated Data

A measurement is right censored when its exact value is unknown but it is known that the value exceeds a specific limit. A censored survival time results from the nature of the sampling process or study design. If a study is continued until all individuals die, complete survival times are available on all subjects and no data are censored. For most follow-up studies, however, the survival time is known only for those individuals who die during the study period. All that is known about the remaining study subjects is that they were alive at the end of the period of observation (i.e., surviving beyond a specific point). The exact time of death is censored (missing). Individuals with right censored survival experience would contribute additional survival time to the total time observed if the study had continued. Figure 11–1 shows two views of the same set of hypothetical survival times for eight individuals (three right censored) collected over a 25-week period. The survival times are: 4, 5^+, 20, 2^+, 15, 12, 8^+, and 10. The "$+$" is a notational convention indicating those individuals who did not die during the study period and are said to be censored (withdrawn) from observation (i.e., 5^+, 2^+, and 8^+).

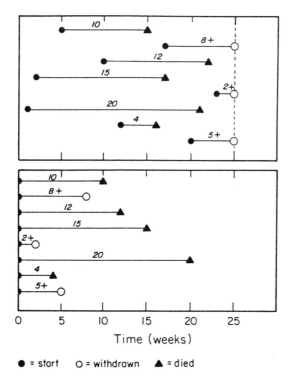

● = start   ○ = withdrawn   ▲ = died

Figure 11–1. Eight hypothetical survival times are shown by time entered the study and by length of follow-up

For contrast, a truncated observation is a measurement that is missing completely. When the sampling process is conducted so that specific types of observations will never be included in the sample, the data are truncated. A classic example of truncated data occurs in genetic studies, where a sample is derived from a list of affected individuals (index cases). A series of families is identifed from a list of cases, such as a registry of patients with a specific disorder. Every family sampled will necessarily have one or more affected individuals. Families that do not contain an affected individual will not be identifed and sampled, producing a set of truncated data. Such a sample is truncated because the nature of the sampling process excludes relevant individuals who belong to families without an index case. For both censored and truncated data the analysis must account for the missing information to produce unbiased summary descriptions.

A distinction between two kinds of censoring is important. An individual can be censored for a particular reason relating to survival. For example, a patient's condition may worsen and, therefore, that individual is removed from the study. This kind of censoring is called informative since the reason for withdrawal from the observation relates to the outcome. The second type of censoring is called noninformative and results when a patient or observation is censored for reasons that have nothing to do with the outcome being studied. That is, the process that causes an observation to be censored is entirely unrelated to the reasons for failure. The probability of failure will then be the same for the censored (unobserved) individuals and for the noncensored (observed) individuals. It is this noninformative right censoring that is assumed in the following and called simply censoring.

Two other types of censoring are worth mentioning: left censoring and interval censoring. Left censoring occurs when an observation enters a study in such a way that the event or failure has already occurred (for example, if a study requires patients to return every six months after treatment to remove a tumor). The exact time of reoccurrence is not known when a patient returns after the first six months and a tumor has already recurred; the follow-up time is said to be left censored. All that is known about the time of reoccurrence is that the tumor occurred before six months. Interval censoring occurs when the failure is known to occur within an interval of time, but the exact time of occurrence is unknown. Continuing the tumor example, if a patient returns a second time after 12 months and the tumor has reoccurred, then the exact time of the event (reoccurrence) is not known, but it must have occurred between six months and a year. The analysis of data with left or interval censoring also requires specific statistical tools, but they will not be discussed here.

Mean Survival Time: Parametric Estimate

The exponential survival time model is completely defined by one parameter, and if it is realistic to assume that an exponential structure underlies the collected data, then it is relatively simple to estimate this single parameter. Consider a data set concerning 10 individuals with acute lung cancer [1] who were followed for different lengths of time (days) until their death or withdrawal from observation (Table 11–2).

An estimated average mortality rate is the number of observed deaths divided by the observed total time at risk. Using the lung cancer follow-up data, the estimated mortality rate λ is

$$\hat{\lambda} = \text{rate} = \frac{\text{number of deaths}}{\text{total time-at-risk}} = \frac{d}{\sum_{i=1}^{n} t_i} = \frac{7}{308} = 0.0227,$$

where d is the number of deaths among the n individuals in the sample

Table 11–2. Lung cancer follow-up data

Person	Status	Days
1	Died	2
2	Censored	72
3	Died	51
4	Censored	60
5	Died	33
6	Died	27
8	Died	14
8	Died	24
9	Died	4
10	Censored	21
Total	Died = 7	308

and t_i is the observed follow-up time for both complete and censored observations ($d = 7$ complete and $n - d = 3$ censored survival times yield a total time at risk of $\sum t_i = 308$ person-days). An estimate of the variance of the estimate λ is

$$\text{variance } (\lambda) = S_\lambda^2 = \frac{\lambda^2}{d}, \tag{11.18}$$

giving an estimated standard error for $\lambda = 0.0227$ of $S_{\hat\lambda} = 0.0086$. The estimates λ and variance (λ) can be derived from maximum likelihood considerations (see Appendix E for a brief general discussion). A natural estimate of the exponential survival curve is then $\hat{S}(t) = e^{-\lambda t}$ and for the lung cancer data, $\hat{S}(t) = e^{-0.0227t}$.

It is worth noting that the transformed estimate $\log(\lambda)$ has an approximate variance of $1/d$ (variance$(\log[\lambda]) = 1/d$). Removing the dependence of the variance on the parameter λ improves the use of the normal distribution as a way of testing conjectures about the rate (λ) and constructing confidence intervals. For the lung cancer data, $\log(\lambda) = \log(0.0227) = -3.784$, and an approximate 95% confidence interval for $\log(\lambda)$ is therefore $-3.784 \pm 1.96\sqrt{1/7}$, giving $(-4.525, -3.043)$, and $(e^{-4.525}, e^{-3.043}) = (0.011, 0.048)$ is then an approximate 95% confidence interval for the rate λ.

Also of interest is the mean survival time, which is estimated by the total observed time lived by all individuals at risk divided by the number who died (the reciprocal of λ) or

$$\text{mean survival time} = \bar{t} = \frac{\sum\limits_{i=1}^{n} t_i}{d} = \frac{1}{\lambda}. \tag{11.19}$$

For the lung cancer data, the mean survival time is $\bar{t} = 308/7 = 44$ days. Mean survival time is related to the reciprocal of a rate, as similarly noted for a life table [expression (9.9)].

The denominator used to calculate the mean survival time is the number of deaths rather than the total number of persons under observation (deaths $d = 7$, not individuals where $n = 10$). The reason relates to the fact that the total survival time is biased (too small) because the total time observed $\sum t_i$ includes individuals who did not die (censored) during the follow-up period. For the lung cancer example, the three patients who were withdrawn from observation would have added more survival time to the total time at risk if the follow-up period had been longer.

A constant hazard rate implies that at any point in time all living individuals have the same expected amount of survival time remaining. The expected amount of time remaining to a specific individual is a function only of the hazard rate λ and not the previous survival time. It is, therefore, consistent to assign to all individuals with incomplete survival times (censored number $= n - d$) the same additional amount of lifetime (represented as T). These "complete" survival times $(t_i + T)$ are then used to estimate the mean survival time as if no censoring occurred. The lung cancer "complete data" adjusted for the censored survival times are given in Table 11–3. The mean survival time based on "complete" survival times, like most estimated mean values, is the total time divided by all individuals observed. Using these "complete data" to calculate the mean survival time gives

$$\bar{t} = \frac{\sum t_i + (n - k)\bar{t}}{n} = \frac{308 + 3\bar{t}}{10},$$

Table 11–3. Lung cancer follow-up data with adjustment for incomplete follow-up

Person	Status	Days
1	Died	2
2	Adjusted	72 + T
3	Died	51
4	Adjusted	60 + T
5	Died	33
6	Died	27
7	Died	14
8	Died	24
9	Died	4
10	Adjusted	21 + T
Total	10	308 + 3T

where $\bar{t}$ estimates the expected survival time T, and solving for $\bar{t}$ produces the same estimate as before

$$\bar{t} = \frac{\sum t_i}{d} = \frac{308}{7} = 44 \text{ days.}$$

The estimate only makes sense if the survival experience of the population sampled can be, at least approximately, described by an exponential survival curve. An estimate of the variance of the estimated mean survival time $\bar{t}$ is given by

$$\text{variance}(\bar{t}) = S_{\bar{t}}^2 = \frac{\bar{t}^2}{d}. \tag{11.20}$$

For the estimate $\bar{t} = 44$ days, the estimated standard error is

$$S_{\bar{t}} = \frac{44}{\sqrt{7}} = 16.630.$$

Mean Survival Time: Nonparametric Estimate

To understand the calculation of the mean survival time without a parametric model, consider first the situation where each individual studied is followed until failure (i.e., no censored survival times). A hypothetical data set of complete survival times might look like: 4, 5, 20, 2, 15, 12, 8, and 10 (weeks). The basis for describing the survival experience nonparametrically is the probability of failure within a specific time interval.

The Kaplan–Meier or product-limit nonparametric estimate of the survival probabilities is based on constructing intervals so that only one death occurs in each. Therefore, the probability of death is simply calculated. If q_i represents the probability of death in the ith interval, then q_i is estimated by one divided by the number of individuals at risk in that interval. If several individuals have identical survival times, then the estimated probability of a single death is multiplied by the number of deaths. For the hypothetical data, each of $n = 8$ intervals (one for each death) is characterized by an estimate of q_i, and these probabilities along with the conditional probabilities of surviving the interval $(p_i = 1 - q_i)$ are given in Table 11–4.

The quantity of most interest is the probability of surviving from the start of the first interval until the end of the kth interval. This survival probability (P_k) is estimated by the product of the

Table 11–4. Hypothetical follow-up data: no censoring

k	Interval	$\hat{q}_k$	$\hat{p}_k$	$\hat{P}_k = \prod \hat{p}_i$	$S_{\hat{P}_k}$
1	0–2	1/8	7/8	7/8	0.117
2	2–4	1/7	6/7	6/8	0.153
3	4–5	1/6	5/6	5/8	0.171
4	5–8	1/5	4/5	4/8	0.177
5	8–10	1/4	3/4	3/8	0.171
6	10–12	1/3	2/3	2/8	0.153
7	12–15	1/2	1/2	1/8	0.117
8	15–20	1/1	0/1	0/8	—

conditional probabilities of surviving each interval, called the product-limit estimate, and is

$$\hat{P}_k = \hat{p}_1 \hat{p}_2 \cdots \hat{p}_k = \prod_{i=1}^{k} \hat{p}_i. \tag{11.21}$$

Little difference exists between the product-limit survival probabilities and the similar values computed from a life table. The life table estimates are based on fixed interval widths, where the product-limit estimates are not; otherwise the resulting survival probabilities estimate the estimated survival curve and play the same role in the analysis of survival data.

For complete data

$$\hat{P}_k = \prod_{i=1}^{k} \hat{p}_i = \frac{n-1}{n}\frac{n-2}{n-1}\frac{n-3}{n-2}\cdots\frac{n-k}{n-k+1} = \frac{n-k}{n} = 1 - \frac{k}{n}, \tag{11.22}$$

which is identical to calculating the survival probability directly. That is, k individuals died before or during the kth interval, resulting in an estimate of the probability of death before k complete intervals of time of k/n, and the probability of surviving beyond the kth interval is $1 - k/n$.

The observed number of deaths has a binomial distribution under the assumption that the probability of death is the same for the series of independent individuals observed within the study period. The usual variance associated with a binomial distribution can be applied to the estimate $\hat{P}_k$, giving an estimated variance of $\hat{P}_k(1 - \hat{P}_k)/n$ for complete data. For the illustrative data, the probability of surviving 12 weeks (intervals 1, 2, ..., 6) is $\hat{P}_6 = 1 - 6/8 = 2/8 = 0.250$, and the estimated variance of $\hat{P}_6$ is 0.0234. The value $\hat{P}_6$ is also $(7/8) \times (6/7) \times (5/6) \times (4/5) \times (3/4) \times (2/3) = 5040/20160 = 2/8 = 0.250$.

The mean survival time in the complete follow-up case is simply the total time lived divided by the number of observed individuals $(n = d)$ and, as usual,

$$\bar{t} = \frac{\displaystyle\sum_{i=1}^{n} t_i}{n}. \tag{11.23}$$

The same expression written in terms of the estimated survival probabilities $\hat{P}_i$ is

$$\bar{t} = \sum_{i=1}^{n} t_i(\hat{P}_{i-1} - \hat{P}_i), \quad \text{where} \quad P_0 = 1. \tag{11.24}$$

Expression (11.24) is more complicated but is useful when complete follow-up times are not available because, as will be seen, the $\hat{P}_i$ values can be estimated in an unbiased way from censored survival data. The mean survival time, calculated either way [(expressions (11.23) or (11.24)] for the hypothetical data, is $\bar{t} = 9.5$ weeks. Also, when no individuals are censored or lost, the variability of the mean survival time is measured by the usual estimate for the standard error of a mean $(S_{\bar{t}} = S_t/\sqrt{n})$, where $S_t^2 = \sum (t_i - \bar{t})^2/(n - 1)$. For the example data, $S_{\bar{t}} = 2.138$. Product-limit estimation applied to complete data leads to familiar results, but when survival times are censored expressions (11.21) and (11.24) continue to produce unbiased values for the survival probabilities and mean survival time where standard methods are biased.

The product-limit calculations of survival probabilities from incomplete survival data followed much the same pattern as described for the complete data. The probability of death in a specific interval is calculated in the identical manner. All individuals who are not censored or lost contribute to the calculation of the probability of death for that interval. Individuals withdrawn or lost from follow-up are included in the calculations only when they are known to be at risk for the entire interval. Otherwise, they are excluded from further calculations. Another view of the number of individuals at risk (risk set) comes from counting only those persons at risk immediately before a failure. This frequently used definition of a risk set is just another way of stating that all individuals must complete the interval to be at risk when the probability of failure is calculated. Suppose three individuals in the previous data set did not die during the follow-up period, producing the same hypothetical data shown in Figure 11-1 $(4, 5^+, 20, 2^+, 15, 12, 8^+,$ and 10 (weeks); for $n = 8$ individuals with $d = 5 =$ deaths during the study period). The probability estimates associated with these survival times are in Table 11-5.

Table 11–5. Hypothetical follow-up data: censoring

k	Interval	$\hat{q}_k$	$\hat{p}_k$	$\hat{P}_k = \prod \hat{p}_i$	$S_{\hat{P}_k}$
1	0–4	1/7	6/7	0.857	0.132
2	4–10	1/4	3/4	0.643	0.210
3	10–12	1/3	2/3	0.429	0.224
4	12–15	1/2	1/2	0.214	0.188
5	15–20	1/1	0/1	0.000	—

For these censored data the survival probabilities are calculated in the identical manner as complete follow-up data ($\hat{P}_k = \prod \hat{p}_i$). For the hypothetical survival data, the probability of surviving three intervals (12 weeks), for example, is $\hat{P}_3 = 0.429$. That is, $\hat{P}_3 = (6/7) \times (3/4) \times (2/3) = 36/84 = 0.429$.

The product-limit estimate of the survival probability $\hat{P}_k$ is subject to sampling variability, which can be estimated by Greenwood's variance formula or

$$\text{variance}(\hat{P}_k) = \hat{P}_k^2 \sum_{i=1}^{k} \frac{\hat{q}_i}{n_i \hat{p}_i}, \tag{11.25}$$

where n_i represents the number of individuals at risk in the ith interval. For example, $\hat{P}_3 = 0.429$, and an estimate of the variance associated with this estimated survival probability is

$$\text{variance}(\hat{P}_3) = (0.429)^2 \left(\frac{1}{7} \frac{1}{6} + \frac{1}{4} \frac{1}{3} + \frac{1}{3} \frac{1}{2} \right) = 0.050.$$

Greenwood's expression for the variance of an estimated survival probability involves a cumulative sum which slightly complicates the calculation. An alternative, simpler approximation [2] is

$$\text{variance}(\hat{P}_k) = q_k \hat{P}_k^2 (1 - \hat{P}_k). \tag{11.26}$$

This alternative variance is most effective when $\hat{P}_k$ is close to zero but is generally conservative (tends to give estimates that are inflated). For this reason Greenwood's estimate of the variance is probably better for general use.

An estimated hazard function is easily calculated from a product-moment survival table such as Table 11–5. For the kth interval, the estimated hazard rate is

$$\text{hazard rate} = \hat{h}_k = \frac{d_k}{n_k(t_k - t_{k-1})}. \tag{11.27}$$

Or, if all recorded failures occur at different times,

$$\text{hazard rate} = \hat{h}_k = \frac{1}{n_k(t_k - t_{k-1})}. \tag{11.28}$$

For example, $\hat{h}_3 = 1/[3(12 - 10)] = 0.167$ from Table 11–5. The symbol u_k is the number of individuals in the risk set associated with interval k. Expression (11.27) is not new. It is simply a rewriting of the approximation given by expression (11.13).

Mean Survival Time from Censored Data

When censored values are present, the direct calculation of a mean produces an estimate that is likely too small, as already noted. The previous expression for the mean, however,

$$\bar{t} = \sum_{i=1}^{d} t_i(\hat{P}_{i-1} - \hat{P}_i), \quad \text{where} \quad \hat{P}_0 = 1 \tag{11.29}$$

can be used when estimates of the survival probabilities are available. Expression (11.32) is sometimes given in a different form as

$$\bar{t} = \sum_{i=1}^{d} \hat{P}_{i-1}(t_i - t_{i-1}), \quad \text{where} \quad t_0 = 0. \tag{11.30}$$

Both expressions produce identical estimated mean values. The value d is again the number of deaths observed or intervals in a sample of n individuals $(d \le n)$. If the data do not contain censored values $(d = n)$, then $\hat{P}_{i-1} - \hat{P}_i = 1/n$ and the expressions for $\bar{t}$ reduce to the usual calculation of a mean value. When censored values are present, the mean $\bar{t}$ is a weighted average of the observed survival times. Expression (11.30) has a clear geometric interpretation. It is the area under the estimated survival curve calculated by summing a series of rectangles whose areas are the height times the width of each interval, or $area_i = \hat{P}_{i-1}(t_i - t_{i-1})$.

The estimated mean survival time from the hypothetical data (4, 5^+, 20, 2^+, 15, 12, 8^+, and 10) is 12.786 weeks, as shown in Table 11–6. Figure 11–2 shows the estimated survival curve associated with these censored data. Note that $\bar{t}$ is the total area under the product-limit estimated survival curve.

The approximate variance of $\bar{t}$ is somewhat complicated, but is usually produced by "package" programs for survival analysis (see details in [3]). An approximate variance for the mean value estimated

Table 11–6. Calculation of the mean from censored survival data

i	t_i	q_i	$\hat{P}_i$	$\hat{P}_{i-1} - \hat{P}_i$	$t_i(\hat{P}_{i-1} - \hat{P}_i)$	$t_i - t_{i-1}$	$\hat{P}_{i-1}(t_i - t_{i-1})$
1	4	0.143	0.857	0.143	0.571	4	4.000
2	10	0.250	0.643	0.214	2.143	6	5.143
3	12	0.333	0.429	0.214	2.571	2	1.286
4	15	0.500	0.214	0.214	3.214	3	1.286
5	20	1.000	0.000	0.214	4.286	5	1.071
Mean	—	—	—	—	12.786	—	12.786

from censored data is given by

$$\text{variance}(\bar{t}) = S_{\bar{t}}^2 = \sum_{i=1}^{d-1} \frac{q_i^2}{p_i} A_i^2, \quad \text{where} \quad A_i = \bar{t} - \sum_{j=1}^{i} P_{j-1}(t_j - t_{j-1}). \quad (11.31)$$

For the hypothetical data, the estimated standard error associated with $\bar{t}$ is $S_{\bar{t}} = 2.108$. More complete descriptions of the properties of this variance are given elsewhere [3]. Incidentally, if no censoring is present, the estimate of the variance of the estimated mean [expression (11.31)] reduces to $\text{variance}(\bar{t}) = \sum (t_i - \bar{t})^2/n^2$, indicating a slight bias because the denominator should be $n(n - 1)$ to yield the usual unbiased estimate of the variance of $\bar{t}$.

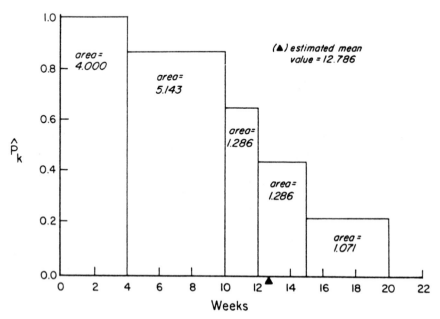

Figure 11–2. Survival curve for the hypothetical eight data values

Table 11–7. Kidney cancer
data: survival probabilities

Interval	$\hat{P}_i$
0–1	0.597
1–2	0.539
2–3	0.503
3–4	0.442
4–5	0.442

Survival probabilities from almost any survival curve can be used to estimate the mean survival time. The kidney cancer data (Table 9–7) provide an example. The survival probabilities for 6 years of follow-up (Table 9–8) are given in Table 11–7. These $n = 126$ patients give an estimated mean survival time $\bar{t} = \sum \hat{P}_i = 2.523$ years because $t_i - t_{i-1} = 1$. The estimated standard error of $\bar{t}$ is 0.236.

The lung cancer data provide another example. The survival probabilities calculated from the ten survival times given previously (Table 11–2) are shown in Table 11–8, and the estimated mean survival time is $\bar{t} = 34.550$ days with an estimated standard error of 8.165. This calculation is slightly complicated by the fact that the longest survival time (72 days) is a censored value (to be discussed).

The average number of years lived from birth calculated from a complete life table is an application of the mean survival time [expression (11.30)]. That is,

$$\bar{t} = \sum \hat{P}_{i-1}(t_i - t_{i-1}) \approx e_0 - 0.5, \tag{11.32}$$

where e_0 is the expected years of life from birth. The approximation occurs because of the indeterminate last age interval in a life table.

Table 11–8. Lung cancer
data: survival probabilities

Interval	$\hat{P}_i$
0–2	0.900
2–4	0.800
4–14	0.700
14–24	0.583
24–27	0.467
27–33	0.350
33–51	0.233
51–72	0.000

For a complete life table, the age interval width is one year or $(l_1 - l_{i-1}) = x - (x - 1) = 1$ (except the last interval); therefore,

$$\bar{t} \approx \sum P_x = \sum \frac{l_x}{l_0} = \frac{1}{l_0} \sum (L_x - 0.5d_x) = \frac{T_0 - 0.5l_0}{l_0}, \quad \text{giving} \quad \bar{t} \approx e_0 - 0.5.$$

An alternative to the mean is the median time of survival. The median survival time can be estimated by linear interpolation within the interval containing the survival probability $P = 0.50$. From the censored hypothetical data set (Table 11–5), the estimated median survival time is

$$\text{median} = 10 + \frac{2(0.643 - 0.5)}{0.643 - 0.429} = 11.336 \text{ weeks,}$$

where the median value is contained in the interval 0.429 to 0.643.

Goodness-of-Fit

Most analyses require a fundamental choice:

> Should a parametric model be used with advantages in efficiency but possible losses due to "wrong model bias," or should a nonparametric approach be selected that incurs some loss of efficiency but does not require an often problematic statistical structure?

Specifically this question might be, does a sample of follow-up data come from a population with exponential survival structure? The answer to such questions clearly dictates subsequent analytic directions. A first step in deciding between parametric and nonparametric methods of analysis is the investigation of the goodness-of-fit of possible parametric choices. One type of goodness-of-fit procedure, involving the comparison of two cumulative distributions, can be formalized with a statistical test (e.g., chi-square or Kolomogorov test [4]), but a simple graphic display often provides sufficient information to choose satisfactorily between parametric and nonparametric approaches. The following is a description of a general graphic technique, but it is only one of the many possibilities for dealing with the question of whether a data set supports a specific parametric model.

Goodness-of-Fit: Cumulative Distributions

Two cumulative distributions must be defined. A population cumulative distribution describes the probability that a sampled value is less than a specified value x_i by

$$Q_i^* = F(x_i) = P(X \le x_i), \tag{11.33}$$

where F represents a parametric function. The value Q_i^* is the probability associated with the value x_i. The function F is based primarily on theoretical considerations. For example, the population cumulative distribution function associated with the exponential model is $F(x_i) = 1 - S(x_i) = 1 - e^{-\lambda x_i}$. The cumulative distribution $F(x_i)$ would then represent the probability of death before time x_i.

The analogous sample estimated cumulative distribution function is

$$Q_i = \frac{\text{the number of observations} \leq x_i}{n} = \frac{i}{n}, \qquad (11.34)$$

where $x_1, x_2, \ldots, x_n$ is an ordered sample of n independent observations. Goodness-of-fit is measured by comparing the theoretically derived population distribution function with the sample derived cumulative distribution function. That is, the probability Q_i^* is compared to the probability Q_i at each observed value x_i. If the theoretically derived and the empirically derived cumulative distribution functions are similar, the parametric form $F(x_i)$ may be helpful as a description of the data. Conversely, if these two distributions differ, the parametric representation will likely be misleading. The plots of Q_i against Q_i^* are called quantile (percentile) plots or simply $Q - Q$ plots.

Normal Distribution Case

The theoretical and empirical cumulative distributional functions and their comparison are illustrated with a sample of 20 observations thought to be normally distributed. An ordered sample of data, in terms of standardized values $\hat{z}_i = (x_i - \bar{x})/S$, is given in Table 11–9 (column 2). These values generate the Q_i^* values (column 4) based in the standard normal distribution. Also shown are the sample cumulative distribution probabilities $(Q_i$, column 3) associated with the $\hat{z}_i$ values.

Cumulative probabilities from the sample should be similar to cumulative probabilities derived from a standard normal distribution when the sampled population is normally distributed. The goodness-of-fit evaluation involves comparing theoretical cumulative normal probabilities derived from the $\hat{z}_i$ values with those directly derived from the sample without a parametric assumption. The logic is that when the sampled population has normal distribution, a probability calculated from $\hat{z}_i$ based on the theoretical normal cumulative distribution (Q_i^*) should be similar to the probability associated with $\hat{z}_i$ based on

Table 11–9. Goodness-of-fit: normal distribution

	$\hat{z}_i$	Q_i	$Q_i^* = F(\hat{z}_i)$
1	-1.49	0.05	0.068
2	-1.21	0.10	0.113
3	-1.19	0.15	0.117
4	-1.06	0.20	0.145
5	-1.01	0.25	0.156
6	-0.87	0.30	0.192
7	-0.68	0.35	0.248
8	-0.63	0.40	0.264
9	-0.07	0.45	0.472
10	0.01	0.50	0.504
11	0.01	0.55	0.504
12	0.04	0.60	0.516
13	0.07	0.65	0.528
14	0.15	0.70	0.560
15	0.15	0.75	0.560
16	0.26	0.80	0.603
17	0.42	0.85	0.663
18	0.76	0.90	0.776
19	1.33	0.95	0.908
20	1.47	1.00	0.929

the sample cumulative distribution (Q_i). For $z_i = -1.49$, the cumulative probability based on the normal distribution is 0.068 (i.e., $Q_i^* = P(Z < -1.49) = 0.068$ from tables or a computer program). The probability based on the sample cumulative distribution associated with $\hat{z}_i = -1.49$ is 0.05 ($Q_1 = 1/n = 1/20 = 0.05$). The comparisons of Q_i with Q_i^* (column 3 with column 4 in Table 11–9) for the 20 observations are shown in Figure 11–3 (left side). The points (Q_i, Q_i^*) will form an approximate straight line (45°) when the population sampled is normal.

Exponential Distribution Case

Testing the goodness-of-fit for the exponential distribution is straightforward, because the theoretical distribution function F is expressed by

$$Q_i^* = F(t_i) = 1 - S(t_i) = 1 - e^{-\lambda t_i} \quad \text{(theoretical probability).} \quad (11.35)$$

Table 11–10 contains a set of computer-generated random "data," ordered from low to high and thought to have an exponential distribution (column 2). A goodness-of-fit comparison is again made between the probabilities Q_i and Q_i^*. For example, $Q_{16}^* = 1 - e^{-0.046(32.28)} = 0.771$ (theoretical; based on the exponential distribution and the estimate $\hat{\lambda} = 1/21.230 = 0.046$) and $Q_{16} = 16/20 = 0.80$

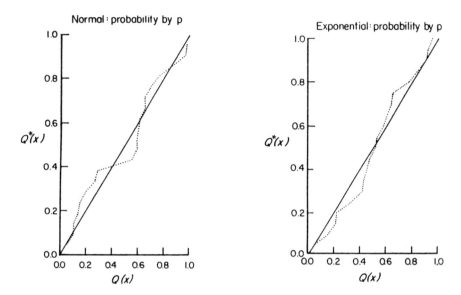

Figure 11–3. Goodness-of-fit plots for the normal and exponential distribution (percentile and probabilities)

Table 11–10. Goodness-of-fit: exponential distribution

	t_i	Q_i	$Q_i^* = F(t_i)$
1	0.94	0.05	0.042
2	3.68	0.10	0.154
3	5.25	0.15	0.213
4	5.48	0.20	0.221
5	8.81	0.25	0.331
6	11.95	0.30	0.420
7	12.31	0.35	0.429
8	13.28	0.40	0.454
9	14.16	0.45	0.475
10	15.80	0.50	0.513
11	16.54	0.55	0.529
12	18.86	0.60	0.577
13	20.38	0.65	0.605
14	22.19	0.70	0.636
15	22.84	0.75	0.647
16	32.38	0.80	0.771
17	40.68	0.85	0.843
18	50.66	0.90	0.901
19	55.10	0.95	0.919
20	67.70	1.00	0.954

(empirical; based only on the observed sample). Figure 11–3 (right side) shows the comparison for the 20 values of Q_i and Q_i^* in Table 11–10 (Q_i, column 3 versus Q_i^*, column 4).

> Aside: Percentile plots are a general technique that allows an evaluation of the goodness-of-fit of a set of data to a theoretical model by the comparison of cumulative distributions. A simple graphic technique that applies specifically to the exponential survival distribution involves plotting a function of the survival distribution. If the survival curve is $S(t) = e^{-\lambda t}$, then
>
> $$\log(-\log(S[t]) = \log(\lambda) + \log(t). \qquad (11.36)$$
>
> That is, when the individual survival times are sampled from an exponential distribution, plotting the transformation $\log(-\log[S(t)])$ against the logarithm of the survival time will deviate from a straight line only because of random variation. Values for $S(t)$ can be estimated using a product-limit estimate or a life table. The "log-log" transformation suggests a more general survival model given by
>
> $$\log(-\log[S(t)]) = \log(\lambda) + b \log(t), \quad \text{then} \quad S(t) = e^{-\lambda t^b}, \qquad (11.37)$$
>
> which is a special case of the Weibull distribution, another mathematical model (two-parameter) used to analyze specific types of survival data [5].

TWO SAMPLE DATA

Studies are designed and data collected so that the mortality or disease experience of two groups can be compared. A study to evaluate two treatments provides an example of this two-sample situation [cited in 7]:

> A clinical trial to evaluate the efficacy of maintenance chemotherapy for acute myelogenous leukemia (AML) was conducted by Embury et al. at Stanford University. After reaching a state of remission through treatment by chemotherapy, the patients who entered the study were randomized into two groups. The first group received maintenance chemotherapy; the second or control group did not. The objective of the trial was to see if maintenance chemotherapy prolonged the time until relapse, that is, increased the length of remission.
>
> Preliminary data collected during the course of the trial follow (in weeks):
>
>
>
> Maintained group ($n = 11$):
> 9, 13, 13[+], 18, 23, 28[+], 31, 34, 45[+], 48, 161[+]
>
> Nonmaintained group ($n = 12$):
> 5, 5, 8, 8, 12, 16[+], 23, 27, 30, 33, 43, 45.
>
>

Table 11–11. Survival probabilities associated with relapse of acute myelogenous leukemia: maintained group

k	Interval	q_k	p_k	$\hat{P}_k = \prod p_i$	$S_{\hat{P}_k}$
1	0–9	1/11	10/11	0.909	0.087
2	9–13	1/10	9/10	0.818	0.116
3	13–18	1/8	7/8	0.716	0.140
4	18–23	1/7	6/7	0.614	0.153
5	23–31	1/5	4/5	0.491	0.164
6	31–34	1/4	3/4	0.368	0.163
7	34–48	1/2	1/2	0.184	0.153
8	>48	1/1	0	0	—

Table 11–12. Survival probabilities associated with relapse of acute myelogenous leukemia: nonmaintained group

k	Interval	q_k	p_k	$\hat{P}_k = \prod p_i$	$S_{\hat{P}_k}$
1	0–5	2/12	10/12	0.833	0.108
2	5–8	2/10	8/10	0.667	0.136
3	8–12	1/8	7/8	0.583	0.142
4	12–23	1/6	5/6	0.486	0.148
5	23–27	1/5	4/5	0.389	0.147
6	27–30	1/4	3/4	0.292	0.139
7	30–33	1/3	2/3	0.194	0.122
8	33–43	1/2	1/2	0.097	0.092
9	43–45	1/1	0	0	—

The product-limit estimates of the survival probabilities ($\hat{P}_k$ values) for these two groups (note: "survival" means time to relapse) are given in Table 11–11 and 11–12. The estimated survival curves are shown in Figure 11–4 for both nonparametric (product-limit—$\hat{P}_k$) and parametric (exponential assumption—$\hat{S}[t] = e^{-\lambda t}$) approaches.

If the longest follow-up period ends with a patient being withdrawn, then the product-limit derived mean value is biased (too small). That is, the final interval is undefined and the longest survival time does not contribute, because each interval used in the calculation must contain at least one death. Intervals are defined by the time of death. The maintained AML data should, therefore, be adjusted to avoid this bias, because the patient who survived the longest (161 weeks) was in remission at the end of the study period, censored. A conventional practice is to consider the longest survival time as ending in a death (or in the AML case, relapse). In this way the survival time contributes

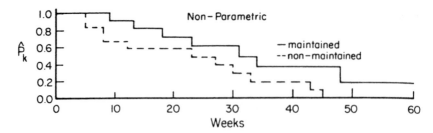

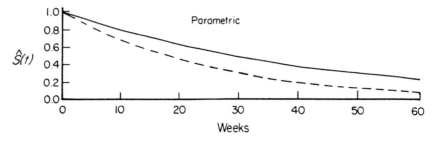

Figure 11–4. Two-sample AML remission data for the maintained and nonmaintained groups—nonparametric and parametric plots of the survival curves

to the total time at risk and a lesser bias is incurred when this artificial endpoint is necessary. The nonparametric estimated mean survival times for these two groups are then [from expression (11.29) or (11.30)]: for maintained = 52.645 (estimated standard error = 19.828) and for nonmaintained = 22.708 (estimated standard error = 4.181). This difference between mean survival times yields weak, at best, evidence of a difference between the two therapies. The large amount of variation in times to relapse associated with the maintained group interferes with assessing the observed difference of about 30 weeks.

For the leukemia data example, the one patient who survived 161 weeks dominates the comparison. The disproportionate influence is seen by comparing the mean and median survival times. The estimated median survival times, maintained = 30.415 weeks and nonmaintained = 21.412 weeks, respectively, differ by far less than the 30 weeks between mean values (difference = 9.003), because extreme survival times have little impact on the median. These median values are estimated by linear interpolation of the product-limit survival curve. Sometimes the median survival time is estimated by using the endpoint of the interval containing the 50th percentile (maintained = 31 weeks and nonmaintained = 23 weeks—a difference of 8 weeks).

Table 11–13. Summary: leukemia data survival times (weeks)

	Mean		Median	
	Maintained	Nonmaintained	Maintained	Nonmaintained
Parametric	60.429	23.182	41.886	16.068
Nonparametric	52.645	22.708	30.415	21.412

A parametric estimate is, in principle, more efficient than a nonparametric approach, but at the cost of making additional assumptions about the structure of the data. If the survival experience of these two groups of leukemia patients is modeled by an exponential survival curve, then parametric estimated mean survival times are: maintained = 60.429 weeks (estimated standard error = 22.840 and nonmaintained = 23.182 weeks (estimated standard error = 6.989). Parametric estimation also does not provide sufficient statistical precision to infer the observed difference in mean survival times is unlikely to be a chance occurrence. The estimated median survival time, based on the exponential distribution, is $\bar{t} \log(2)$ and for the AML data are: maintained = 41.886 weeks and nonmaintained = 16.068 weeks. The estimates from the AML data are summarized in Table 11–13.

The trade-off between parametric and nonparametric analyses is illustrated by these estimates. The choice between the two approaches is rarely clear and relies primarily on the judgment of the investigator, supported by goodness-of-fit analysis.

Evaluation of Two-Sample Data

A formal nonparametric evaluation of differences in survival times between groups is accomplished by a chi-square procedure almost identical to the traditional Mantel–Haenszel chi-square technique [expression (7.53)].

Similar to the product-limit (Kaplan–Meier) estimate, the data are sorted into strata based on times of each death (t_i). The process produces a set of 2×2 tables, one for each recorded death, where all individuals under observation are classified as treatment or control and survived or died (i.e., d = number of deaths = number of strata—one stratum for each death if all survival times differ). Specifically, each time of death generates a standard 2×2 table such

Table 11–14. 2×2 table generated for each stratum

t_i	Died	Survived	Total
Treatment	a_i	b_i	$a_i + b_i$
Control	c_i	d_i	$c_i + d_i$
Total	$a_i + c_i$	$b_i + d_i$	n_i

Table 11–15. AML follow-up data summary

i	Interval	a_i	b_i	c_i	d_i	n_i
1	0–5	0	11	2	10	23
2	5–8	0	11	2	8	21
3	8–9	1	10	0	8	19
4	9–12	0	10	1	7	18
5	12–13	1	9	0	7	17
6	13–18	1	7	0	6	14
7	18–23	1	6	1	5	13
8	23–27	0	6	1	4	11
9	27–30	0	5	1	3	9
10	30–31	1	4	0	3	8
11	31–33	0	4	1	2	7
12	33–34	1	3	0	2	6
13	34–43	0	3	1	1	5
14	43–45	0	3	1	0	4
15	45–48	1	1	0	0	2

as Table 11–14. The AML data produces 15 ($d = 15$ strata) 2×2 tables (Table 11–15 and Figure 11–5 displays these 15 tables).

The analysis of an association between two binary variables (died/survived and treatment/control), while controlling for the confounding influence of a third variable (time), is a typical use of the Mantel–Haenszel chi-square procedure. The difference between the analysis of a series of 2×2 tables generated by survival data and the usual application of the Mantel–Haenszel procedure is that survival data tables (strata) are not independent. Individuals who survive are included in subsequent tables, introducing a dependency among the tables. The lack of independence is not critical and a chi-square summary remains an accurate evaluation of treatment/survival association. The censored survival times contribute to the time at risk until withdrawn from observation and, like the product-limit estimator, the association between treatment and outcome is not biased by the incomplete follow-up. That is, the number at risk n_i is sequentially

t=5	death	alive	total
M	0	11	11
NM	2	10	12
total	2	21	23

t=18	death	alive	total
M	1	7	8
NM	0	6	6
total	1	13	14

t=33	death	alive	total
M	0	4	4
NM	1	2	3
total	1	6	7

t=8	death	alive	total
M	0	11	11
NM	2	8	10
total	2	19	21

t=23	death	alive	total
M	1	6	7
NM	1	5	6
total	2	11	13

t=34	death	alive	total
M	1	3	4
NM	0	2	2
total	1	5	6

t=9	death	alive	total
M	1	10	11
NM	0	8	8
total	1	18	19

t=27	death	alive	total
M	0	6	6
NM	1	4	5
total	1	10	11

t=43	death	alive	total
M	0	3	3
NM	1	1	2
total	1	4	5

t=12	death	alive	total
M	0	10	10
NM	1	7	8
total	1	17	18

t=30	death	alive	total
M	0	5	5
NM	1	3	4
total	1	8	9

t=45	death	alive	total
M	0	3	3
NM	1	0	1
total	1	3	4

t=13	death	alive	total
M	1	9	10
NM	0	7	7
total	1	16	17

t=31	death	alive	total
M	1	4	5
NM	0	3	3
total	1	7	8

t=48	death	alive	total
M	1	1	2
NM	0	0	0
total	1	1	2

Figure 11–5. Full display of the AML data by known times of remission for maintained and nonmaintained groups in a series of 2 × 2 tables

reduced in each stratum by the number who died (usually one), the number who are censored, and those lost from observation to form the number of individuals at risk in the next stratum (n_{i+1}). Again, censored observations are included only where they are present for the entire interval.

The two-sample analysis consists of testing for an association between treatment/control status and disease outcome among a series of strata based on time of death. The expected number of deaths when no treatment/survival association exists for each stratum (table) is

$$\text{expected} = \hat{A}_i = \frac{(a_i + b_i)(a_i + c_i)}{n_i}, \tag{11.38}$$

and the estimated variance for the observed number of deaths in the treatment group (a_i) is

$$\text{variance}\,(a_i) = \frac{(a_i + b_i)(a_i + c_i)(b_i + d_i)(c_i + d_i)}{n_i^2(n_i - 1)}. \tag{11.39}$$

Table 11–16. AML follow-up data

i	Interval	a_i	$\hat{A}_i$	Variance
1	0–5	0	0.956	0.476
2	5–8	0	1.048	0.474
3	8–9	1	0.579	0.244
4	9–12	0	0.556	0.247
5	12–13	1	0.588	0.242
6	13–18	1	0.571	0.245
7	18–23	1	1.077	0.456
8	23–27	0	0.545	0.248
9	27–30	0	0.556	0.247
10	30–31	1	0.625	0.234
11	31–33	0	0.571	0.245
12	33–34	1	0.667	0.222
13	34–43	0	0.600	0.240
14	43–45	0	0.750	0.188
15	45–48	1	1.000	0.000
Total	—	7	10.689	4.008

These two estimates are the same as those used for the Mantel–Haenszel chi-square test of association [expressions (7.51) and (7.52)]. The expected values and the variances for the illustrative AML data are shown in Table 11–16. A weighted chi-square statistic is then calculated as

$$X^2 = \frac{\left\{ \sum\limits_{i=1}^{k} w_i(a_i - \hat{A}_i) \right\}^2}{\sum\limits_{i=1}^{k} w_i^2 \, \text{variance} \, (a_i)},$$

to summarize and assess the differences $a_i - \hat{A}_i$. The value X^2 has an approximate chi-square distribution with one degree of freedom under the hypothesis of no association between treatment/control status and survival in all strata. Large values of X^2, therefore, imply an association between treatment and survival. When $w_i = 1$, X^2 is formally the Mantel–Haenszel chi-square statistic and sometimes called the log-rank test. The term log-rank is a bit obscure, because the development used here involves neither logarithms nor ranks. It arises from an alternative derivation. Others have suggested alternative weights: $w_i = n_i$ (Gehan, cited in [6]) and $w_i = \sqrt{n_i}$ (Tarone and Ware, cited in [6]). Gehan's suggestion emphasizes the early observed values more heavily than the Mantel–Haenszel statistic, while the Tarone–Ware suggestion is intermediate. All three are different weighings for comparisons of the number of observed deaths (7 in the AML example)

Table 11–17. Chi-square values for the three chi-square tests

	w_i	Chi-square	p-value
Mantel–Haenszel	1	3.396	0.065
Tarone–Ware	$\sqrt{n_i}$	2.981	0.084
Gehan	n_i	2.723	0.099

to the number expected when the treatment and survival time are unrelated (10.689 from the AML data). The three chi-square values for the AML data are shown in Table 11–17.

The chi-square analysis of the AML data indicates, on the basis of borderline evidence, that the treatment may influence survival.

The Mantel–Haenszel statistic is similar to another procedure also based on a chi-square statistic [6]. Both procedures give basically the same results for the comparison of two groups. The advantage of the additional test is that it can be generalized to situations where more than two treatments (k) are considered, producing a series of $2 \times K$ tables. Like the Mantel–Haenszel procedure, expected values are estimated based on postulating independence between treatment/control status and outcome. The total expected number of deaths among the treatment individuals $(\hat{A})$ is estimated (notation from Table 11–14) by a sum of the estimated values from each table or

$$\text{total number of deaths expected} = \hat{A} = \sum \hat{A}_i = \sum \frac{(a_i + b_i)(a_i + c_i)}{n_i}.$$

Similarly, the total number of expected deaths among the controls is estimated by

$$\text{total number of deaths expected} = \hat{C} = \sum \hat{C}_i = \sum \frac{(a_i + c_i)(c_i + d_i)}{n_i}.$$

The parallel observed values are $a = \sum a_i$ (total observed deaths among the treated individuals) and $c = \sum c_i$ (total observed deaths among the control individuals). Comparing these expected values to the observed values, a chi-square statistic becomes

$$X^2 = \frac{(a - \hat{A})^2}{\hat{A}} + \frac{(c - \hat{C})^2}{\hat{C}}.$$

The test statistic X^2 has an approximate chi-square distribution with one degree of freedom when treatment/control status is unrelated to survival outcome. Using again the AML data, $a = 7$ and $c = 11$ and the corresponding expected values are $\hat{A} = 10.689$ and

$\hat{C} = 7.311$. The chi-square statistic is then $X^2 = (7 - 10.689)^2/10.689 + (11 - 7.311)^2/7.311 = 3.135$, yielding a p-value $= 0.077$. Note that this X^2 statistics is smaller than the similar value calculated using the Mantel–Haenszel approach. The Mantel–Haenszel technique will always produce a smaller chi-square statistic. If more than two groups are compared, then a series of expected values generated under the hypothesis that the treatments are independent of survival are compared to the observed values again with a chi-square statistic.

The Wilcoxon Test and the Gehan Generalization

A modification of the Wilcoxon test provides an alternative to the Mantel–Haenszel approach to evaluate observed differences in survival times between two groups. First, consider a review of the situation where incomplete survival data are not involved.

Like the two-sample t-test, the Wilcoxon two-sample test is designed to assess differences between two independent samples of observations. The Wilcoxon test, however, is nonparametric and is valid regardless of the distribution of the sampled populations or the size of the collected sample. For clarity, one sampled group is called the "control" and the other the "treatment." The first step is to replace the data values y_{ij} (again y_{ij} represents a measurement from the ith group on the jth individual) by their ranks (R_{ij}; rank 1 = lowest value, rank 2 = next lowest, etc., where $i = 1 = $ control and $i = 2 = $ treatment groups), disregarding group membership. If the sample consists of n_1 control and n_2 treatment observations, then the "data" become the integers 1, 2, 3, . . . , n, where $n = n_1 + n_2$. A summary statistic that reflects differences between treatment and control groups is the sum of the ranks associated with the treatment observations ($R = \sum R_{ij}$—or the sum over j for the group $i = 2$). If there is no systematic differences between groups, the sum of the treatment ranks should be proportional to the number of treatment observations (n_2). Specifically, the expected sum of the ranks for the treatment group is

$$\text{expected sum of treatment ranks} = ER = n_2 \left[\frac{n + 1}{2} \right], \qquad (11.40)$$

which is n_2 times the average rank. For example, if the treatment and control groups have the same number of observations, then the sum of the ranks for each group should be about equal when the groups differ only because of random variation ($ER = n(n + 1)/4$, where $n_1 = n_2 = n/2$). If the two samples systematically differ, then the sum of the treatment ranks will likely be extreme (differ from the expected).

The null hypothesis of no difference between treatment and control groups is assessed by comparing the observed value R with the null hypothesis generated value ER. This comparison, as usual, requires an expression for the variance of R, which is

$$\text{variance}(R) = n_1 n_2 \frac{n+1}{12} \tag{11.41}$$

when no systematic difference exists between the treatment and control groups.

A seemingly different process for calculating a summary rank statistic involves counting the number of values less than each ordered observation and counting the number of values greater than each ordered observation. The sum of the differences (D_{ij}) between these counts associated with the n_2 treatment observations also serves as a test statistic $(D = \sum D_{ij})$.

An example will make the process clear. A group of women with a history of having large newborn infants reporting pregnancy complications $(n_2 = 9)$ is compared to a set of controls $(n_1 = 10)$ for levels of glucose determined by glucose tolerance tests. These data (ordered from low to high) are shown in Table 11–18. Each observation produces a D_{ij} value. For the test statistic $D = \sum D_{ij}$, like R, extreme values lead to rejecting the hypothesis that no difference exists

Table 11–18. Results from glucose tolerance tests

Group	y_{ij}	Rank = R_{ij}	Lower than y_{ij}	Greater than y_{ij}	D_{ij}
No complications	100	1	0	18	−18
No complications	110	2	1	17	−16
No complications	117	3	2	16	−14
No complications	119	4	3	15	−12
Complications	120	5	4	14	−10
No complications	122	6	5	13	−8
No complications	127	7	6	12	−6
Complications	128	8	7	11	−4
Complications	132	9	8	10	−2
No complications	133	10	9	9	0
No complications	135	11	10	8	2
Complications	140	12	11	7	4
No complications	141	13	12	6	6
Complications	143	14	13	5	8
No complications	151	15	14	4	10
Complications	162	16	15	3	12
Complications	177	17	16	2	14
Complications	181	18	17	1	16
Complications	184	19	18	0	18

between the two compared groups. Either R or D can equally be used to evaluate observed differences between the two groups, because these two statistical measures are related. The exact relationship is $D = 2R - n_2(n + 1)$ and, therefore, variance$(D) = 4$ variance(R). Incidentally, the relationship between D and R shows that $ED = 0$ (i.e., $ED = 2ER - n_2(n - 1) = 0$). Also note that the D_{ij} values are symmetrically distributed around zero when the null hypothesis is true.

The sum of the pregnancy complications ("treatment") ranks is $R = \sum R_{ij} = 5 + 8 + 9 + 12 + 14 + 16 + 17 + 18 + 19 = 118$. The expected value of $R(ER)$ is 90. Correspondingly, the sum of the differences in counts associated with the "treatment" is $D = \sum D_{ij} = -10 - 4 - 2 + 4 + 8 + 12 + 14 + 16 + 18 = 56$. A statistical significance test of either nonparametric measure is

$$z = \frac{R - ER}{\sqrt{\text{variance}(R)}} = \frac{D - 0}{\sqrt{\text{variance}(D)}}, \tag{11.42}$$

where z has an approximately standard normal distribution when sample sizes are at least moderately large (say, both n_1 and $n_2 >$ about 10) and no systematic differences exist between the treatment and control groups. Tables of the exact distribution of R are available for small sample sizes [7]. For the example data, the test using D is $z = 56/\sqrt{600} = 2.286$ producing an approximate p-value of 0.22. The test of R is, of course, identical because the probabilities associated with D are the same as those associated with R. An alternative way to calculate the variance of D is

$$\text{variance}(D) = \frac{n_1 n_2 \sum_{i=1}^{2} \sum_{j=1}^{n_i} D_{ij}^2}{n(n - 1)} \quad (\textstyle\sum\sum D_{ij}^2 = 2{,}280 \text{ for the example data}).$$

$$\tag{11.43}$$

The D version of the Wilcoxon test statistic and its variance are introduced because they generalize [8] to the comparison of two groups containing censored survival times.

Gehan [8] applied the Wilcoxon two-sample rank test to evaluate differences between samples that include censored survival times. The Gehan generalization of the Wilcoxon procedure employs the values D_{ij} rather than the ranks. The number of survival times that are known to be less than each ordered observation are counted. Similarly, the number of survival times when they are known to be greater than each ordered observation are counted. The difference D_{ij} is then calculated for each survival time (censored and noncensored). The partial information from the censored values is incorporated into the test statistic by this counting process. For example, if an individual is withdrawn from a study after 13 weeks (13^+), it is known that this person's survival time exceeds all individuals who died in less than 13 weeks. The test statistic is, as before, the sum of the differences $(D = \sum D_{ij})$ associated with the treatment survival times, and the expected value remains zero under the null hypothesis. The variance is given by expression (11.43). Consider again the AML data ordered without regard to treatment/control status, displayed in Table 11–19. The sum of the D_{ij} values associated with the $n_2 = 11$ maintained individuals is $D = \sum D_{ij} = -14 - 10 + 7 - 6 - 3 + 11 + 5 + 9 + 17 + 16 + 18 = 50$ and the variance$(D) = 11(12)(3503)/(23)(22) = 913.826$, producing $z = (50 - 0)/\sqrt{913.826} = 1.654$ giving a p-value of 0.098.

The Gehan chi-square test produces a somewhat higher p-value (0.097) than the Mantel–Haenszel procedure for assessing the association between survival and treatment (p-value $= 0.065$, Table 11–17) but the results are almost identical to the Gehan weighted chi-square test (p-value $= 0.099$, Table 11–17). The Gehan chi-square test and

Table 11–19. Results from maintenance chemotherapy trial

Group	t_{ij}	Lower than t_{ij}	Greater than t_{ij}	D_{ij}
Nonmaintained	5	0	21	-21
Nonmaintained	5	0	21	-21
Nonmaintained	8	2	19	-17
Nonmaintained	8	2	19	-17
Maintained	9	4	18	-14
Nonmaintained	12	5	17	-12
Maintained	13	6	16	-10
Maintained	13^+	7	0	7
Nonmaintained	16^+	7	0	7
Maintained	18	7	13	-6
Nonmaintained	23	8	12	-4
Maintained	23	8	11	-3
Nonmaintained	27	10	10	-0
Maintained	28^+	11	0	11
Nonmaintained	30	11	8	3
Maintained	31	12	7	5
Nonmaintained	33	13	6	7
Maintained	34	14	5	9
Nonmaintained	43	15	4	11
Nonmaintained	45	16	3	13
Maintained	45^+	17	0	17
Maintained	48	17	1	16
Maintained	161^+	18	0	18

the Gehan/Wilcoxon test are related, giving similar results in assessing a treatment influence on the disease outcome or, in symbols, $z^2 \approx X^2$. Specifically, for the AML data $z^2 = (1.654)^2 = 2.736$ and $X^2 = 2.723$. In all but exceptional situations, both the Gehan version of the chi-square test and the Gehan–Wilcoxon rank test give results that do not substantially differ.

12 A Model for Survival Data: Proportional Hazards Model

It is rarely sufficient to demonstrate that one group of individuals has a significantly longer mean survival time than another. Pursuit of plausible explanations for observed differences between groups is also important in understanding survival experience. Survival time, like risk measured by a probability, is affected by a number of interrelated factors. For example, factors such as age, severity of disease, past health status, and race provide concomitant information that likely improves the description of survival data. The investigation of the role of these explanatory variables usually requires postulating a statistical model that relates the survival time (e.g., time until failure) to a series of measurements thought to influence an individual's survival. The analysis of these explanatory variables is conducted in much the same manner as the assessment of the risk variables in a logistic regression analysis. Of course, a statistical model linking a series of explanatory variables to survival time will, at best, approximate the unknown underlying situation. One is never assured that a mathematical structure is "biologically" correct. Alternative approaches, however, are rarely possible without large amounts of data, making a statistical model a basic tool in the investigation of a series of variables relevant to survival time. The success of a model-based approach depends on choosing a model that adequately reflects the relationships within the data set. The choice of an appropriate statistical structure is an art, requiring knowledge of the mathematical properties of the model and a clear understanding of the phenomenon under investigation. One useful approach to survival data is the application of the proportional hazards model. This chapter explores this complex model in simple terms with the dual purpose of illustrating the technique and providing insight into the process of modeling survival experience. Also included are five applications of the proportional hazards model to survival data. The multivariate analysis of survival data is a mathematically sophisticated topic, and texts are devoted entirely to the statistical analysis of failure-time data (e.g., [1], [2], and [3]). This chapter is a brief introduction.

Simplest Case

The simplest application of a proportional hazards model (sometimes called the Cox model, after the statistician D. R. Cox who originated the analytic approach) involves the comparison of two treatment groups made up of individuals with varying survival times, some of which may be censored. A small hypothetical data set of 12 subjects is given in Table 12–1. These data consist of two treatment groups (A and B) of six individuals with a total of three incomplete survival times.

Before employing a proportional hazards model to evaluate treatment differences between groups A and B, it is useful to apply the chi-square assessment of an association [expression (7.53)] between two treatments and a disease outcome to this small data set. When the analysis involves simply two comparison groups, the Mantel-Haenszel approach relates to the proportional hazards model as will be seen. The hypothetical data classified into a series of 2 × 2 tables based on the nine known times of death gives Table 12–2. The same data are fully displayed in Figure 12–1. The chi-square statistic for evaluating an association in a series of 2 × 2 tables is, once again,

$$X^2 = \frac{\left\{\sum\limits_{i=1}^{k}(a_i - \hat{A}_i)\right\}^2}{\sum\limits_{i=1}^{k}\text{variance}\,(a_i)} \quad \text{and} \quad X^2 = \frac{(2.743)^2}{1.428} = 5.269, \quad (12.1)$$

Table 12–1. Hypothetical data

Treatment A	5	8	12	22^+	37	41
Treatment B	23	40	43	51^+	53^+	62

Table 12–2. Hypothetical data displayed in 2 × 2 tables: Summary

Time (t)	a_i	$a_i + b_i$	n_i	$\hat{A}_i$	$a_i - \hat{A}_i$	Variance (a_i)
5	1	6	12	6/12	6/12	396/1,584 = 0.250
8	1	5	11	5/11	6/11	300/1,210 = 0.248
12	1	4	10	4/10	6/10	216/900 = 0.240
23	0	2	8	2/8	−2/8	84/448 = 0.188
37	1	2	7	2/7	5/7	60/294 = 0.204
40	0	1	6	1/6	−1/6	25/180 = 0.139
41	1	1	5	1/5	4/5	16/100 = 0.160
43	0	0	4	0/4	0	0/48 = 0.000
62	0	0	1	0/1	0	—
Total	5	—	—	2.257	2.743	1.428

t=5	death	alive	total
A	1	5	6
B	0	6	6
total	1	11	12

t=23	death	alive	total
A	0	2	2
B	1	5	6
total	1	7	8

t=41	death	alive	total
A	1	0	1
B	0	4	4
total	1	4	5

t=8	death	alive	total
A	1	4	5
B	0	6	6
total	1	10	11

t=37	death	alive	total
A	1	1	2
B	0	5	5
total	1	6	7

t=43	death	alive	total
A	0	0	0
B	1	3	4
total	1	3	4

t=12	death	alive	total
A	1	3	4
B	0	6	6
total	1	9	10

t=40	death	alive	total
A	0	1	1
B	1	4	5
total	1	5	6

t=62	death	alive	total
A	0	0	0
B	1	0	1
total	1	0	1

Figure 12–1. Full display of the hypothetical data by known times of death for group A and group B in a series of 2 × 2 tables

yielding a p-value of 0.022 for the $k = 9$ tables. The data show evidence of a nonrandom difference in survival time associated with the two treatments A and B.

Aside: The expected value and the estimated variance of a_i in the situation where no survival times are identical can be simplified over the previous more general expressions (11.38) and (11.39) as

$$\text{expected} = \hat{A}_i = \frac{a_i + b_i}{n_i}$$

and

$$\text{variance } (a_i) = \frac{(a_i + b_i)(c_i + d_i)}{n_i^2}. \tag{12.2}$$

The proportional hazards model, in its simplest form, postulates that the hazard function associated with the survival times in group A relates to the hazard function associated with the survival times in group B by a multiplicative constant or

$$\lambda_B(t) = c\lambda_A(t) \quad \text{or} \quad \frac{\lambda_B(t)}{\lambda_A(t)} = c, \tag{12.3}$$

where $\lambda_A(t)$ and $\lambda_B(t)$ represent hazard functions for groups A and B, respectively. Unlike the exponential model, these hazard rates can vary depending on time t.

The constant c can be estimated from survival data. For example, continuing to use the hypothetical data, $\hat{c} = 0.168$ is the estimated constant of proportionality for the hazard rates associated with treatments A and B. That is, the hazard rate in group B is estimated to be about six times smaller than in group A or $\lambda_B(t) = 0.168 \, \lambda_A(t)$. The estimate is, like the logistic regression case, found by a maximum likelihood estimation procedure and requires a complex computer algorithm. In most cases the collected survival data are too sparse to estimate reliably the hazard functions themselves; however, the estimate of the constant c provides an efficient summary measure of the difference in survival experience between two groups. A special property of the proportional hazards model is that the estimate of the proportionality constant (c) does not require the actual form of the hazard function to be specified. The comparison of the relative survival between the two groups can be analyzed without knowledge or assumptions about the functional form of the hazard functions $\lambda_A(t)$ or $\lambda_B(t)$, as long as they are proportional.

Additionally, the estimation of the constant c makes use of both the complete and the incomplete observations in the data set. Not unlike the product-limit estimate of the survival probabilities, information from the censored observations is utilized where it is relevant and ignored by the estimation process when it is not to form an unbiased estimate of c.

In terms of survival curves, the property of proportionality of hazard functions translates to

$$S_B(t) = [S_A(t)]^c, \tag{12.4}$$

where $S_A(t)$ and $S_B(t)$ represent the survival curves for groups A and B. The general relationship between survival curves when the hazard functions are proportional is dealt with in a following section [expression (12.14)].

If one survival curve is known or estimated, then the other is directly related when the hazard functions are proportional. For example, if for members of group A (Table 12–1) $S_A(t_0) = 0.6$ at a specific time t_0, then

$$\hat{S}_B(t_0) = [S_A(t_0)]^{\hat{c}} = (0.6)^{0.168} = 0.918 \tag{12.5}$$

explicitly gives the probability of survival for a member from group B in terms of the probability of survival of a member of group A. Note that $S_B(t)$ will always be greater than $S_A(t)$ when $\lambda_B(t)$ is less than $\lambda_A(t)$, which is not surprising because a smaller hazard rate implies a higher probability of survival. That is, the survival curve $S_A(t)$ will always be below the survival curve $S_B(t)$ for all values of t, because $\hat{c} = 0.168 < 1$.

Several methods can be used to evaluate statistically the estimate $\hat{c}$. To test the null hypothesis that the hazard functions are the same (H_0: $c = 1$), an effective technique is to compare two likelihood statistics. The first is derived under the conditions that $\lambda_B(t) = \lambda_A(t)$ and the second under the hypothesis that $\lambda_B(t) = c\lambda_A(t)$. For the illustrative data, these two likelihoods statistics are $L_0 = 31.997$ for $c = 1$ and $L_1 = 27.148$ for $c \neq 1$, produced as part of the maximum likelihood procedure. The difference $L_0 - L_1 = 4.849$ has an approximate chi-square distribution with one degree of freedom when $c = 1$, producing a p-value of 0.028. The degrees of freedom are the difference in the number of parameters between the compared models.

Alternatively, a statistical test of $\hat{c}$ in terms of the log $(\hat{c})$ is equally effective, or

$$z = \frac{\log(\hat{c}) - \log(c)}{S_{\log(\hat{c})}} \tag{12.6}$$

and z has an approximate standard normal distribution when $c = 1$ or $\log(c) = 0$. For example, from the hypothetical data, the logarithm of $\hat{c}$ is $\log(0.168) = -1.785$ with a variance $[\log(\hat{c})] = 0.745$ (estimated as part of the maximum likelihood procedure). Therefore, $z = -1.785/\sqrt{0.745} = -2.067$, and the corresponding p-value is 0.039. Again showing statistical evidence that the survival experience is likely different between groups A and B.

The Mantel-Haenszel chi-square test gives results similar to the difference between likelihood statistics, particularly when large sample sizes are involved (e.g., $X^2 = 5.286$ with p-value $= 0.022$ [expression (12.1)] compared to $L_0 - L_1 = 4.849$ with a p-value $= 0.028$, for the hypothetical data). The fact that the log-likelihood and chi-square approaches are related indicates that the proportional hazards model can be viewed as a process that stratifies the survival data on the time of failure and combines information from each stratum to estimate the overall constant of proportionality c, measuring the difference between two proportional hazard functions. Also similar to the Mantel-Haenszel chi-square procedure, the proportional hazards approach is non-parametric in the sense that no need exists to specify the form of the hazard functions or survival curves to assess the relative influence of two treatments or to compare two groups and, as mentioned, produces estimates of the model parameters that are not biased by the presence of censored data.

AML Example

The data introduced in Chapter 11 concerning two treatments for acute myelogenous leukemia (AML) [4] can be analyzed using the conjecture that the hazard functions associated with treatments, maintained (M) and nonmaintained (NM), are proportional. The estimated constant of proportionality is $\hat{c} = 0.405$. Therefore, $\lambda_M(t) = \hat{c}\lambda_{NM}(t) = 0.405\lambda_{NM}(t)$. The hazard rates reflecting the risk of a relapse in the maintained group of leukemia patients are estimated to be considerably smaller than the hazard rates associated with the subjects not receiving the special chemotherapy (a 2.5-fold difference). The difference in likelihood statistics produces $L_{c=1} - L_{c\neq1} = 85.796 - 82.500 = 3.296$, which has an approximate chi-square distribution with one degree of freedom and yields a p-value of 0.069. Assuming proportional hazard rates, the comparison of likelihood statistics produces borderline evidence of a systematic difference between these two treatments. This result is expectedly similar to the chi-square analysis of the same data ($X^2 = 3.396$ with a p-value $= 0.065$, Table 10–18).

To explore these data further, it is assumed that the survival experience is adequately described by an exponential function for the nonmaintained group. This special case of proportional hazard functions gives

$$S_M(t) = \{S_{MN}(t)\}^{0.405} = \{e^{-\lambda_{NM}t}\}^{0.405}, \tag{12.7}$$

where λ_{NM} is the constant hazard rate for the nonmaintained group. Although this relationship results from a further and perhaps unrealistic assumption, it allows a simple and direct comparison of the two survival experiences. For example, Figure 12–2 is based on

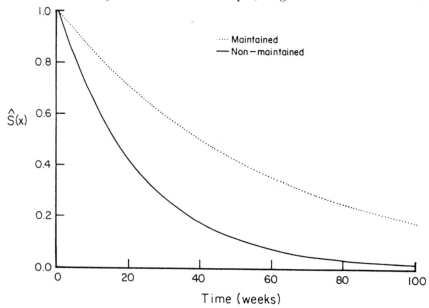

Figure 12–2. Survival curves for the AML data for the maintained and non-maintained groups

expression (12.7) and the estimated parameter $\hat{\lambda}_{NM} = 1/\bar{t} = 1/23.182 = 0.043$, giving $\hat{\lambda}_M = 0.405(0.043) = 0.0174$. A value of λ_M estimated directly from the 11 AML observations is $1/\bar{t} = 1/60.429 = 0.0165$, which agrees closely with the estimate using the proportional hazards model. Equally, the ratio of the survival rates calculated directly from the AML data can be compared to the proportional hazards estimate. The exponential model produces hazard rates of $\lambda_{NM} = 0.043$ weeks (nonmaintained) and $\lambda_M = 0.0165$ weeks (maintained), giving a ratio based on these estimates of $\lambda_M/\lambda_{MN} = 0.383$. The proportional hazards ratio based on the proportional hazards model is, again, $\hat{c} = 0.405$; the two approaches agree, implying that the assumption of a constant hazard function for this leukemia remission data is not unreasonable.

General Case

A general additive proportional hazards model with k explanatory variables is written as

$$\lambda_j(t; x_{1j}, x_{2j}, \ldots, x_{kj}) = \lambda_0(t)\, c_j = \lambda_0(t)\, e^{\sum_{i=1}^{k} b_i x_{ij}}. \tag{12.8}$$

The value $\lambda_j(t; x_{1j}, x_{2j}, \ldots, x_{kj})$ represents the hazard rate for the jth group or person with specific explanatory values at time t relative to $\lambda_0(t)$, an arbitrary "baseline" hazard rate also at time t. The value x_{ij} represents one of a series of measures on each group or individual, and the coefficient b_i determines the influence of that measurement on survival time. The model allows the proportionality constant c_j to be factored into a series of multiplicative components each associated with the influence of a specific explanatory variable. The rate ratio c_j can be viewed as

$$c_j = e^{\sum_{i=1}^{k} b_i x_{ij}} = (e^{b_1 x_{1j}})(e^{b_2 x_{2j}})(e^{b_3 x_{3j}}) \cdots (e^{b_k x_{kj}}). \tag{12.9}$$

The relative contribution to survival time of each x_{ij} is measured by $(e^{b_i})^{x_{ij}}$. The quantity e^{b_i} is called the relative hazard for the ith explanatory variable.

A common and useful practice is to "center" the x variables so that the proportional hazards model becomes

$$\lambda_j(t; x_{1j}, x_{2j}, \ldots, x_{kj}) = \lambda_0(t)\, e^{\sum_{i=1}^{k} b_i(x_{ij} - \bar{x}_i)}, \tag{12.10}$$

where $\bar{x}_i$ is the mean of the ith explanatory variable based on all n observations. For this form of the model, the "baseline" hazard function $\lambda_0(t)$ represents the hazard rate where all x variables are at their mean values (the "average" hazard function). Two alternative forms of the proportional hazards model are

$$\log\left\{\frac{\lambda_j(t)}{\lambda_0(t)}\right\} = \sum_{i=1}^{k} b_i(x_{ij} - \bar{x}_i) \quad \text{or} \quad \log[\lambda_j(t)] = \log[\lambda_0(t)] + \sum_{i=1}^{k} b_i(x_{ij} - \bar{x}_i),$$

(12.11)

showing more directly the way the explanatory variables (x_{ij}) relate to the ratio of hazard functions. The first part of expression (12.11) shows that the logarithm of the ratio of proportional hazard functions does not depend on time but only on the explanatory variables x_{ij}. The second part shows the proportional hazards model in a form analogous to a linear multiple regression model with an "intercept" term that depends on follow-up time separated from a weighted sum of explanatory variables that does not depend on follow-up time. In both cases, the role of the explanatory variables (x_{ij}) is explored by means of estimated b_i coefficients in much the same way as the coefficients from a multivariable linear or logistic regression analysis.

The proportional hazards model is an effective way of accounting for the confounding influence of time in the analysis of follow-up data. The basic model [expression (12.8)] requires that the explanatory variables do not change over the time of the study. The influence of time and the explanatory variable are separate components of the model [expression (12.11)], which is another way of saying that the constant of proportionality c_j is unaffected by time. However, the proportional hazards model can be modified so that the explanatory variables also depend on time. A treatment could vary during the follow-up period, or characteristics of individuals such as blood pressure or cholesterol can certainly change during the follow-up period. The analysis of risk in the presence of such time-dependent explanatory variables is complex and is reviewed elsewhere (e.g., [1] or [2]).

The hazard function and the survival curve are related; as mentioned, high hazard rates lead to low survival probabilities and conversely. Formally,

$$\lambda(t) = -\frac{dS(t)/dt}{S(t)} \quad \text{translates to} \quad S(t) = e^{-\int_0^t \lambda(u)du}. \quad (12.12)$$

When two hazard functions $(\lambda_j(t)$ and $\lambda_0(t))$ are proportional such that

$$\lambda_j(t) = \lambda_0(t)\, e^{\sum b_i x_{ij}}, \quad (12.13)$$

then

$$S_j(t) = e^{-\int_0^t \lambda_j(u)du} = \left[e^{-\int_0^t \lambda_0(u)du}\right]^{e^{\sum b_i x_{ij}}} \quad \text{giving} \quad S_j(t) = [S_0(t)]^{e^{\sum b_i x_{ij}}}. \quad (12.14)$$

In the special case where the survival curve is exponential (i.e., $S_0(t) = e^{-\lambda_0 t}$), then

$$S_j(t) = [e^{-\lambda_0 t}]^{e^{\sum b_i x_{ij}}}. \tag{12.15}$$

The proportional hazards model is called semiparametric—it is made-up of a nonparametric piece and a parametric piece. The nonparametric property stems from the fact that the hazard functions remain as general functions, and it is not necessary to describe this part of the model in a parametric form. However, the relationship between the explanatory variables and the survival times is described parametrically. Specifically, the role of each covariable is measured by a parameter (b_i), which is also a fundamental part of the pro-portional hazards model.

Two Properties of Proportional Hazards Survival Curves

When two hazard functions are proportional, the survival curves will not cross. Consider, for example, the survival curve given by

$$S_0(t) = 1 - \frac{t}{100}, \quad \text{where} \quad 0 \leq t \leq 100 \tag{12.16}$$

and, as before, $\lambda_0(t) = 1/(100 - t)$ [expression (1.22)]; further, suppose that two groups (1 and 2) have proportional hazard functions where:

$$\lambda_1(t) = 2\lambda_0(t) \quad \text{and} \quad \lambda_2(t) = 4\lambda_0(t) \quad \text{then} \quad S_2(t) = [S_1(t)]^2. \tag{12.17}$$

These two survival curves do not cross, but it is not obvious from the plots of survival curves or hazard functions that the hazard rates are proportional (Figure 12–3, top). The transformation $\log(-\log[S(t)])$ is useful. For proportional hazards functions, this transformation produces survival curves that are parallel and differ because of the presence of explanatory variables. Figure 12–3 (bottom left) shows the transformed functions of $S_1(t)$ and $S_2(t)$. If the transformed values of $S_1(t)$ and $S_2(t)$ are parallel, the plot of one against the other is a single straight line (Figure 12–3, bottom right).

The form of the proportional hazards model guarantees that the survival curves do not cross. Since

$$S_i(t; x_1, x_2, \ldots, x_k) = \{S_j(t; x_1', x_2', \ldots, x_k')\} e^{\sum b_i (x_i - x_i')}, \tag{12.18}$$

then

$$e^{\sum b_i (x_i - x_i')} \geq 1 \quad \text{implies} \quad S_i(t) \leq S_j(t) \tag{12.19}$$

and

$$e^{\sum b_i (x_i - x_i')} \leq 1 \quad \text{implies} \quad S_i(t) \geq S_j(t) \tag{12.20}$$

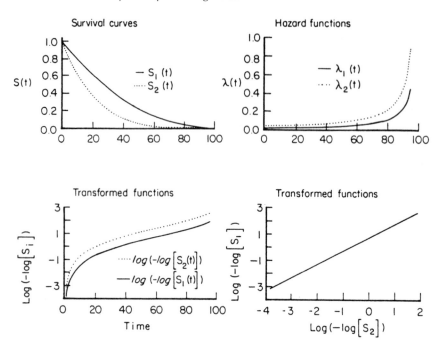

Figure 12–3. Comparisons of two hypothetical survival curves $S_1(t)$ and $S_2(t)$ based on $\lambda_0(t) = 1/(100 - t)$

for all values of t, which mathematically requires that the two survival curves do not intersect. The fact that the survival curves do not cross and simplifying transformation exists, is important in the difficult task of deciding if the relationships within a data set are meaningfully represented by a proportional hazards model. A plot of the survival curves and the "log-log" transformation of the survival curves is a good place to start the goodness-of-fit evaluation of a proportional hazards model. One further note: the fact that the survival curves do not cross when the hazard functions are proportional does not mean that estimated survival curves will not cross. Estimates, subject to variation, can fluctuate to an extent where plots cross (see Figure 12–6) even when the underlying hazard function are proportional.

Proportional Hazards Model: Application I

Illustration: CD4 Counts and Serum β_2-microglobulin

A bivariate proportional hazards model allows two important questions to be explored: Do the two risk factors have independent influences and if so, what are their individual contributions to survival time? These two issues arise in the study of HIV-positive patients and the relationship of two predictors of AIDs—CD4 counts and serum β_2-microglobulin levels. Studies have shown levels of both measures correlate with progressively severe degrees of illness. A two-variable proportional hazards model describing the time to AIDS ("survival") allows the evaluation of these two measures as a prognostic tool for AIDS among HIV-infected individuals.

The proportional hazards model

$$\lambda_j(t; x_1, x_2) = \lambda_0(t)\, e^{b_1(x_{1j}-800) + b_2(x_{2j}-200) + b_3(x_{1j}-800)(x_{2j}-200)} \quad (12.21)$$

addresses the issue of the independence of effects. Note that $\lambda_0(t)$ is the hazard function for individuals with CD4 counts $= 800$ and levels of serum β_2-microglobulin $= 200$. Estimates from this statistical structure allow evaluation of the degree of interaction observed in the data. In a fashion almost identical to the bivariate logistic analysis, the key parameter is b_3, which reflects the magnitude of the interaction between the variables x_1 and x_2.

Data from the San Francisco Men's Health Study [5] provide $n = 348$ seropositive men who have been examined and interviewed every six months so that their time from diagnosis to AIDS (in months) can be accurately determined. The CD4 counts and β_2-microglobulin levels where measured when HIV-positive participants entered the study. Applying a bivariate proportional hazards model [expression (12.21)] to these data gives the estimates in Table 12–3, where x_{1j} represents the CD4 count and x_{2j} represents the β_2-microglobulin level measured on the jth study participant.

The impact of the interaction can be assessed by postulating that the coefficient b_3 is zero and, as usual, $z = \hat{b}_3/S_{\hat{b}_3} = -0.604$ is viewed as a random fluctuation from zero with an approximate standard normal distribution, giving an associated p-value of 0.546.

Alternatively, the interaction model can be contrasted with the addditive model (b_3 set to zero) where

$$\lambda_j(t; x_1, x_2) = \lambda_0(t)\, e^{b_1(x_{1j}-800) + b_2(x_{2j}-200)}. \quad (12.22)$$

Table 12–3. Estimated coefficients for CD4 counts and β_2-microglobulin levels from a proportional hazards analysis including an interaction term

	Term	Coefficient	Std. Error	p-value	Hazard Ratio
CD4	b_1	-0.00149	0.00125	<0.001	0.999
β_2	b_2	0.00348	0.00038	0.016	1.003
CD4 $\times$ β_2	b_3	-0.0000023	0.0000038	0.546	0.999

-2Loglikelihood $= 1995.591$; number of model parameters $= 3$.

Table 12–4. Estimated coefficients for CD4 counts and β_2-microglobulin levels from a proportional hazards analysis excluding the interaction term—an additive model

	Term	Coefficient	Std. Error	p-value	Hazard Ratio
CD4	b_1	−0.00162	0.00033	<0.001	0.998
β_2	b_2	0.00404	0.00082	<0.001	1.004

−2Loglikelihood = 1995.952; number of model parameters = 2.

Estimates from the additive model where CD4 count and serum β_2-microglobulin are considered as independent contributors to time to AIDS are given in Table 12–4.

The difference in likelihood statistics measures the impact of including an interaction term in the model and is $L_0 - L_1 = 1995.952 - 1995.591 = 0.361$ (one degree of freedom and a p-value $= 0.548$), again showing no evidence of an interaction between CD4 counts and β_2-microglobulin levels.

The additive model allows an estimate of the joint but independent effects of these two measures of risk. Estimated hazard ratios are given by

$$\text{estimated hazard ratio} = e^{-0.00162(x_1 - 800) + 0.00404(x_2 - 200)},$$

where the comparison is relative to an individual with a CD4 count of 800 and β_2-microglobulin level of 200 and yields the values given in Table 12–5.

Another issue concerns the confounding effects of these variables. Assessment of the confounding influence of a variable or variables using a proportional hazards model is not different in principle from the usual approach to assessing confounding. Two estimates are compared: one estimated from an additive model including and one estimated from an additive model excluding the confounding variable or variables. When the β_2-microglobulin variable (x_2) is deleted from the bivariate proportional hazards model, the estimate of the coefficient associated with the CD4 counts is $\hat{b}_1 = -0.00202$, which is somewhat different

Table 12–5. Estimated hazard ratios from the proportional hazards model for three levels of CD4 counts (x_1) and three levels of β_2-microglobulin (x_2)

	$x_2 = 200$	$x_2 = 300$	$x_2 = 400$
$x_1 = 800$	1.000	1.498	2.245
$x_1 = 500$	1.626	2.433	3.646
$x_1 = 300$	2.243	3.361	5.037

from the estimate when the influence of β_2-microglobulin is retained in the model where $\hat{b}_1 = -0.00162$ (about a 23% difference). Similarly, the confounding influence of CD4 counts on β_2-microglobulin can be seen from the proportional hazards model excluding CD4 counts where $\hat{b}_2' = 0.00517$, which again is rather different from the estimate from the bivariate model where $\hat{b}_2 = 0.00404$. This analysis illustrates a perhaps subtle distinction. Independence of variables (additivity) refers to the relationship between risk factors and outcome; confounding refers to the impact of a variable or variables on the relationship between another variable and its influence on the outcome.

Proportional Hazards Model: Application II

Illustration: Leukemia Survival

Data [6] collected to investigate the relationship between survival of acute myelogenous leukemia patients, white blood cell (WBC) counts and a white cell morphologic characteristic can be explored using a proportional hazards model. The morphologic characteristic is the presence or absence of Auer rods, termed AG-positive and AG-negative. The survival times (in weeks) and the white blood cell count for AG-positive and AG-negative patients are given in Table 12–6.

Table 12–6. Survival times and white blood cell counts

	AG-Positive				AG-Negative	
	Weeks	WBC		Weeks	WBC
1	65	2,300	18	65	3,000
2	156	750	19	17	4,000
3	100	4,300	20	7	1,500
4	134	2,600	21	16	9,000
5	16	6,000	22	22	5,300
6	108	10,500	23	3	10,000
7	121	10,000	24	4	19,000
8	4	17,000	25	2	27,000
9	39	5,400	26	3	28,000
10	143	7,000	27	8	31,000
11	56	9,400	28	4	26,000
12	26	32,000	29	3	21,000
13	22	35,000	30	30	79,000
14	1	100,000	31	4	100,000
15	1	100,000	32	43	100,000
16	5	52,000	33	56	4,400
17	65	100,000			

These survival times are complete (no censoring; all patients died), producing 17 *AG*-positive and 16 *AG*-negative observations. A simple correlation coefficient shows that the *WBC* count is related to survival time (correlation $= -0.33$). This correlation and the generally recognized fact that *WBC* count is associated with the length of leukemia survival imply that the *WBC* count should be included in the description of the relationship between *AG*-status and survival time. A proportional hazards model is one way to investigate the influence of *AG*-status on survival (binary variable) while accounting for the influence of *WBC* level ("continuous" variable). The model relating *WBC* count and *AG*-status to survival time (including the possibility of an interaction) is

$$\lambda_{AG}(t; x_1, x_2) = \lambda_0(t)\, e^{b_1 x_1 + b_2 x_2 + b_3 x_1 x_2}. \tag{12.23}$$

The relationship between the *AG*-positive and *AG*-negative survival curves is then

$$S_{AG-}(t; x_1, x_2) = \{S_{AG+}(t; x_1', x_2')\}^{e^{b_1(x_1 - x_1') + b_2(x_2 - x_2') + b_3(x_1 x_2 - x_1' x_2')}}, \tag{12.24}$$

where x_1 is an indicator $(0, 1)$ of *AG*-status, and x_2 is the *WBC* count. As before, underlying this approach is the assumption that the hazard rates associated with the survival of leukemia patients are accurately described by two proportional hazard functions. The estimated parameters for this model under two conditions are given in Tables 12–7 and 12–8—interaction and additive effects.

Table 12–7. Leukemia and WBC count: Interactions present
Full Model

	Term	Coefficient	Std. Error	*p*-value	Hazard Ratio
AG-status	$\hat{b}_1$	1.816	0.583	0.002	6.144
WBC	$\hat{b}_2$	0.0000415	0.000017	0.015	1.000
WBC × *AG*-status	$\hat{b}_3$	−0.0000209	0.0000105	0.047	1.000

$-2\text{LogLikelihood} = 136.731$; number of model parameters $= 3$.

Table 12–8. Leukemia and WBC count: Interactions absent
Interaction Excluded

	Term	Coefficient	Std. Error	*p*-value	Hazard Ratio
AG-status	$\hat{b}_1$	1.115	0.445	0.012	3.049
WBC	$\hat{b}_2$	0.0000082	0.0000053	0.121	1.001

$-2\text{LogLikelihood} = 140.663$; number of model parameters $= 2$.

It is likely that the relationship between WBC count and survival pattern is not the same for the AG-positive and AG-negative groups, which means that the coefficients $\hat{b}_1$ and $\hat{b}_2$ do not exclusively characterize the roles of the two explanatory variables, AG-status and WBC count. The test of the interaction coefficient $(b_3 = 0?)$ and the comparison of likelihood statistics $(z = \hat{b}_3/S_{\hat{b}_3} = 1.990$ and the difference $= 140.663 - 136.731 = 3.932$, degrees of freedom $= 1)$ produce small p-values (both are 0.047), indicating the definite possibility of a different relationship between WBC count and survival for the two types of AG-status. The additive model (Table 12–8), therefore, is not likely a useful tool in assessing the impact of the two explanatory variables. The presence of interaction, as usual, limits the amount of possible summarization. Specifically, $\hat{b}_1$ and $\hat{b}_2$ do not simply reflect independent influences of the AG-status and the WBC counts on survival.

For these data, survival curves for a series of WBC counts (2,500, 20,000, 50,000, and 100,000) are estimated separately (one set for

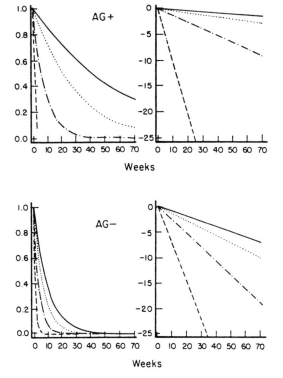

Figure 12–4. Survival curves and the logarithm of the survival curves based on the proportional hazards model for $AG+$ and $AG-$ leukemia patients.

AG-positive and one set for AG-negative) under the more restrictive condition that the hazard rates are constant. The curves plotted in Figure 12–4 for both AG-positive and AG-negative cell types are based on the exponential survival curve $\hat{S}_{AG^+}(t) = e^{-\hat{\lambda}t}$, where $\hat{\lambda}$ is estimated from the weeks of survival given for the AG-positive patients (the logarithms of these survival curves are also shown). The lack of similarity between these curves (interaction) for the two cell characteristics is clear. Survival in the AG-positive group depends more critically on white blood cell count than the AG-negative group. For a specific WBC count, the survival curve for the AG-positive patients is generally above the comparable AG-negative curve. Combining the data from the two cell types would produce an average effect, obscuring the fact that survival and white blood cell counts behave differently depending on AG-status.

Proportional Hazards Model: Application III

Illustration: Lung Cancer Survival Data

Preliminary observations from a clinical trial [7] provide an illustrative set of 131 lung cancer survival times as well as the ages of the patient (explanatory variable). The data are divided into two groups based on the patient's measured vital capacity. One group has 95 patients with "high" vital capacity ratios and the other 36 patients with "low" vital capacity ratios. The vital capacity groups, survival time (in days), and patient's age are given in Tables 12–9 and 12–10.

Figure 12–5 (top) shows the product-limit estimates of the survival curves associated with these two vital capacity groups. The "high" vital capacity group apparently has better survival experience. Figure 12–5 (bottom) shows a definite influence of age on the pattern of survival for these patients. The two vital capacity groups subdivided by age into those less than or equal to 65 and those greater than 65 years old produce distinct survival patterns. A summary of mean survival times additionally indicates that age influences survival (Table 12–11).

Two expected problems arise when survival data are classified into subgroups. The choice of the bounds for the categories adds an arbitrary element to the analysis that can influence final interpretations. More important, the number of observations in some categories becomes small (e.g., "low", age > 65 contains nine individuals and only six complete observations). This reduction in sample size leads to increased variation and difficulty in interpretation. The lack of clarity

Table 12–9. Lung cancer data: "High" vital capacity

			Complete				
Time	Age	Time	Age	Time	Age	Time	Age
0	74	1	74	1	63	3	78
4	66	5	40	9	65	19	51
21	73	30	62	36	68	39	50
40	56	48	64	51	72	61	58
89	64	90	41	90	69	92	76
113	73	127	64	131	51	138	75
139	56	143	50	159	60	168	74
170	71	180	69	189	56	192	68
201	64	212	58	223	70	229	76
238	63	265	65	275	63	292	55
317	65	322	55	350	54	357	73
380	51						
			Censored				
Time	Age	Time	Age	Time	Age	Time	Age
62	66	75	44	77	60	81	38
83	59	83	42	84	67	86	62
88	53	92	59	98	55	104	62
116	62	129	35	131	43	162	45
167	56	173	54	178	63	179	69
184	69	184	67	194	58	256	57
263	46	269	63	338	47	344	52
347	59	349	61	350	66	362	56
362	60	364	63	364	58	364	58
365	66	368	70	368	39	372	58
388	59	388	68	400	64	524	59
528	63	545	63	546	55	552	52
555	57	558	63					

Note: The first 45 survival times are complete (died within the study period) and the following 50 are censored.

in Figure 12–5 comes, to a large extent, from increased variation associated with the estimated age-group specific survival curves.

The mean ages of patients in the two groups differ ("high" = 57.63 years and "low" = 60.13 years) and age is undoubtedly related to survival, implying adjustment (via a proportional hazards model) will help identify differences between the two compared groups attributable to influences other than age. The assumption of proportional hazards allows adjustment for the influence of age and provides a systematic evaluation of "high" and "low" capacity groups while avoiding the problems incurred by stratifying the data into several age categories. Large gains in efficiency are achieved because the entire data set, all 131 observations, is focused on the estimation of two parameters.

Table 12-10. Lung cancer data: "Low" vital capacity

				Complete			
Time	Age	Time	Age	Time	Age	Time	Age
0	55	2	75	2	73	2	65
6	61	17	74	22	51	23	66
54	67	56	51	61	36	63	54
64	54	69	70	146	53	155	47
161	46	233	41	248	61	283	53
				Censored			
Time	Age	Time	Age	Time	Age	Time	Age
47	56	73	55	86	48	89	65
91	58	169	58	172	62	177	53
183	48	188	52	194	67	266	53
266	53	267	52	351	71	372	71

Note: The first 20 survival times are complete (died within the study period) and the following 16 are censored.

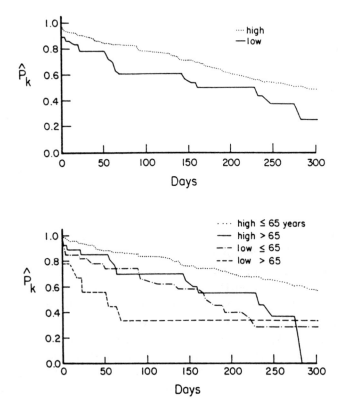

Figure 12-5. Product-limit estimates of the survival curves for two groups of lung cancer patients by vital capacity and by age

Table 12–11. Summary: lung cancer mean survival time

		n_i	Censored	Mean	Std. Error
"High"	Age ≤ 65	68	41	229.5	19.3
"High"	Age > 65	27	9	156.7	23.8
"Low"	Age ≤ 65	27	13	132.4	17.4
"Low"	Age > 65	9	3	120.4	46.9
	Total	131	66	187.0	12.7

Application of a proportional hazards model to these lung cancer data requires making the influence of age and group membership components of the model, thus producing the potential to separate and measure each variable's influence on the observed differences in survival times. That is, the overall ratio of hazard functions is factored into a piece measuring the influence of age and a piece measuring the influence of vital capacity on survival (additive model). Such an additive proportional hazards model is

$$\lambda_j(t; x_{1j}, x_{2j}) = \lambda_0(t) c_j = \lambda_0(t) e^{b_1 x_{1j} + b_2(x_{2j} - \bar{x}_2)} = \lambda_0(t) [e^{b_1 x_{1j}}][e^{b_2(x_{2j} - \bar{x}_2)}],$$
$$(12.25)$$

where x_{1j} is a binary variable indicating "high" ($x_{1j} = 0$) or "low" ($x_{1j} = 1$) vital capacity groups and x_{2j} is the reported age of the jth patient. Maximum likelihood estimates and likelihood statistics associated with this model are given in Table 12–12.

Contrasting the additive bivariate model (age and group included) to the model with age excluded (reduced model) shows noticeable confounding bias. The coefficient associated with the group membership (b_1) changes from 0.637 to 0.540 when age is excluded from the model or, in terms of the relative hazard, the change is 1.891 to 1.716. Also, the statistical evaluation of the model excluding age shows that age has a strong influence on the survival time. The difference in likelihood statistics $L_{b_2=0} - L_{b_2 \neq 0} = 546.976 - 540.552 = 6.424$ has an approximate chi-square distribution when age is not related to survival ($b_2 = 0$) with one degree of freedom (the difference in the number of parameters needed to specify the two models) and yields a p-value of 0.011. Both the extent of the confounding bias and the strength of association indicate, not surprisingly, that age plays an important role in the survival of these patients and should be included in the model.

The influence of the "high" versus "low" vital capacity can be similarly assessed. The comparison of the likelihood statistics

Table 12–12. Proportional Hazards Model: lung cancer data

Group and Age Included

	Term	Coefficient	Std. Error	p-value	Hazard Ratio
Group	$\hat{b}_1$	0.637	0.275	0.020	1.891
Age	$\hat{b}_2$	0.038	0.015	0.013	1.039

-2LogLikelihood $= 540.552$; number of model parameters $= 2$.

Age Excluded

	Term	Coefficient	Std. Error	p-value	Hazard Ratio
Group	$\hat{b}_1$	0.540	0.274	0.049	1.716

-2LogLikelihood $= 546.976$; number of model parameters $= 1$.

Vital Capacity Group Excluded

	Term	Coefficient	Std. Error	p-value	Hazard Ratio
Age	$\hat{b}_2$	0.034	0.016	0.027	1.035

-2LogLikelihood $= 545.486$; number of model parameters $= 1$.

(bivariate versus reduced model) produces a statistical evaluation of the influence of the vital capacity classification (difference between likelihood statistics is $L_{b_1 = 0} - L_{b_1 \neq 0} = 545.486 - 540.552 = 4.934$). This difference has a chi-square distribution with one degree of freedom when vital capacity is unrelated to survival (i.e., $b_1 = 0$) yielding a p-value of 0.026. Like age, the classification of individuals by vital capacity is likely associated with survival. The increase in the likelihood statistic, furthermore, cannot be attributed to influences of age, because a measure of the age-effect is maintained in both the bivariate and reduced analyses (x_2 is included in both models).

An alternative evaluation of the coefficients from the proportional hazards model comes from the usual Wald-statistic of $z_i = \hat{b}_i / S_{\hat{b}_i}$, which has an approximate normal distribution with mean $= 0$ and variance $= 1$ when the ith variable is unrelated to survival (i.e., $b_i = 0$). Age ($z_2 = 2.533$ giving a p-value $= 0.013$) and group membership ($z_1 = 2.316$ giving a p-value $= 0.020$) show the expected agreement with the likelihood approach.

Confidence intervals for the estimated coefficients from the proportional hazard model are constructed in the usual way (e.g., $\hat{b}_i \pm 1.96\, S_{\hat{b}_i}$ for an approximate 95% confidence interval), and confidence intervals for the relative hazard are then ($e^{\hat{b}_{lower}}, e^{\hat{b}_{upper}}$). For example, the approximate 95% confidence interval based on the estimated age-coefficient $\hat{b}_2 = 0.038$ is $\hat{b}_{lower} = 0.038 - 1.96(0.015) = 0.009$ and $\hat{b}_{upper} = 0.038 + 1.96(0.015) = 0.067$ and the corresponding confidence interval based on the relative hazard of $e^{\hat{b}_2} = 1.039$ is $(e^{0.009}, e^{0.067})$ or (1.009, 1.070). The analogous 95% confidence interval for the relative hazard $e^{\hat{b}_1} = 1.891$ associated with the vital capacity variable is (1.103, 3.241).

This analysis implies that a useful estimated proportional hazards model is

$$\lambda_j(t; x_{1j}, x_{2j}) = \lambda_0(t)\, e^{0.637x_{1j} + 0.038(x_{2j} - 59.45)}, \tag{12.26}$$

where the mean age for all 131 patients is $\bar{x}_2 = 59.45$ years.

To explore further the lung cancer survival data, assume that the "high" vital capacity group (Table 12–9) provides an adequate estimate of $S_0(t)$. The product-limit estimated survival curve $\hat{S}_0(t)$ is given in Table 12–13 and is also depicted in Figure 12–6.

The survival curves for the "high" and "low" vital capacity groups (ignoring age)

$$\text{high capacity: } \hat{S}_0(t) \quad \text{versus} \quad \text{low capacity: } \{\hat{S}_0(t)\}^{1.716}$$

Table 12–13. Lung cancer data—$\hat{S}_0(t)$

Obs	Days	$\hat{S}_0(t)$	Obs	Days	$\hat{S}_0(t)$
1	1	0.968	23	139	0.720
2	3	0.958	24	143	0.707
3	4	0.947	25	159	0.694
4	5	0.937	26	168	0.680
5	9	0.926	27	170	0.666
6	19	0.916	28	180	0.652
7	21	0.905	29	189	0.637
8	30	0.895	30	192	0.622
9	36	0.884	31	201	0.606
10	39	0.874	32	212	0.590
11	40	0.863	33	223	0.575
12	48	0.853	34	229	0.559
13	51	0.842	35	238	0.544
14	61	0.832	36	265	0.527
15	89	0.820	37	275	0.510
16	90	0.808	38	292	0.493
17	90	0.796	39	317	0.476
18	92	0.784	40	322	0.459
19	113	0.771	41	350	0.439
20	127	0.759	42	357	0.418
21	131	0.746	43	380	0.380
22	138	0.733	—	—	—

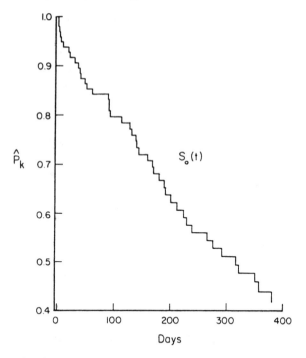

Figure 12–6. Product-limit estimates of the survival curve for lung cancer patients with "high" vital capacity, $\hat{S}_0(t)$

are plotted in Figure 12–7 (top). To show the influence of age, the survival curves

high capacity: $\{\hat{S}_0(t)\}^{e^{0.038(x_2 - \bar{x}_2)}}$ versus   low capacity: $\{\hat{S}_0(t)\}^{e^{0.637 + 0.038(x_2 - \bar{x}_2)}}$

are also shown in Figure 12–7 (bottom) for age 55 ($x_2 = 55$) and age 75 ($x_2 = 75$). A model representing the relationship of age and group membership to survival time uses the data with great efficiency and produces a clear and easily interpreted picture (Figure 12–5 contrasted with Figure 12–7). The price is, as usual, the insecurity that the model does not adequately represent the actual structure underlying data.

Ratios of Hazard Functions from the Proportional Hazards Model

The ratio of two hazard functions (relative hazard) summarizes the survival experience of two groups or individuals and is a particularly meaningful description of two proportional hazard functions. The ratio of hazard rates is analogous to ratios of average mortality or incidence rates except that these rates are instantaneous measures and

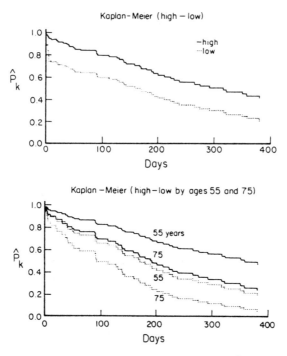

Figure 12–7. Estimates of the survival curves for two groups of lung cancer patients by vital capacity and by age based on proportional hazards model

can be adjusted for the influence of the explanatory variables. For the proportional hazards model the difference in survival between two groups or individuals is measured by

$$\frac{\lambda_1(t; x_1, x_2, \ldots, x_k)}{\lambda_2(t; x'_1, x'_2, \ldots, x'_k)} = e^{\sum b_i(x_i - x'_i)}, \tag{12.27}$$

where x_i and x'_i represent different levels of the ith explanatory variable.

When two groups differ by a single variable (i.e., are identical for all but one variable, say x_i), then for $x_i \neq x'_i$

$$\frac{\lambda_1(t; x_1 = x'_1, x_2 = x'_2, x_3 = x'_3, \ldots, x_k = x'_k)}{\lambda_2(t; x'_1, x'_2, x'_3, \ldots, x'_k)} = e^{b_1(x_1 - x'_1)} e^{b_2(x'_2 - x'_2)} \ldots e^{b_k(x'_k - x'_k)}$$

$$= e^{b_i(x_i - x'_i)} \tag{12.28}$$

allowing survival to be compared for different levels of a single explanatory variable with the remaining variables held constant. In other words, the relative hazard associated with a particular variable represents an assessment of the influence on survival from a specific variable while the other $k - 1$ explanatory variables have equal values in the groups or the individuals being compared. A similar interpretation was made for the adjusted coefficients in the logistic regression model. A primary goal of multivariate analysis is the isolation of individual effects. Expression (12.28) shows that an additive proportional hazards model has exactly this property.

The ratio of hazard functions is analogous to an odds ratio measure estimated from an additive logistic model. The value e^{b_i} indicates the relative influence of a measurement on survival independent of other explanatory variables, when an additive model is used to represent the relationships between explanatory variables and the hazard rate. The relative hazard, for example, associated with vital capacity group membership is $e^{0.637} = 1.891$. That is, the hazard rate in the "low" vital capacity group is a little less than twice that of the "high" vital capacity group for any specific age. Similarly, the influence of age on the hazard rates for these lung cancer patients, regardless of group membership, is $e^{0.038(age_2 - age_1)}$, where age_1 and age_2 are compared. For example, if $age_1 = 55$ and $age_2 = 75$, then the relative hazard is $e^{0.038(20)} = 2.138$. Or, the lung cancer patients age 75 are at about twice the risk (measured by a hazard rate) as patients age 55 within either vital capacity group.

The additive nature of a proportional hazards model dictates that group membership and age do not interact. Therefore, a 55-year-old member of the "high" vital capacity group compared to a 75-year-old member of the "low" vital capacity group yields a hazard ratio of $e^{0.637 + 0.038(20)} = 1.891(2.138) = 4.043$, illustrating a specific partitioning of the overall hazard ratio (4.043) into relative components (vital capacity group status $= 1.891$ and age $= 2.138$).

Proportional Hazards Model: application IV

Illustration: Histology-Specific Lung Cancer Data

A series of 137 patients with advanced lung cancer categorized by cancer histology [8] provides an opportunity to apply a proportional hazards model that requires distinct categories be specified. The data consist of individual survival times (days) classified by one of four lung cancer histology categories (squamous cell, small cell, adenocarcinoma, and large cell) and by a new or standard treatment ($x_{1j} = 0$ for the standard treatment and $x_{1j} = 1$ for the new treatment). Three other explanatory variables are also recorded for each patient: a general medical status index (x_{2j}), months from diagnosis to the start of the study (x_{3j}), and age (x_{4j}). These data are given in Tables 12–14 and 12–15.

Table 12–14. Lung cancer by type: new treatment

Squamous Cell				Small Cell				Adenocarcinoma				Large Cell			
Time	x_{2j}	x_{3j}	x_{4j}	Time	x_{2j}	x_{3j}	x_{4j}	Time	x_{2j}	x_{3j}	x_{4j}	Time	x_{2j}	x_{3j}	x_{4j}
999	90	12	54	25	30	2	69	24	40	2	60	52	60	4	45
122	80	6	60	103$^+$	70	22	36	18	40	5	69	164	70	15	68
87$^+$	80	3	48	21	20	4	71	83$^+$	99	3	57	19	30	4	39
231$^+$	50	8	52	13	30	2	62	31	80	3	39	53	60	12	66
242	50	1	70	87	60	2	60	51	60	5	62	15	30	5	63
991	70	7	50	2	40	36	44	90	60	22	50	43	60	11	49
111	70	3	62	20	30	9	54	52	60	3	43	340	80	10	64
1	20	21	65	7	20	11	66	73	60	3	70	133	75	1	65
587	60	3	58	24	60	8	49	8	50	5	66	111	60	5	64
389	90	2	62	99	70	3	72	36	70	8	61	231	70	18	67
33	30	6	64	8	80	2	68	48	10	4	81	378	80	4	65
25	20	36	63	99	85	4	62	7	40	4	58	49	30	3	37
357	70	13	58	61	70	2	71	140	70	3	63	—	—	—	—
467	90	2	64	95	70	1	61	186	90	3	60	—	—	—	—
201	80	28	52	80	50	17	71	84	80	4	62	—	—	—	—
1	50	7	35	51	30	87	59	19	50	10	42	—	—	—	—
30	70	11	63	29	40	8	67	45	40	3	69	—	—	—	—
44	60	13	70	25	70	2	6	80	40	4	63	—	—	—	—
283	90	2	51	—	—	—	—	—				—	—	—	—
15	50	13	40	—	—	—	—	—				—	—	—	—

The rigorous determination of whether or not a proportional hazards model is an accurate representation of the data is not presented. Statistical tests to assess the assumption of proportionality are part of several "package" computer programs (see [9], for example), and plotting estimated survival curves can help indicate the adequacy or, particularly, the inadequacy of a statistical model. The relationship among survival curves, as mentioned, is the key to exploring the choice of a proportional hazards model.

To begin to understand the role of the explanatory variables in influencing differences in survival times among the lung cancer patients, an additive proportional hazards model is proposed that includes all five explanatory variables. The model is not fundamentally different from the one described in the previous case [expression (12.8)] except that a set of design variables is used to indicate histologic categories. That is, three design variables (z_1, z_2, and z_3) are used to identify four histologic groups: $z_1 = 1$ if the cancer type is small cell with $z_2 = z_3 = 0$; $z_2 = 1$ if the cancer type is adenocarcinoma with $z_1 = z_3 = 0$; $z_3 = 1$ if the cancer type is large cell, with $z_1 = z_2 = 0$; and squamous cell carcinoma is established as the baseline for comparison

Table 12–15. Lung cancer by type: standard treatment

Squamous Cell				Small Cell				Adenocarcinoma				Large Cell			
Time	x_{2j}	x_{3j}	x_{4j}	Time	x_{2j}	x_{3j}	x_{4j}	Time	x_{2j}	x_{3j}	x_{4j}	Time	x_{2j}	x_{3j}	x_{4j}
72	60	7	69	30	60	3	61	8	20	19	61	177	50	16	66
411	60	5	64	384	60	9	42	92	70	10	60	162	80	5	62
228	60	3	38	4	40	2	35	35	40	6	62	216	50	15	52
126	60	9	63	54	80	4	63	117	80	2	38	553	70	2	47
118	70	11	65	13	60	4	56	132	80	5	50	278	60	12	63
10	20	5	49	123+	40	3	55	12	50	4	63	12	40	12	68
82	40	10	69	97+	60	5	67	162	80	5	64	260	80	5	45
110	80	29	68	153	60	14	63	3	30	3	43	200	80	12	41
314	50	18	43	59	30	2	65	95	80	4	34	156	70	2	60
100+	70	6	70	117	80	3	46	—	—	—	—	182+	90	2	62
42	60	4	81	16	30	4	53	—	—	—	—	143	90	8	60
8	40	58	63	151	50	12	69	—	—	—	—	105	80	11	66
144	30	4	63	22	60	4	68	—	—	—	—	103	80	5	38
25+	80	9	52	56	80	12	43	—	—	—	—	250	70	8	53
11	70	11	48	21	40	2	55	—	—	—	—	100	60	13	37
—	—	—	—	18	20	15	42	—	—	—	—	—	—	—	—
—	—	—	—	139	80	2	64	—	—	—	—	—	—	—	—
—	—	—	—	20	30	5	65	—	—	—	—	—	—	—	—
—	—	—	—	31	75	3	65	—	—	—	—	—	—	—	—
—	—	—	—	52	70	2	55	—	—	—	—	—	—	—	—
—	—	—	—	287	60	25	66	—	—	—	—	—	—	—	—
—	—	—	—	18	30	4	60	—	—	—	—	—	—	—	—
—	—	—	—	51	60	1	67	—	—	—	—	—	—	—	—
—	—	—	—	122	80	28	53	—	—	—	—	—	—	—	—
—	—	—	—	27	60	8	62	—	—	—	—	—	—	—	—
—	—	—	—	54	70	1	67	—	—	—	—	—	—	—	—
—	—	—	—	7	50	7	72	—	—	—	—	—	—	—	—
—	—	—	—	63	50	11	48	—	—	—	—	—	—	—	—
—	—	—	—	392	40	4	68	—	—	—	—	—	—	—	—
—	—	—	—	10	40	23	67	—	—	—	—	—	—	—	—

by $z_1 = z_2 = z_3 = 0$. An additive proportional hazards model incorporating the five explanatory variables is

$$\lambda_j(t) = \lambda_0(t)\,e^{c_1 z_{1j} + c_2 z_{2j} + c_3 z_{3j} + b_1 x_{1j} + b_2(x_{2j} - \bar{x}_2) + b_3(x_{3j} - \bar{x}_3) + b_4(x_{4j} - \bar{x}_4)}. \quad (12.29)$$

The lung cancer data analyzed using three sets of conditions produces the maximum likelihood estimates of the model parameters given in Table 12–16.

The comparison of the full model to the model with the months from diagnosis (x_3) and age (x_4) variables removed (reduced model) shows that these two variables add little to the understanding of the survival times of the lung cancer patients. Comparison of the respective likelihood statistics (difference $= 918.101 - 916.335 = 1.766$

Table 12–16. Histology-specific lung cancer data

Full Model

	Term	Coefficient	Std. Error	p-value	Hazard Ratio
Indicator 1	$\hat{c}_1$	0.884	0.268	<0.001	2.421
Indicator 2	$\hat{c}_2$	1.170	0.296	<0.001	3.223
Indicator 3	$\hat{c}_3$	0.372	0.280	0.184	1.450
Treatment	$\hat{b}_1$	−0.385	0.205	0.061	0.680
Status	$\hat{b}_2$	−0.033	0.006	<0.001	0.968
Months	$\hat{b}_3$	0.001	0.008	0.913	1.001
Age	$\hat{b}_4$	−0.012	0.009	0.188	0.988

−2LogLikelihood = 916.335; number of model parameters = 7.

Age and Months Excluded

	Term	Coefficient	Std. Error	p-value	Hazard Ratio
Indicator 1	$\hat{c}_1$	0.848	0.264	<0.001	2.334
Indicator 2	$\hat{c}_2$	1.134	0.293	<0.001	3.109
Indicator 3	$\hat{c}_3$	0.361	0.279	0.195	0.716
Treatment	$\hat{b}_1$	−0.334	0.199	0.094	1.400
Status	$\hat{b}_2$	−0.031	0.005	<0.001	0.970

−2LogLikelihood = 918.101; number of model parameters = 5.

Age, Months, and Histologies Excluded

	Term	Coefficient	Std. Error	p-value	Hazard Ratio
Treatment	$\hat{b}_1$	−0.239	0.182	0.190	0.787
Status	$\hat{b}_2$	−0.033	0.005	<0.001	0.967

−2LogLikelihood = 936.722; number of model parameters = 2.

with degrees of freedom = 2 gives a p-value = 0.414) yields no statistical evidence that these two explanatory variables are useful in the study of the survival of these patients. Also, only negligible confounding of the influences of treatment status and histology appears associated with age and diagnosis measurements. The medical status index (x_1) is, however, worth including in the analysis ($z = -5.952$ with a p-value < 0.001). The same is true of the variables that separate the data into histologic types. The model excluding histologic type $(c_1 = c_2 = c_3 = 0)$ substantially increases the likelihood statistic over the three-variable model (Table 12–16), producing a significant difference in likelihood statistics (difference = 936.722 − 918.101 = 18.621 with three degrees of freedom yielding a p-value < 0.001). Also, histologic type is a confounder of the treatment effect ($\hat{b}_1 = -0.334$ when histology is included and this parameter changes to $\hat{b}_1' = -0.239$ when histology is excluded). Last, the treatment variable coefficient ($\hat{b}_1 = -0.334$) indicates that treatment status is marginally important in explaining the differences in survival times between these two groups of patients when adjusted for medical status and for histologic type. The value $z = \hat{b}_1/S_{\hat{b}_1} = -0.334/0.199 = -1.678$ produces a p-value of 0.094 when the medical status index and the histologic types are maintained in the model.

To explore these data further, assume that the hazard rates are at least approximately constant over the range of the follow-up period. This additional assumption yields a model in terms of survival probabilities where

$$S_j(t) = \left\{e^{-\lambda_0 t}\right\} e^{0.848z_{1j} + 1.134z_{2j} + 0.361z_{3j} + 0.334x_{1j} - 0.031(x_{2j} - \bar{x}_2)}$$

for specified histologies, medical status, and treatment. Under the constant hazard rate assumption, the expression for the proportional hazards model can be manipulated to produce estimated mean survival times as

$$\bar{t}_k = \bar{t}_0 \, e^{-\sum b_i x_{ik}}. \tag{12.30}$$

The value $\bar{t}_k$ is the estimated mean survival time for group k relative to an arbitrary value $\bar{t}_0$. The value $\bar{t}_0$ is the mean survival time associated with "baseline" category. Setting $\bar{t}_0$ to 138.57 days (the average survival time for patients with squamous cell carcinoma receiving the standard treatment with average level of medical status) yields a series of estimated values for $\bar{t}_k$ under selected conditions. Some examples are given in Table 12–17.

A comparison of these tables and the values within each table describes the relative influence of the explanatory and treatment variables on mean survival time. These tables represent an application of the estimated relative hazard ratios applied to a baseline value (138.57 days) under the assumption that the hazard rates are at least approximately constant and illustrate one of many ways a statistical model can be used to describe the issues under study.

Dependence on Follow-Up Time

A proportional hazards model does not require the relationship between follow-up time and survival to be specified in detail. The estimated relative hazard measures the influence of each explanatory variable on survival as long as the hazard functions are proportional. It is instructive to illustrative the situation where dependency exists

Table 12–17. Lung cancer mean survival times—no treatment and medical status influence

	Squamous	Small	Adeno	Large
Standard	138.57	52.58	46.08	118.08
New	138.57	52.58	46.08	118.08

Model: $\bar{t}_k = \bar{t}_0 e^{-(0.969z_{1k} + 1.101z_{2k} + 0.160z_{3k})}$.

Lung cancer mean survival times—treatment but no medical status influence

	Squamous	Small	Adeno	Large
Standard	138.57	46.68	44.85	108.69
New	177.04	59.64	57.30	138.85

Model: $\bar{t}_k = \bar{t}_0 e^{-(1.088z_{1k} + 1.128z_{2k} + 0.243z_{3k} + 0.245x_{1k})}$.

Lung cancer mean survival times—both treatment and medical status influence

	Squamous	Small	Adeno	Large
Standard	130.92	52.97	43.46	137.95
New	225.96	66.48	58.63	135.93

Model: $\bar{t}_k = \bar{t}_0 e^{-(0.848z_{1k} + 1.134z_{2k} + 0.361z_{3k} + 0.334x_{1k} - 0.031(\bar{x}_{2k} - \bar{x}_2))}$.
Note: x_{2k} is set equal to the mean score for the kth group medical status group $(\bar{x}_{2k})$.

between follow-up time and a survival measure. Two perspectives provide a brief discussion. A model showing the dependency of the odds ratio on follow-up time is presented, followed by a comparison of the logistic regression (no consideration of follow-up time) to the proportional hazard regression (accounting for the possible dependency on follow-up time) using the WCGS data.

Odds Ratio Model

Consider two groups with exponential survival with constant hazard rates given by λ_1 and $\lambda_2 (\lambda_1 < \lambda_2)$. The survival probabilities associated with these two groups are

$$S_1(t) = e^{-\lambda_1 t} \quad \text{and} \quad S_2(t) = e^{-\lambda_2 t}. \tag{12.31}$$

The odds ratio measuring the relative differences in survival for these two groups at a specific follow-up time t is

$$or(t) = \frac{S_1(t)/[1 - S_1(t)]}{S_2(t)/[1 - S_2(t)]} = \frac{S_1(t)[1 - S_2(t)]}{S_2(t)[1 - S_1(t)]} = \frac{e^{\lambda_2 t} + 1}{e^{\lambda_1 t} + 1}.$$

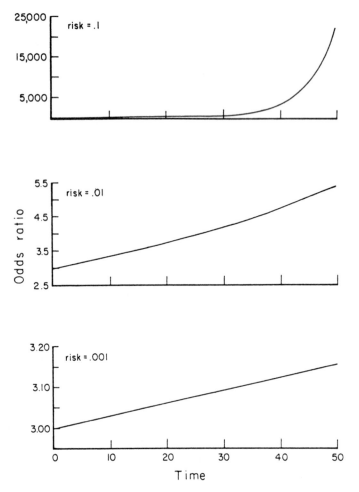

Figure 12–8. Odds ratio plotted against time for two groups that experience exponential survival $(\lambda_2/\lambda_1 = 3)$

To illustrate, Figure 12–8 shows $or(t)$ for $\lambda_1 = 0.1$, 0.01, and 0.001 with $\lambda_2/\lambda_1 = 3$ (note the extremely different scales on the vertical axes in Figure 12–8).

As follow-up time increases, the odds ratio increases. This increase is large (very large) for a hazard rate of above 0.1 (top of Figure 12–8). The structure of the odds ratio is such that it is forced to become infinite and difficult to interpret as follow-up time increases. However, for small and more typical hazard rates (in the neighborhood of 0.001), follow-up time has a less dramatic impact on the odds ratio (bottom of Figure 12–8). For hazard rates in the range normally experienced by human populations the odds ratio increases over time in an essentially linear pattern with a slope proportional to the difference between the two hazard rates. That is,

$$or(t) \approx \frac{\lambda_2}{\lambda_1}[1 + 0.5t(\lambda_2 - \lambda_1)]$$

for $\lambda_i < 0.005$. The dependency of the odds ratio on follow-up time for constant hazard rates is relatively simple. More complicated cases are easily envisioned. Postulating constant hazard rates, however, shows that the magnitude of an odds ratio depends on follow-up time. The degree of the association between group membership and disease outcome is a function of time as well as hazard rates (λ_1, λ_2), which complicates the interpretation of the odds ratio calculated as a measure of risk, even in this simple case. In other words, risk measured by an odds ratio is confounded by follow-up time for exponentially distributed survival times, as long as $\lambda_1 \neq \lambda_2$.

Western Collaborative Group Study Data

The Western Collaborative Group Study (WCGS) produced a prospective cohort data set that includes the time from admission to the study to the time of a coronary event or withdrawal—follow-up times for 3,154 individuals (see Appendix A). Of these participants, 257 coronary events occurred, and the remaining 92% of the sample was either lost to follow-up (16%) or withdrawn from follow-up disease-free (censored) when the study ended. The proportional hazards model applied to these data shows the influence of eight risk factors on the risk of coronary events while accounting for confounding influences of time over the follow-up period. Table 12–18 gives estimated coefficients

Table 12–18. A comparison of the proportional hazards model and the logistic model (WCGS data)

Factor	"Cox" Model		Logistic Model	
	$\hat{b}_i$	Std. Error	$\hat{b}_i$	Std. Error
Age	0.063	0.011	0.065	0.012
Height	0.015	0.031	0.016	0.033
Weight	0.007	0.004	0.008	0.004
Systolic bp	0.014	0.006	0.018	0.006
Diastolic bp	0.008	0.010	−0.002	0.010
Cholesterol	0.009	0.001	0.011	0.002
Smoking	0.021	0.004	0.021	0.004
A/B	0.671	0.137	0.653	0.145

for the proportional hazards model compared to those produced by the multiple logistic model (Table 8–13) applied to the same data.

The two analyses hardly differ. The multiple logistic model estimates are derived from data pooled or averaged over time, whereas the proportional hazards model takes time into account. That is, a logistic analysis does not utilize information on time of survival (follow-up); a response that occurs early in a study is given the same weight as a later response. If follow-up time is related to outcome and to the other explanatory factors, adjusting for its confounding influence is necessary. The results from a proportional hazards model differ from those of a logistic model depending on the extent to which time is a confounder. Additionally, the follow-up period must be long enough that survival times are known for a substantial proportion of the sample (complete survival times) before a logistic and proportional hazard regression will appreciably differ.

Time does not significantly influence the WCGS data for these two reasons. Coronary events occurred only among a small proportion (8%) of the study subjects (92% of the subjects "survived"), producing little information on the association of follow-up time and disease outcome. Also, the eight risk variables, measured only once at the beginning of the study, are not strongly related to time to a coronary event.

Appendix A

DESCRIPTION OF THE WCGS DATA SET

The Western Collaborative Group Study (WCGS) recruited middle-aged men (ages 39 to 59) associated with ten California companies and collected data on 3,154 individuals during the years 1960–61. These subjects were selected to study the relationship between behavior pattern and the risk of coronary heart disease (CHD). A number of other risk factors were also measured to provide the best possible assessment of risk from behavior type. Analyzed here is a subset of eight of these risk factors. They are: age, height, weight, systolic blood pressure, diastolic blood pressure, cholesterol level, amount smoked, and behavior type. Behavior type is classified into two categories (called type-A or type-B) from a tape-recorded interview developed for the purpose and administered by trained interviewers. A precise definition of type-A and type-B behavior is complicated and equivocal. In general terms, type-A behavior is characterized by a sense of time urgency, aggressiveness, and ambition. A type-A individual is typically thought of as a competitive personality. The type-B behavior is essentially the converse, manifesting itself in a relaxed, noncompetitive, less hurried individual. A total of 1,589 type-A and 1,565 type-B individuals were identified.

The outcome variable was the presence of coronary heart disease determined by an independent medical referee. Clinical coronary disease occurred in 257 subjects during 9 years of follow-up, producing a crude incidence of CHD of about 11.1 per 1,000 subjects at risk per year. The men lost to follow-up (504) were considered to be non-CHD cases and were about evenly split between type-A and type-B individuals. A total of 92.5% of all possible person-years of follow-up was completed.

Of particular note is the time of CHD event or withdrawal from the study recorded as the number of days of follow-up for each individual participating in the study. The average follow-up was about 7.35 years. The WCGS and data are completely described in a number of places (e.g., [1], [2], and [3]), and a report on 22 years of follow-up has been recently published [4].

The ten variables employed in the text and their mean values at baseline are

Table A–1. List of variables in the WCGS data subset

Variable	Units	Mean	Std. Deviation	Minimum	Maximum
Age	Years	46.279	5.524	39	59
Height	Inches	69.778	2.529	60	78
Weight	Pounds	169.954	21.100	78	320
Systolic BP	mm Hg	128.633	15.112	98	230
Diastolic BP	mm Hg	82.016	9.727	58	150
Cholesterol	mg/100 ml	226.372	43.420	103	645
Smoking	Cigarettes/day	11.601	14.518	0	99
Behavior type	A or B	—	—	0	1
Time	Days	2,683.859	666.524	18	3,430
CHD event	0 or 1	—	—	0	1

The long-term follow-up of WCGS participants [4] indicates that the relationship between behavior type and coronary heart disease is not simple. Behavior type showed a strong association with the incidence of CHD. However, no similar association was found using 22-year heart disease mortality data. The predictive association of behavior and incidence as well as the absence of an association with mortality are not likely to be totally explained by artifact or bias [4]. An explanation may lie in the possibility that behavior type is related to recovery from nonfatal heart disease. The details of this conjecture and a discussion of the associations among a series of risk variables with coronary heart disease mortality are given elsewhere [4]. The WCGS data illustrate a number of statistical approaches to epidemiologic issues and are used to explore the original observation that behavior type is associated with coronary heart disease incidence.

Appendix B

BINOMIAL AND POISSON DISTRIBUTIONS

The binomial and Poisson distributions are basic to many aspects of data analysis, and it is worthwhile to review some of the properties of these distributions. Complete descriptions are found in most introductory statistics texts (e.g., [5]).

A binomially distributed variable is made up of a series of variables with two outcomes. That is,

1. The binary variable X_i is either 1 or 0 with probabilities p or $1 - p$, respectively;
2. Each X_i variable is statistically independent; and
3. The probability p is the same for all X_i.

The binomial variable X is the sum of n values of X_i or

$$X = X_1 + X_2 + \cdots + X_n. \tag{B.1}$$

More simply, X represents the count of the number of times X_i equals 1. The binary character of X_i makes the X variable applicable to a wide range of data with two outcome possibilities—alive or dead, male or female, case of control, and, in general, event A or event not A.

The probabilities associated with a specific value of X, denoted as k, are given by the expression

$$P(X = k) = \binom{n}{k} p^k (1 - p)^{n-k} \quad \text{where} \quad k = 0, 1, 2, \ldots, n. \tag{B.2}$$

The term $\binom{n}{k}$ is the number of different ways k values of 1 can occur among n values of 0 and 1. The quantity $p^k(1 - p)^{n-k}$ is the probability of a specific configuration of 1's and 0's. The product is the probability that k values of X_i will equal 1 and $n - k$ values will equal 0 and, therefore, the sum X equals k. A direct result of these binomial probabilities is that the expected value of X for a series of n events is

$$\text{expected binomial value} = np \tag{B.3}$$

Table B–1. Binomial distribution*, $n = 10$ and $p = 0.4$

k	0	1	2	3	4	5	6	7	8	9	10
$P(X = k)$	0.006	0.040	0.121	0.215	0.251	0.201	0.111	0.042	0.011	0.002	0.000

$*P(X = k) = \binom{10}{k}(0.4)^k(1 - 0.4)^{10-k}.$

and the variance associated with the binomial variable X is

$$\text{variance}(X) = np(1 - p). \tag{B.4}$$

To illustrate, consider the case for $n = 10$ and $p = 0.4$, shown in Table B–1. The expected value is $np = 10(0.4) = 4$ and the variance is $np(1 - p) = 10(0.4)(0.6) = 2.4$.

A related distribution, called the Poisson distribution (named after the French mathematician Simeon Denis Poisson), can be justified from the following considerations:

$$P(X = k) = \binom{n}{k}p^k(1 - p)^{n-k} = \frac{n(n - 1)(n - 2)\cdots(n - k + 1)}{k!} \, p^k\left(1 - \frac{np}{n}\right)^{n-k}$$

$$\tag{B.5}$$

and

$$P(X = k) = \frac{1\left(1 - \dfrac{1}{n}\right)\left(1 - \dfrac{2}{n}\right)\cdots\left(1 - \dfrac{k - 1}{n}\right)}{k!} \, (np)^k\left(1 - \frac{np}{n}\right)^{n-k}. \tag{B.6}$$

If n is large and p is small, then $\left(1 - \dfrac{np}{n}\right)^{n-k} \approx e^{-np}$ giving

$$P(X = k) = \frac{(np)^k e^{-np}}{k!} = \frac{\lambda^k e^{-\lambda}}{k!}. \tag{B.7}$$

Expression (B.7) describes the Poisson probabilities viewed as a limiting case of the binomial distribution. That is, the binomial distribution becomes indistinguishable from the Poisson distribution when n (the number of X_i values) is large and $P(X_i = 1) = p$ is small. The Greek letter $\lambda = np$ is the traditional notation associated with a Poisson distribution.

The Poisson distribution can be derived from other considerations and, like the binomial distribution, plays an important role in analyzing discrete data. The expectation and variance are also derived from the probabilities $P(X = k)$. The expected value of a Poisson distributed variable X is

$$\text{expected Poisson value} = \lambda \qquad \text{(B.8)}$$

with variance of X given by

$$\text{variance}(X) = \lambda. \qquad \text{(B.9)}$$

Situations arise where the variable observed is binary, the number of occurrences n is large, and p is small, implying that the Poisson distribution can be used instead of a binomial distribution as a description of a phenomenon with two outcomes. For example, the probability of k cases of leukemia occurring in a specific or geographic area ($n = $ all possible persons at risk for leukemia and $p = $ the probability that any one person is diagnosed with leukemia) has been modeled by a Poisson distribution (reviewed in [6]). For the application of a Poisson distribution, knowledge of p and n is unnecessary; only the parameter λ must be known or estimated to generate a set of Poisson probabilities. A partial list of phenomena that have been observed to "fit" a Poisson distribution is: deaths by horse kicks, numbers of radioactive decay particles, arrival of patients at a doctor's waiting room, typographical errors, numbers of individuals over 100 years old, occurrences of suicide, telephone calls arriving at a switchboard. . .

Appendix C

THE ODDS RATIO AND ITS PROPERTIES

The odds ratio, central to many epidemiologic analyses, is not the simplest statistical measure of association. This section reviews some of its properties. More complete descriptions exist elsewhere (e.g., [7], [8], or [9]).

The odds are a ratio of two probabilities: the probability an event occurs divided by the probability the event does not occur. (The word *odds* refers to a single entity, but tradition and formal English dictate that the word be treated as a plural noun.) If an event has probability p, then the odds of the event are $p/(1 - p)$. When a series of n binary outcomes are observed where a events occur and b events do not $(n = a + b)$, then the odds are estimated by a/b. For example, if a specific horse finishes among the top three fastest 30 times out of 50 races, then the odds are estimated as 3 to 2 (1.5) the horse will "show."

The odds ratio measures the relative magnitude of two sets of odds occurring under differing conditions. For example,

$$odds(\text{under conditions 1}) = \frac{p_1}{1 - p_1} \tag{C.1}$$

and are estimated by a/b, where a events occur and b events do not occur. Also,

$$odds(\text{under conditions 2}) = \frac{p_2}{1 - p_2} \tag{C.2}$$

and are estimated by c/d, where c events occur and d events do not occur. The symbols p_1 and p_2 represent the probability of occurrence of the events being considered under conditions 1 and 2, respectively. The odds ratio is then

$$odds\ ratio = \frac{p_1/(1 - p_1)}{p_2/(1 - p_2)} = \frac{p_1(1 - p_2)}{(1 - p_1)p_2}. \tag{C.3}$$

Data for the calculation of an odds ratio is typically displayed in a 2×2 table such as Table C–1. An estimate of this odds ratio is

Table C–1. A 2 × 2 table

	Disease	No Disease	Total
Conditions 1 = risk factor present = F	a	b	$a + b$
Conditions 2 = risk factor absent = $\bar{F}$	c	d	$c + d$
Total	$a + c$	$b + d$	n

given by

$$\widehat{or} = \frac{a/b}{c/d} = \frac{ad}{bc}. \tag{C.4}$$

The possible values of an odds ratio run from zero to infinity (∞). The odds ratio measure is symmetric about the value 1.0 in the sense that or represents the same degree of association as $1/or$.

> Aside: An alternate prospective on the odds ratio arises from comparing observed and expected values along the same lines as a standard mortality ratio (SMR, defined in Chapter 1). Using the notation for a 2 × 2 table (Table C–1), the observed number of diseased individuals with a risk factor (F) is a. From the same table, when the risk factor is absent $(\bar{F})$ the number of cases of disease is c and the number of individuals who are disease-free is d. The quantity c/d estimates the ratio of diseased to nondiseased among individuals who do not have the risk factor. If the risk factor has no impact on the disease frequency, the ratio of diseased to nondiseased individuals among those with the risk factor should differ from c/d only because of random variation (i.e., $a/b \approx c/d$). Equating these two ratios gives an expression for the expected number of diseased individuals when the risk factor is unrelated to the disease or
>
> $$\textit{expected number with the disease} = E(A) = b\,\frac{c}{d}$$
>
> The ratio of observed to expected is then
>
> $$\text{``}SMR\text{''} = \frac{a}{E(A)} = \frac{a}{b\,\dfrac{c}{d}} = \frac{ad}{bc} = \widehat{or}.$$
>
> Therefore, an estimated odds ratio can be viewed as a SMR-like quantity from a 2 × 2 table.

Since the odds ratio is generally estimated from a sample of data, it will vary from sample to sample. An estimate of this sampling variation is

$$\text{variance}(\widehat{or}) = \widehat{or}^{2}\left[\frac{1}{a} + \frac{1}{b} + \frac{1}{c} + \frac{1}{d}\right]. \tag{C.5}$$

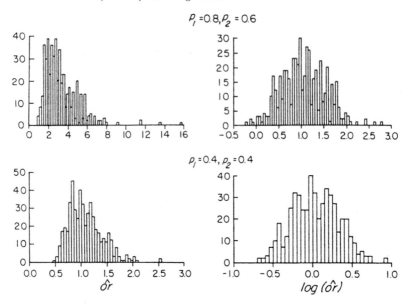

Figure C–1. Histograms of the odds ratio and log-odds for two sets of conditions

Figure C–1 (top left) shows a simulated distribution of 500 values of the odds ratio calculated from samples of size $n = 50$ collected under two conditions ($p_1 = 0.8$ and $p_2 = 0.6$). The distribution of these estimated odds ratios is skewed to the right. The mean of the distribution is 3.170, showing that the directly estimated odds ratio is biased (the expected odds ratio is $(0.8)(0.4)/(0.2)(0.6) = 2.667$). To reduce this bias by producing a more symmetric distribution, the logarithm of the odds ratio is used. A simulated distribution of $\log(\widehat{or})$ is also shown in Figure C–1 (top-right) also for $p_1 = 0.8$ and $p_2 = 0.6$. The distribution is clearly more symmetric with the mean value = 1.037 where $\log(or) = \log(2.667) = 0.981$ is expected. The estimated sample variance associated with the estimate $\log(\widehat{or})$ is

$$\text{variance}[\log(\widehat{or})] = \frac{1}{a} + \frac{1}{b} + \frac{1}{c} + \frac{1}{d}. \tag{C.6}$$

The values of $\log(or)$ range from $-\infty$ to ∞. When the mean value is 0.0, $\log(or)$ is equivalent to $-\log(or)$ as a measure of association. Simulated distributions of $\widehat{or}$ and $\log(\widehat{or})$ are also shown (Figure C–1, bottom) for the case where the two conditions generating the odds are not different (i.e., $p_1 = p_2 = 0.4$).

Other bias-reducing transformations have been suggested for the odds ratio. Two examples are

$$\widehat{or}_H = \frac{(a + 1/2)(d + 1/2)}{(b + 1/2)(c + 1/2)} \tag{C.7}$$

(H for Haldane's [10] suggestion) with estimated variance

$$\text{variance}(\widehat{or}_H) = \frac{1}{a + 1/2} + \frac{1}{b + 1/2} + \frac{1}{c + 1/2} + \frac{1}{d + 1/2} \tag{C.8}$$

and

$$\widehat{or}_{SS} = \frac{ad}{(b + 1)(c + 1)} \tag{C.9}$$

(SS for small sample odds ratio) [11]. A useful property of these two estimates is that the odds ratio remains defined when $b = 0$ or $c = 0$, which is not the case for $\widehat{or}$.

Properties

Some of the properties of or and $\widehat{or}$ derived from a 2 × 2 table are:

1. The odds ratio is invariant to interchanging rows and columns, although interchanging a row only or a column only changes or to $1/or$.
2. Multiplying the rows and/or the columns by positive constants does not change the value of or.
3. The odds ratio has a probabilistic interpretation (as described).
4. The odds ratio approximates the relative risk:

$$\text{relative risk} = \frac{\text{probability of the disease with the factor present}}{\text{probability of the disease with the factor absent}}$$

$$= \frac{P(D|\text{factor})}{P(D|\text{no factor})} \approx \widehat{or},$$

where the frequency of the disease is rare among those with and without the factor.
5. The logarithm of the odds ratio produces a more or less symmetric distribution that can usually be approximated accurately with a normal distribution.

The last property is perhaps the most useful because it allows approximate statistical tests and confidence intervals to be easily constructed based on the normal distribution. The exact properties of the odds ratio have been derived but are complex and difficult to compute. Using the normal distribution as an approximation is simple and sufficiently accurate for most situations.

A null hypothesis of the form H_0: $or = or_0$ can be assessed by reference to a standard normal distribution with the test statistic

$$z = \frac{\log(\widehat{or}) - \log(or_0)}{\sqrt{\text{variance}(\log(\widehat{or}))}}, \tag{C.10}$$

where the value for or_0 is usually chosen to be 1.0. An odds ratio of one implies that the probability of occurrence of the event under study is the same for both conditions 1 and 2 ($p_1 = p_2$). The value z has an approximate standard normal distribution with mean $= 0$ and variance $= 1$ when $or = or_0$.

An $(1 - \alpha)$-level confidence interval can also be constructed using a normal distribution as an approximation for the distribution of the logarithm of the estimated odds ratio or

$$\text{upper} = \log(\widehat{or}) + z_{1-\alpha/2}\sqrt{\text{variance}(\log(\widehat{or}))} \quad \text{and} \tag{C.11}$$

$$\text{lower} = \log(\widehat{or}) - z_{1-\alpha/2}\sqrt{\text{variance}(\log(\widehat{or}))}, \tag{C.12}$$

where $z_{1-\alpha} =$ the $(1 - \alpha)$th percentile of a standard normal distribution. The probability that the parameter $\log(or)$ is found between these upper and lower bounds is approximately $1 - \alpha$. These limits can be directly transformed to provide a $(1 - \alpha)$-level confidence interval of the odds ratio itself. The probability is approximately $1 - \alpha$ that the "true" odds ratio or is found in the interval $(e^{\text{lower}}, e^{\text{upper}})$. That is, it is unlikely that the odds ratio underlying the observed data (estimated by $\widehat{or}$) will be less than e^{lower} or greater than e^{upper}.

Appendix D

PARTITIONING THE CHI-SQUARE STATISTIC

Suppose the focus of an analytic technique is on a series of independent measures of association, symbolized by M_i, that take on the value 0 when no association exists (null hypothesis). A parallel series of weights w_i are defined as

$$w_i = \frac{1}{\text{variance}(\hat{M}_i)}, \tag{D.1}$$

where $\hat{M}_i$ represents an estimate of M_i. Then, under rather general considerations,

$$X_i^2 = \frac{\hat{M}_i^2}{\text{variance}(\hat{M}_i)} = w_i \hat{M}_i^2 \tag{D.2}$$

has an approximate chi-square distribution with one degree of freedom when the null hypothesis $M_i = 0$ is true.

Three properties of the statistic M_i are:

1. A summary measure of association for k estimates of M_i is

$$\bar{M} = \frac{\sum\limits_{i=1}^{k} w_i \hat{M}_i}{\sum\limits_{i=1}^{k} w_i} \tag{D.3}$$

and

$$X_A^2 = \frac{\bar{M}^2}{\text{variance}(\bar{M})} = \frac{\left(\sum\limits_{i=1}^{k} w_i \hat{M}_i\right)^2}{\sum\limits_{i=1}^{k} w_i} \qquad (A \text{ for association}) \tag{D.4}$$

has an approximate chi-square distribution with one degree of freedom when the null hypothesis is true (i.e., $M_i = 0$ for $i = 1, 2, \ldots, k$), and the k measures of association M_i are independent.

2. The total chi-square statistic is

$$X^2 = \sum_{i=1}^{k} X_i^2 = \sum_{i=1}^{k} w_i \hat{M}_i^2 \tag{D.5}$$

and has an approximate chi-square distribution with $k - 1$ degrees of freedom when all k values of $\hat{M}_i$ are random deviations from 0 (no association exists in all k situations).

3. A chi-square statistic that measures the heterogeneity among the k measures of association is

$$X_H^2 = X^2 - X_A^2 = \sum_{i=1}^{k} w_i (\hat{M}_i - \bar{M})^2 \quad (H \text{ for heterogeneity}) \tag{D.6}$$

and X_H^2 has an approximate chi-square distribution with $k - 2$ degrees of freedom when all k measures of associations M_i are the same. Formally, X_H^2 is used to assess deviations from the null hypothesis that $M_1 = M_2 = \cdots = M_k = M$.

A summary of these chi-square statistics is found in Table D–1. The total chi-square statistic X^2 is partitioned into two pieces, X_A^2 and X_H^2. The chi-square statistic X_A^2 evaluates the measure of association $\bar{M}$ resulting from combining the M_i values over k situations. This summary measure is most meaningful when each of the k components measure the same degree of association. The chi-square statistic X_H^2 reflects the degree of heterogeneity among the k measures of association.

Application: 2 × K Table

If $\hat{M}_i = \hat{b}_i = (y_i - \bar{y})/(x_i - \bar{x})$, then $w_i = (x_i - \bar{x})^2/\text{variance}(y)$ gives

$$\bar{M} = \hat{b}_{y|x} \quad \text{and} \quad X_A^2 = X_L^2 = \frac{\hat{b}_{y|x}^2}{\text{variance}(\hat{b}_{y|x})}.$$

Also, $X_H^2 = X_{NL}^2$ measures nonlinearity. Both X_L^2 and X_{NL}^2 are further

Table D–1. Partitioned values of a chi-square statistic

Summary	Chi-Square	Degrees of Freedom
Association	$X_A^2 = \bar{M}^2/\text{variance}(\bar{M})$	1
Heterogeneity	$X_H^2 = \sum_{i=1}^{k} w_i(\hat{M}_i - \bar{M})^2$	$k - 2$
Total	$X^2 = \sum_{i=1}^{k} w_i \hat{M}_i^2$	$k - 1$

defined in Chapter 6 and play key roles in connection with the analysis of a $2 \times K$ table.

Application: Mantel-Haenszel Chi-Square Statistic

If $M_i = (a_i - \hat{A}_i)/\text{variance}(a_i)$, then $w_i = \text{variance}(a_i)$ giving

$$
\bar{M} = \frac{\sum\limits_{i=1}^{k} a_i - \sum\limits_{i=1}^{k} \hat{A}_i}{\sum\limits_{i=1}^{k} \text{variance}(a_i)} \quad \text{and} \quad X_A^2 = X_{MH}^2 = \frac{\left(\sum\limits_{i=1}^{k} a_i - \sum\limits_{i=1}^{k} \hat{A}_i\right)^2}{\sum\limits_{i=1}^{k} \text{variance}(a_i)},
$$

which is the Mantel-Haenszel chi-square statistic used in Chapters 6, 11, and 12 to assess the association reflected in a series of 2×2 tables.

Appendix E

MAXIMUM LIKELIHOOD ESTIMATION

Once a statistical model is postulated, estimates of specific parameters are necessary before it becomes a useful tool in the analysis of a data set. A statistically optimum estimation technique is the method of maximum likelihood.

> Aside: Maximum likelihood estimation is one of the many statistical contributions of British geneticist/statistician Ronald Aylmer Fisher (1890–1962). R. A. Fisher ranks among the great scientists of the twentieth century. He began his career in genetics and went on to develop much of modern statistics to solve genetic and agricultural problems. His temperament was sometimes controversial, but his dominance in fields of genetics and statistics is never questioned. His work provided the research world with the confidence interval, experimental design, analysis of variance, as well as a large number of concepts in theoretical statistics. At the same time he laid down much of the mathematical foundation for Darwin's theory of evolution. Fisher's early books, *Statistical Methods for Research Workers* (1925) and *The Genetical Theory of Natural Selection* (1930), were revolutionary in their impact and remain classics today.

In simple terms, a maximum likelihood estimate of a parameter is that value that is most likely for the sampled data. In a sense, things are turned around. The data are considered fixed, and questions are asked about the possible values of the parameter. That is, for a specific set of observations, which of all possible values of the parameter is the most likely to have produced the observed data? An example illustrates. Consider a model consisting of a single parameter that determines the values of variables X and Y. The probability that $X = 1$ is p and $X = 0$ is $1 - p$. Similarly, it is postulated that the same parameter is associated with Y (i.e., $P(Y = 1) = p$ and $P(Y = 0) = 1 - p$). Additionally, X and Y are statistically independent, giving the statistical structure shown in Table E–1. Say the data in Table E–2 were observed.

The probability that such a sample occurred is related to a likelihood function where

$$\text{likelihood function} = [p^2]^{36}[p(1-p)]^{14}[(1-p)p]^{34}[(1-p)^2]^{16}. \quad (E.1)$$

This likelihood value is a small number but nevertheless reflects the probabilities associated with the model for any parameter p for the observed data set. Each value of p produces a different likelihood. The maximum likelihood principle states that the estimate of p will be that value that maximizes the likelihood (denoted as $\hat{p}$). The data (36, 14, 34, and 16) are fixed, and the value of p is varied until the maximum value of the likelihood is found. Estimation reduces to searching for this value. Rather than dealing with extremely small likelihood values, it is conventional to take the logarithm of the likelihood for ease of manipulation. The value of p that maximizes the logarithm of the likelihood, maximizes the likelihood. A few values of the loglikelihood [expression (E.1)] for different parameters p are given in Table E–3.

The loglikelihood is a continuous function of p and is shown in Figure E–1. The maximum value is attained at $p = 0.6$, giving a maximum likelihood estimate of $\hat{p} = 0.6$, using the illustrative data and model. This estimate can also be found by employing techniques from calculus. In fact, the maximum likelihood estimate for this simple case is identical to the natural estimate of the number of times X or Y equals one divided by the total number of observations or $\hat{p} = 120/200 = 0.6$.

The mechanics of finding maximum likelihood estimates becomes more tedious as the number of parameters in the model increases, but the process does not change in principle. Consider a two-parameter

Table E–1. Model

	$X = 1$	$X = 0$	Total
$Y = 1$	p^2	$(1-p)p$	p
$Y = 0$	$p(1-p)$	$(1-p)^2$	$1-p$
Total	p	$1-p$	1

Table E–2. Data

	$X = 1$	$X = 0$	Total
$Y = 1$	36	14	50
$Y = 0$	34	16	50
Total	70	30	100

Table E–3. Loglikelihood values from the data in Table E–2

p	Loglikelihood
$p = 0.2$	$L = -177.7$
$p = 0.3$	$L = -139.7$
$p = 0.4$	$L = -117.6$
$p = 0.5$	$L = -105.4$
$p = 0.6$	$L = -101.3$
$p = 0.7$	$L = -105.8$
$p = 0.8$	$L = -122.3$
$p = 0.9$	$L = -163.6$

situation. Twin births are either monozygotic (m) or dizygotic (d). Although zygosity of a twin pair is not generally recorded, twin births can be categorized by the sex of the pair: male-male, male-female, and female-female. A model describing the relationship between zygosity and sex of the twin pair and an application of the maximum likelihood estimation technique produces an estimate of the frequency of the two zygotic types of twins. The following model is postulated:

$$P(\textit{male-male pair which is monozygotic}) = p$$

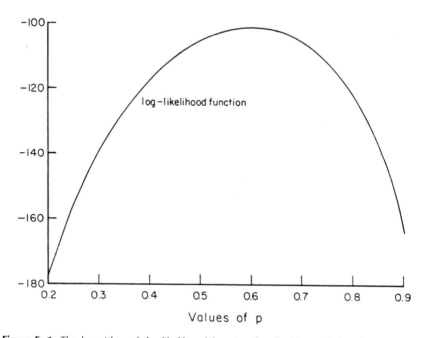

Figure E–1. The logarithm of the likelihood function for the binomial data for a range of the possible values of the parameter p

and

$$P(\text{male-male pair which is dizygotic}) = p^2$$

and the probability of a male-male twin pair is a mixture of these two zygotic types or

$$P(\text{male-male}) = pm + p^2 d, \tag{E.2}$$

where $d = 1 - m$ is the frequency of monozygotic twin pairs. Similarly, the probabilities associated with the other two types of twin pairs are

$$P(\text{female-male}) = 2p(1 - p)d$$

and

$$P(\text{female-female}) = (1 - p)m + (1 - p)^2 d. \tag{E.3}$$

The complete twin model and a data set of 109 twin pairs are shown in Table E–4. The likelihood function associated with this twin model depends on two parameters (p and d) and is given by

$$likelihood = [p(1 - d) + p^2 d]^{32}[2p(1 - p)d]^{41}[(1 - p)(1 - d) + (1 - p)^2 d]^{36}. \tag{E.4}$$

This two-dimensional likelihood function is shown in Figure E–2, A search of the likelihood function indicates that the maximum occurs at $p = 0.482$ and $d = 0.753$. Therefore, the values that maximize the likelihood associated with the specific data (32, 41, and 36) are the maximum likelihood estimates $\hat{p} = 0.482$ and $\hat{d} = 0.753$. No other pair of values produces a larger value of likelihood function or logarithm of the likelihood function for the observed data. These two values $\hat{p}$ and $\hat{d}$ are the most likely among all possible values of p and d for the given set of twin data.

The maximum likelihood estimates for multiparameter models are typically estimated by computer techniques. The definition of the maximum likelihood estimate, however, is the same. To estimate k parameters of a model, say $\theta_1, \theta_2, \theta_3, \ldots, \theta_k$, the maximum likelihood estimate of the k values is such that $likelihood$ $(\theta_1, \theta_2, \theta_3, \ldots, \theta_k)$ is

Table E–4. Maximum likelihood estimation: Data and model for a set of two pair data

Pair Type	Male-Male	Female-Male	Female-Female	Total
Model	$pm + p^2 d$	$2p(1 - p)d$	$(1 - p)m + (1 - p^2)d$	1.0
Observed number	32	41	36	109

Likelihood function – Twin data (four views)

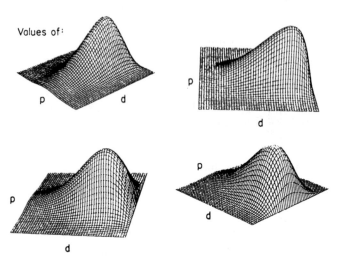

Figure E–2. Four views of the bivariate loglikelihood function for the estimates of the two parameters (p, d) from the twin data

maximum or

$$\text{likelihood}(\hat{\theta}_1, \hat{\theta}_2, \hat{\theta}_3, \ldots, \hat{\theta}_k) \geq \text{likelihood}(\theta_1, \theta_2, \theta_3, \ldots, \theta_k)$$

for all possible values of the set of k parameters. The interpretation is also the same; the estimates $\hat{\theta}_1, \hat{\theta}_2, \hat{\theta}_3, \ldots, \hat{\theta}_k$ is that set of parameters that makes the sampled data most likely to have occurred.

The maximum likelihood process also produces an estimate of the variation associated with the estimated parameters. The variance of a maximum likelihood estimate is related to the likelihood function and is calculated by sometimes rather complicated manipulations. Estimated variances, however, are part of maximum likelihood estimation computer programs, making these estimated variances widely available. For example, the estimates $\hat{p} = 0.482$ and $\hat{d} = 0.753$ from the twin data have estimated variances of variance$(\hat{p}) = 0.00143$ and variance$(\hat{d}) = 0.00862$, respectively. A measure of the reliability is always an important part of the interpretation of an estimated value.

Another property of maximum likelihood estimation is that a function of a maximum likelihood estimate is itself a maximum likelihood estimate. It is often the case that maximum likelihood estimates are expressed in different forms or are used to estimate other relevant quantities. For example, if an estimate of the proportion of male-male pairs is desired, the maximum likelihood estimate is $\hat{p}\hat{m} + \hat{p}^2\hat{d} = 0.482(0.247) + (0.482)^2(0.753) = 0.294$, or the number of male-male pairs is estimated by $109(0.294) = 32.046$ and is also the maximum likelihood estimate because both estimates are based on the maximum likelihood estimates $\hat{p} = 0.482$ and $\hat{d} = 0.753$. In general, if $\hat{\theta}$ is a maximum likelihood estimate, then $f(\hat{\theta})$ is also a maximum likelihood estimate (e.g., if $\hat{b}$ is a maximum likelihood estimate, so is $e^{\hat{b}}$). A more extensive description of the theory and practice of maximum likelihood estimation is part of a mathematical statistics course (e.g., see [12]).

Likelihood Function

The likelihood function, which is an essential part of the maximum likelihood process, is a valuable summary of a model's "fit" to the data. Comparison of likelihood values under differing conditions allows an evaluation of different statistical models. The twin data will continue to serve as an example. The likelihood associated with the estimates $\hat{p} = 0.482$ and $\hat{d} = 0.753$ is 1.72×10^{-52}. This extremely small number is proportional to the probability of the occurrence of the observed data for these specific values of the parameters. The occurrence of the observed set of data (32 male-male pairs, 41 male-female pairs, and 36 female-female pairs) is not likely, but this probability can be compared to other similar probabilities. For example, say it is postulated that $p = 0.5$ where the observed value $\hat{p} = 0.482$ is considered a result of sampling variation (H_0: $p = 0.5$) while the proportion of dizygotic twins (d) remains 0.753. The likelihood under the condition that $p = 0.5$ is 1.53×10^{-52}—an expected decrease over the previous maximum value because the likelihood is maximum at $p = 0.482$ and any other value of p will produce some decrease. Is a difference of this magnitude expected by chance alone? A result from mathematical statistics is helpful for comparing likelihood values. The difference between the logarithms of two likelihood values multiplied by -2 has an approximate chi-square distribution when the two conditions being compared are identical and the observed loglikelihoods differ only because of random variation (null hypothesis is true). The degrees of freedom are equal to the difference in the number of estimated parameters associated with each of the models compared. For the twin data, if $\hat{p} = 0.482$, then $-2\text{loglikelihood} = L_1 = 238.381$ and if $p = 0.5$, then $-2\text{loglikelihood} = L_0 = 238.616$—$d$ remains 0.753 for both models. The difference $L_0 - L_1 = 238.616 - 238.381 = 0.235$ has an approximate chi-square distribution with one degree of freedom when $\hat{p}$ differs from 0.5 by chance, producing a significance probability of

p-value $= 0.628$. That is, no evidence exists in the data to support the notion that the probability of a male among twin births is different from the probability of a female twin ($p = 0.5$). Additionally, suppose it is postulated that the same proportion of dizygotic twins are born as monozygotic twins ($d = m = 0.5$ and $p = 0.5$). The value of -2loglikelihood associated with this conjecture is $L_0 = 247.069$. Comparison of the loglikelihood values gives $L_0 - L_1 = 247.069 - 238.381 = 8.69$, which has an approximate chi-square distribution with two degrees of freedom when the fit of the two models (i.e., loglikelihoods) differs by chance. An increase of 8.69 is not likely (p-value $= 0.013$), showing that the hypothesis of equally frequent sex and zygotic types is not consistent with the observed data.

In general, one set of conditions generates loglikelihood value L_1; a more restrictive set of conditions generates a second loglikelihood value L_0, and the increase $[-2 \log(L_0)] - [-2 \log(L_1)] = X^2$ measures the impact of the restricted set of conditions via a chi-square distribution. The difference between loglikelihood values is a quantitative assessment (with a chi-square distribution) that indicates whether two models differ because of a systematic influence (small p-value) or whether the more complicated model capitalizes on only random variation to produce a smaller loglikelihood value (large p-value). The evaluation of "nested" models by comparing loglikelihoods is a basic tool in multivariate statistical analysis.

Problems

Chapter 1   Measures of Risk: Rates and Probabilities

1. A population is sampled to determine the probability of illness. A total of N days are recorded where it is determined that an individual is ill, well, or status is unknown. That is,

y days ill + n days well + k days status unknown = N total days $(y + n + k = N)$.

Two possibilities for estimating the probability a person from this population is ill are:
Strategy (i): Ignore the k days where the status is unknown.
Strategy (ii): Assume that the probability of illness is the same for days when the status is known and unknown (i.e., days where status is unknown occur at random).
Demonstrate that strategy (i) and strategy (ii) are equivalent.

2. Four schemes for collecting data to estimate the average length of stay in an institution are:
(i) Complete follow-up: For each individual entering an institution the length of stay is determined from beginning to end.
(ii) Retrospective follow-up: A series of institutionalized patients is identified at a specific time, and the amount of time each person has been institutionalized is ascertained.
(iii) Partial follow-up: The entire stay is recorded from admission to discharge from those patients present at the start of sampling, using their admission records and observing them until they are discharged.
(iv) Interval follow-up: A series of institutionalized patients is followed for a specific period of time (some are discharged before and some remain institutionalized at the end of the time period).
Four sets of 1,000 hypothetical observations that would result under these four sampling schemes are:

Weeks	Complete	Retrospective	Partial	Interval
0	135	332	45	344
1	271	288	180	325
2	271	198	271	208
3	180	108	240	92
4	90	48	150	31
5	36	18	72	—
6	12	6	28	—
7	4	2	11	—
8	1	0	3	—
9	0	0	0	—

Note: The distribution of lengths of stay is the same in all four cases; the difference arises from the way the data were collected. Investigate the issue of length bias for these four data-collecting patterns. Estimate the degree of bias in each case for the mean length of stay. How is the estimate of the variance of the distribution of lengths of stay affected by the data-collection schemes.

3. Can a one-year average mortality rate exceed the number of deaths—rate $(R_x) >$ deaths (d_x)?

Chapter 2   Variation and Bias

4. For a one-way classification of data an estimate of σ^2 is denoted S_p^2 and for a two-way classification by S^2. Usually $S^2 < S_p^2$ producing a more efficient analysis of the data while controlling the influence of an extraneous variable. However, occasionally losses are incurred by forming a two-way classification. Find a condition such that a two-way analysis is less efficient than a one-way analysis (i.e., $S^2 > S_p^2$). Hint: $\sum\sum (y_{ij} - \bar{y}_{i.})^2 = \sum\sum (\bar{y}_{.j} - \bar{y})^2 + \sum\sum (y_{ij} - \bar{y}_{i.} - \bar{y}_{.j} + \bar{y})^2$.

5. If two hypotheses are under consideration, show that the overall type I error (one or two type I errors) is less than α if both tests are conducted at a level of $\alpha/2$—(i) if the two tests are independent and (ii) if the two tests are not independent.

Chapter 3   Statistical Power and Sample Size Calculations

6. Derive an expression for the sample size necessary to detect a difference δ between two proportions (i.e., $\delta = p_2 - p_1$) where the sample sizes from each source differ. That is, one source yields r times more data than the other source or $n_1 = rn_2$—find n_1 where r is known.

7. If $H_0: Np_0 = 2$, generate the Poisson distribution associated with this null hypothesis.

$$\text{note:}\quad P(x = k) = \frac{e^{-Np_0}(Np_0)^k}{k!}.$$

Select a critical point so that $P(X > 0) \approx 0.05$. If $H_1: N\rho p_0 = 4$, generate the Poisson distribution under this alternative hypothesis that the relative risk is 2 $(\rho = 2)$ and compute the power [i.e., $P(X > 0 = ?)$]. Use the normal approximation approach to make the same calculation and compare the two results.

8. Consider the null hypothesis that the sample was collected from a normal population with mean 0.0 and variance σ^2 and the alternative that the sample was collected from a normal population with the same variance but with mean μ. Find an expression for the power curve associated with different values of μ where the test statistic is the 95th percentile. That is, H_0 is tested against H_1 using

$$\hat{P} = \bar{y} + 1.96 S_Y.$$

The approximate variance of an estimated percentile is

$$\text{variance}(\hat{P}) \approx \frac{\sigma^2}{n} [1 + (\tfrac{1}{2}) z_{1-\alpha}^2].$$

Compute the efficiency of using the 95th percentile compared to using the mean value $(\bar{y})$ to detect a difference of μ between two normal populations with the same variance for set values of α and β. Define efficiency as k/n, where n is the sample size required using $\bar{y}$ and k is the sample size required when $\hat{P}$ is employed.

Chapter 4   Cohort Data: Description and Illustration

9. When the residual values resulting from a "median polish" are subtracted from the original data, the resulting table perfectly fits an additive model, or

$$n_{ij} = n_{11} + a_i + t_j.$$

For the table

	$j = 1$	$j = 2$	$j = 3$	$j = 4$	$j = 5$
$i = 1$	10	15	18	20	40
$i = 2$	5	8	3	2	10
$i = 3$	6	10	15	17	30

find values $t_1, t_2, t_3, t_4, a_1, a_2,$ and a_3 that produce an additive relationship between the rows and the columns of the table.

Chapter 5   Clustering: Space and Time Data

10. Show that when $P(X = k) = \lambda^k e^{-\lambda}/k!$,

$$P(X = i + 1) = \frac{\lambda}{i + 1} P(X = i).$$

Use this expression to generate the Poisson probabilities starting with $P(X = 0) = e^{-\lambda}$ for $\lambda = 2$.

11. Show that for $F(r) = P(R < r) = 1 - e^{-n\pi r^2/A}$, then

$$\text{median } (r) = 0.470 \sqrt{\frac{A}{n}}.$$

12. Consider the data:

Group I: 11, 18, 21
Group II: 10, 8, 12

(i) t-test: Compute a t-statistic to evaluate the mean difference between groups I and II—find the one-sided p-value.

(ii) Permutation test: List all possible mean differences (there are 20) from the data to evaluate the observed differences between groups I and II—find the one-sided p-value.

3. Prove that the jackknife estimate of the mean and the variance for a sample of n observations is the same as the usual estimates $\bar{x} = \sum x_i/n$ and $S^2 = \sum (x_i - \bar{x})^2/(n - 1)$. Also show that for this case the bias must be zero.

Chapter 6   The Two × K Contingency Table and the Two × Two Table

14. Show that

$$X_L^2 = \frac{\hat{b}_{y|x}^2}{\text{variance }(\hat{b}_{y|x})} = \frac{\hat{b}_{x|y}^2}{\text{variance }(\hat{b}_{x|y})}.$$

15. Demonstrate for a $2 \times K$ table that

$$X_L^2 = (n - 1)\, r_{xy}^2.$$

16. Show that

(i) $\displaystyle\sum_{i=1}^{n} (y_i - \bar{y})^2 = \frac{n_1 n_2}{n}$ when y_i takes on the values 0 and 1 only;

(ii) variance $(\bar{x}_2 - \bar{x}_1) = $ variance $(\hat{b}_{x|y})$; and

(iii) $\dfrac{(\bar{x}_2 - \bar{x}_1)^2}{\text{variance }(\bar{x}_2 - \bar{x}_1)} = \dfrac{\hat{b}_{y|x}^2}{\text{variance }(\hat{b}_{y|x})}.$

17. Consider the following $2 \times K$ table:

	X = 0	X = 1	X = 2	X = 3	X = 4	Total
Y = 0	18	16	24	24	52	134
Y = 1	20	24	60	35	50	189
Total	38	40	84	59	102	323

Compute: X^2, X_L^2, and X_{NL}^2. Find the associated p-values. For the same data compute the ridit $\hat{P}$, where $Y = 1$ is the reference group—also find the associated p-value.

18. Show that if no interaction is observed between a risk factor and a disease for a $2 \times 2 \times 2$ table, then the disease-confounder and confounder–risk-factor relationships also show no interaction. That is,

$$\text{if } \widehat{or}_{FD|C} = \widehat{or}_{FD|\bar{C}}, \quad \text{then} \quad \widehat{or}_{CD|F} = \widehat{or}_{CD|\bar{F}} \quad \text{and} \quad \widehat{or}_{CF|D} = \widehat{or}_{CF|\bar{D}}.$$

19. The relationships among the variables in a $2 \times 2 \times 2$ table for a disease (D), a risk factor (F) and a confounder (C) are given by

$$or_{pooled} = \frac{1 + (or_{CD|F} - 1)\, P(C\,|\,F\bar{D})}{1 + (or_{CD|\bar{F}} - 1)\, P(C\,|\,\overline{FD})} \times or_{FD|\bar{C}}$$

when no interaction exists.

Create a numeric set of data in a $2 \times 2 \times 2$ table and illustrate that this expression links the relationships among F, D and C. Demonstrate that if $or_{CD|\bar{F}} = 1$, then C is not a confounder and demonstrate that if $or_{CF|\bar{D}} = 1$, then C is also not a confounder.

Chapter 7   The Analysis of Contingency Table Data: Logistic Model I

20. If $P(D\,|\,F) = P(D)$, then events represented by F and D are statistically independent. Show statistical independence of F and D also implies that $P(D\,|\,\bar{F}) = P(D)$ for

events represented by $\bar{F}$ and D, where $\bar{F}$ is the complement of event F or $1 - P(F) = P(\bar{F})$.

Further show that $P(D|F) = P(D)$ implies that relative risk $= P(D|F)/P(D|\bar{F}) = 1$ and odds ratio $= or = P(D|F)P(\bar{D}|\bar{F})/P(\bar{D}|F)P(D|\bar{F}) = 1$.

21. Consider the following model and data:

$$\text{log-odds} = a + bf_1 + cf_2 + df_1f_2$$

Disease by factor 1 by factor 2

		Factor 1			No Factor 1	
	Disease	No Disease	Total	Disease	No Disease	Total
Factor 2	10	12	22	80	52	132
No Factor 2	15	48	63	55	70	125
Total	25	60	85	135	122	257

Estimate the coefficients and fill in the rest of the table (these answers can be calculated *easily* by hand).

Logistic Regression: Disease by factor 1 by factor 2

Variable	Term	Coefficient	Std. Error	p-value	Odds Ratio
Constant	$\hat{a}$	???	???	—	—
Factor 1	$\hat{b}$	???	???	???	???
Factor 2	$\hat{c}$	???	???	???	???
Interaction	$\hat{d}$	???	???	???	???

22. Consider the $2 \times 2 \times 2$ table for risk factors A and B:

	$B = 1$		$B = 0$	
	D	$\bar{D}$	D	$\bar{D}$
$A = 1$	$P(D|A=1, B=1)$	$P(\bar{D}|A=1, B=1)$	$P(D|A=1, B=0)$	$P(\bar{D}|A=1, B=0)$
$A = 0$	$P(D|A=0, B=1)$	$P(\bar{D}|A=0, B=1)$	$P(D|A=0, B=0)$	$P(\bar{D}|A=0, B=0)$

Describe the eight probabilities contained in the $2 \times 2 \times 2$ table with a strictly additive logistic model or

$$P(D|A = i, B = j) = \frac{1}{1 + e^{-(a+bi+cj)}}$$

Express the odds ratios or_{11}, or_{01}, and or_{10} in terms of the equivalent probabilities modeled by the logistic function where

$$or_{ij} = \frac{P(D \mid A = i, B = j) \, P(\bar{D} \mid A = 0, B = 0)}{P(\bar{D} \mid A = i, B = j) \, P(D \mid A = 0, B = 0)}.$$

Show that $or_{11} = or_{01} \times or_{10}$ for the additive logistic model and that $or_{11} \neq or_{01} \times or_{10}$ for a nonadditive logistic model.

Chapter 8   The Analysis of Binary Data: Logistic Model II

23. Show that for a simple logistic regression model, x_i and $x_i^* = x_i - \bar{x}$ produce the same value for the coefficient b (i.e., the value of b from the model log-odds $= a + bx$ is not influenced by the transformation). Show that the coefficient b is affected by the same transformation in the quadratic model (i.e., the value of b from the model log-odds $= a + bx + cx^2$ is influenced by the transformation).

24. Consider the linear model:

$$y_{ij} = a + b_1 x_{1j} + b_2 x_{2j} + \gamma z_j + e_{ij}.$$

If z is excluded from the model, the estimate of b_2 is potentially biased. The confounder bias is measured by

$$\text{bias} = \frac{\gamma S_z [r_{z2} - r_{z1} r_{12}]}{S_2 (1 - r_{12}^2)},$$

where S_i is the standard deviation of the ith variable and r_{ij} is the correlation between variables i and j. Identify three sets of conditions where the elimination of variable z does not induce bias in the estimation of b_2 (i.e., z is not a confounding influence).

Chapter 9   The Analysis of Matched Data

25. Consider the following binary data from a matched pairs study.

Strata	Status	F	Strata	Status	F
1	1	0	10	1	0
1	0	1	10	0	1
2	1	0	11	1	0
2	0	1	11	0	1
3	1	0	12	1	1
3	0	1	12	0	0
4	1	1	13	1	1
4	0	0	13	0	1
5	1	1	14	1	1
5	0	0	14	0	0
6	1	1	15	1	0
6	0	0	15	1	0
7	1	1	16	1	1
7	0	0	16	1	1
8	1	0	17	1	1
8	0	1	17	1	0
9	1	0	18	1	1
9	0	0	18	1	0

Construct a summary table from these data of the form:

	Control F	Control $\bar{F}$	Total
Case F	a	b	$a + b$
Case $\bar{F}$	c	d	$c + d$
Total	$a + c$	$b + d$	N

The values a, b, c, and d represent numbers of pairs for the above data, and N is the total number of pairs observed.

Calculate the odds ratio $\widehat{or}$ and its variance.

Based on four different approaches (exact method, small-sample approximation, large-sample approximation, and the asymptotic method), calculate the 95% confidence intervals based in the estimate $\widehat{or}$.

For the model

$$\text{log-odds} = a_i + bF,$$

what is an estimate of b?

Calculate the odds ratio for this same data as if it were a prospective study where observations on cases of disease (Status) and risk factor (F) were not collected in a matched pattern. Also estimate a 95% confidence for this odds ratio.

26. Consider a set of matched data with a case (D) and three controls ($\bar{D}$). The notation for $1:3$ matched data set is summarized in the following table:

	Control F and F and F	Control $\bar{F}$ and F and F	Control $\bar{F}$ and $\bar{F}$ and F	Control $\bar{F}$ and $\bar{F}$ and $\bar{F}$
Case F	n_{13}	n_{12}	n_{11}	n_{10}
Case $\bar{F}$	n_{03}	n_{02}	n_{01}	n_{00}

What is the odds ratio expression for the association between a risk factor F and a disease D? (Hint: Use the Mantel-Haenszel estimate.)

Do the numbers of sets n_{13} and n_{00} play a role in this estimate?

Chapter 10   Life Tables: An Introduction

27. Survival data from a clinical trial are as follows (in days):

Treatment group (n = 12):   Control group (n = 12):

$4, 8, 12^{+}, 19, 25, 28^{+}, 41, 44, 57^{+}, 68, 73^{+}, 97$ $2, 3, 7, 9, 15, 19^{+}, 33, 38, 40, 53^{+}, 54, 65.$

The "$+$" means that the individual was withdrawn alive after being observed for a number of days (censored).

Construct a life table for each group using 5-day intervals. Compute the probability of survival for each interval. Compare the probability of surviving 40 days for the treatment and control groups $(\hat{P}_{40})$. Estimate the hazard function for each interval using different approximations [e.g., $-\log(p_x)$ and q_x] and compare the results.

28. Consider the "two marksmen model" of Berkson and Elveback, where the marksmen shoot alternatively at the targets n times. Show that the net probability for marksmen 1 (Q_1) is approximated by the intuitive estimate (Q_1'), particularly when the crude probabilities q_1 and q_2 are small.

29. Competing risk

	Nonfactor	Factor
Disease $= d_1$	x_1	y_1
Other $= d_2$	x_2	y_2
Population	50,000	50,000

Compute the crude, hazard-based, and intuitive net probabilities of disease for

(i) $x_1 = 2,000$, $x_2 = 2,000$, $y_1 = 500$, $y_2 = 500$.

(ii) $x_1 = 1,000$, $x_2 = 1,000$, $y_1 = 500$, $y_2 = 5,000$.
(iii) $x_1 = 200$, $x_2 = 20$, $y_1 = 100$, $y_2 = 10$.

Chapter 11   Estimates of Risk from Follow-Up Data

30. Create a small numeric example and illustrate that the following two expressions give the same estimated mean value:

$$\bar{t} = \sum_{i=1}^{k} t_i(\hat{P}_{i-1} - \hat{P}_i) \text{ where } \hat{P}_0 = 1 \text{ and } \bar{t} = \sum_{i=1}^{k} \hat{P}_{i-1}(t_i - t_{i-1}), \text{ where } t_0 = 0.$$

Demonstrate algebraically that the two ways of calculating the mean survival times are identical.

Also if no censoring occurs, show that both forms for $\bar{t}$ reduce to the usual estimate of $\bar{t} = \sum t_i/n$.

Show that Greenwood's formula

$$\text{variance}(\hat{P}_k) = \hat{P}_k^2 \sum \frac{q_i}{n_i p_i}$$

reduces to the binomial variance of $P_k(1 - P_k)/n$ when no censoring occurs.

31. Derive an estimate for the median based on a sample from a population with exponential survival (i.e., $S(t) = e^{-\lambda t}$). Also develop an expression for the upper and lower bounds of an approximate 95% confidence interval for this estimated median.

32. Consider the data again:

Treatment group (n = 12):   Control group (n = 12):

$4, 8, 12^+, 19, 25, 28^+, 41, 44, 57^+, 68, 73^+, 97$ $2, 3, 7, 9, 15, 19^+, 33, 38, 40, 53^+, 54, 65$.

(i) Compute $\hat{\lambda}_1$ and $\hat{\lambda}_2$ (based on exponential survival).
(ii) Estimate the survival curves for each group parametrically (based on exponential survival) and nonparametrically (product-moment estimators).

(iii) Compute parametrically the mean survival times from group 1 and group 2 based on exponential survival and nonparametrically based on the product-moment estimators.
(iv) Estimate the median survival times parametrically (based on exponential survival) and nonparametrically.
(v) Use the Mantel-Haenszel chi-square test to evaluate the differences in survival times between treatment and control groups.
(vi) Use the Gehan generalization of the Wilcoxon test to evaluate the differences in survival times between treatment and control groups.
(vii) Demonstrate with the above data that $W = \sum n_i(a_i - \hat{A}_i)$ and $z^2 \approx X^2$ for the Gehan generalization approach compared to the Gehan chi-square test.

Chapter 12   A Model for Survival Data: Proportional Hazards Model

33. Consider the lung cancer survival data

	Days	$S_0(t)$		Days	$S_0(t)$
1	1	0.968	22	139	0.720
2	3	0.958	23	143	0.707
3	4	0.947	24	159	0.694
4	5	0.937	25	168	0.680
5	9	0.926	26	170	0.667
6	19	0.916	27	180	0.652
7	21	0.905	28	189	0.637
8	30	0.895	29	192	0.622
9	36	0.884	30	201	0.606
10	39	0.874	31	212	0.591
11	40	0.863	32	223	0.575
12	48	0.853	33	229	0.560
13	51	0.842	34	238	0.544
14	61	0.832	35	265	0.528
15	89	0.820	36	275	0.511
16	90	0.796	37	292	0.493
17	92	0.784	38	317	0.476
18	113	0.772	39	322	0.459
19	127	0.759	40	350	0.439
20	131	0.746	41	357	0.419
21	138	0.733	42	380	0.380

(i) Show that an adequate description of survival for this group is $\hat{S}_0(t) = 0.936 - 0.0015t$.
(ii) Write an expression for the hazard function associated with the linear model $S_0(t)$ given in the previous problem (i).
(iii) Using this model of $S_0(t)$ create a plot that shows the differences between the "treatment" and "control" (groups = "high" and "low") groups using the coefficients estimated for these data from the proportional hazards model [see Chapter 12, expression (12.23)].
(iv) Similarly show the influence of age on these two groups (plot four curves) employing the linear model.

Bibliography

Chapter 1

1. Kleinbaum, D. G., Kupper, L. L., and Morgenstern, H. *Epidemiologic Research: Principle and Methods.* 1982. Van Nostrand Reinhold, Co., New York.
2. Selvin, S. (1977). Three statistical models for estimating length of stay. Health Services Research (4):322–30.
3. Fleiss, J. L. *Statistical Methods for Rates and Proportions.* 1981. John Wiley and Sons, Inc., New York.
4. Breslow, N. E., and Day, N. E. Statistical Methods in Cancer Research, Volume II, *The Design and Analysis of Cohort Studies.* 1987. Oxford University Press, Oxford, UK.
5. Cochran, W. G. *Sampling Techniques.* 1965. John Wiley and Sons, Inc., New York.
6. Owen, D. B. *Handbook of Statistical Tables.* 1962. Addison-Wesley Publishing Co., Reading, Mass.
7. McNeil, D. R. *Interactive Data Analysis.* 1977. John Wiley and Sons, Inc., New York.
8. Tukey, J. *Exploratory Data Analysis.* 1977. Addison-Wesley, Reading, Mass.
9. *Surveillance, Epidemiology End Results, Incidence and Mortality Data 1973–77.* U.S. Department of Health and Human Resources. NIH 81–2330. National Cancer Institute, Bethesda, Maryland.
10. Cox, D. R. *Analysis of Binary Data.* 1970. Methuen Co., London, UK.

Chapter 2

1. Snedecor, G. W., and Cochran, W. G. *Statistical Methods.* 1974. The University of Iowa State Press, Ames, Iowa.
2. Kleinbaum, D. G., Kupper, L. L., and Morgenstern, H. *Epidemiologic Research: Principle and Methods.* 1982. Van Nostrand Reinhold Co., New York.
3. Kelsey, J. L., Thompson, W. D., and Evans, A. S. *Methods in Observational Epidemiology.* 1986. Oxford University Press, Oxford, UK.
4. Greenland, S., and Robins, J. M. (1985). Confounding and misclassification. Am. J. Epid. (122):495–506.
5. Fuller, W. A., and Hidiroglou, M. A. (1978). Regression estimates after correcting for attenuation. J. Am. Stat. Assoc. (73):99–114.
6. Phillips, A. N., and Davey-Smith, G. (1992). Bias in relative odds estimation owing to imprecise measurement of correlated exposure. Stat. Med. (11):953–61.
7. Ernster, V. L., Mason, L., et. al. (1982). Effects of caffeine-free diet on benign breast disease: A randomized trial. Surgery 91 (3):263–67.
8. Robinson, R. G. (1985). Blood pressure: A contextual analysis of the effects of race, social status and stress. Ph.D. dissertation. University of California, Berkeley.

9. Saracci, R. (1987). The interactions of tobacco smoking and other agents in cancer etiology. Epid. Reviews 9:175–93.

10. Rivard, T. (1985). Master's thesis. University of California, Berkeley.

11. Fleiss, J. *The Design and Analysis of Clinical Experiments.* 1986. John Wiley and Sons, Inc., New York.

12. Miller, R. *Simultaneous Statistical Inference.* 1966. McGraw-Hill, New York.

13. Gardner, M. J., and Altman, D. G. *Statistics with Confidence.* 1989. The Universities Press, London, UK.

14. Robinson, W. S. (1950). Ecological correlations and the behavior of individuals. Am. Social Rev. (15):351–57.

15. Lave, L. B., and Seskin, E. P. *Air Pollution and Human Health.* 1977. The Johns Hopkins Univeristy Press, Baltimore.

16. Keys, A., ed. (1970). Coronary heart disease in seven countries. Am. Heart Assoc. Monograph. No. 29. The American Heart Association, New York.

17. Kasl, S. V. (1970). Mortality and the business cycle: Some questions about research strategies when utilizing macro-social models and ecologic data. Am. J. Public Health (69):784–88.

18. Draper, N. R., and Smith, H. *Applied Regression Analysis.* 1966. John Wiley and Sons, Inc., New York.

Chapter 3

1. Johnson, N. L. *Discrete Distributions.* 1969. John Wiley and Sons, Inc., New York.

2. Fleiss, J. L. *Statistical Methods for Rates and Proportions.* 1981. John Wiley and Sons, Inc., New York.

3. Casagrande, J. T., Pike, M. C., and Smith, P. G. (1978). An improved approximate formula for calculating sample sizes for comparing two binomial distributions. Biometrics (34):483–86.

4. Kleinbaum, D. G., Kupper, L. L., and Morgenstern, H. *Epidemiologic Research: Principle and Methods.* 1982. Van Nostrand Reinhold Co., New York.

5. Kahn, H. A., and Sempos, C. T. *An Introduction to Epidemiologic Methods.* 1989. Oxford University Press, New York.

6. Cox, D. R. (1957). Note on grouping. J. Am. Stat. Assoc. (19):543–49.

Chapter 4

1. Frost, W. H. (1939). The age selection of mortality from tuberculosis in successive decades. Amer. J. Hyg. (4):91–96.

2. Levin, M. L. (1953). The occurrence of lung cancer in man. Acta Unio. Internationalis Contra Cancrum, 531–41.

3. Poskanzer, D., and Schwab, R. S. (1963), Cohort analysis of Parkinson's syndrome. J. Chronic Dis., (16):961–73.

4. Ernster, V. L., Selvin, S., and Winkelstein, W. (1978). Cohort mortality for prostatic cancer among United States non-whites. Science, (200):1165–66.

5. Avila, M. H., and Walker, A. W. (1987). Age dependence of cohort phenomena in breast cancer mortality in the United States. Am. J. Epid. (126):377–84.

6. McNeil, D. *Interactive Data Analysis.* 1977. John Wiley and Sons, Inc., New York.

7. Tukey, J. *Exploratory Data Analysis.* 1977. Addison-Wesley, Reading, Mass.

8. Selvin, S., Levin, L. I., Merrill, D. W., and Winkelstein, W. (1983). Selected epidemiologic observations of cell-specific leukemia mortality in the United States, 1969–1977. Am. J. Epid. (117):140–52.

Chapter 5

1. Lilienfeld, A. M. *Foundations of Epidemiology*. 1976. Oxford University Press, New York.
2. Feller, W. *An Introduction to Probability Theory and Its applications*. 1957. John Wiley and Sons, Inc., New York.
3. Ripley, B. D. *Spatial Statistics*. 1981. John Wiley and Sons, Inc., New York.
4. Selvin, S., Merrill, D. W., Schulman, J. et. al. (1988). Transformations of maps to investigate clusters of disease. Soc. Sci. Med. (26):215–21.
5. Schulman, J., Selvin, S., and Merrill, D. W. (1988). Density equalized map projections: A method for analyzing cluster around a fixed point. Stat. Med. (7):491–505.
6. Schulman, J. (1987). The statistical analysis of density equalized maps. Ph.D. thesis, University of Calfornia, Berkeley.
7. Knox. G. (1964). The detection of space/time interaction. Applied Stat. (13):25–29.
8. Knox, G. (1964). Epidemiology of childhood leukemia in Northumberland and Durham. Brit. J. Prev. Soc. Med. (18):17–24.
9. Mantel, N. (1967). The detection of disease clustering and a generalized regression approach. Cancer Res. (27):209–20.
10. Shaw, G. M. *Private communication*.
11. Shaw, G. M. (1987). A comparison of techniques for the detection of spatial and temporal/spatial disease clustering. Ph.D. thesis, University of California, Berkeley.
12. Kaldor, J., Harris, J. A., Glazer, E., et. al. (1984). Statistical association between cancer incidence and major-cause mortality and estimated exposure to emissions from petroleum and chemical plants. Environ. Health Prospect (45):319–32.
13. California Department of Health Services. Epidemiology study of the incidence of cancer as related to industrial emissions in Contra Costa County, California. Environmental Protection Agency, 1982 (Report no. r806393-01).
14. Efron, B. *The Jackknife, the Bootstrap and Other Resampling Plans*. 1982. Society for Industrial and Applied Mathematics, Bristol, England.
15. Diaconis, P., and Efron, B. (1983). Computer-methods in statistics. Scientific American (248):116–30.

Chapter 6

1. Everitt, B. S. *The Analysis of Contingency Table Data*. 1977. Chapman and Hall, London, UK.
2. Bishop, M. M. Y., Feinberg, S. E., and Holland, P. W. *Discrete Multivariate Analysis: Theory and Practice*. 1975. The MIT Press, Cambridge, Mass.
3. Kahn, H. A., and Sempos, C. T. *An Introduction to Epidemiologic Methods*. 1989. Oxford University Press, New York.
4. MacMahon, B., et. al. (1981). Coffee consumption and pancreatic cancer. New England J. of Medicine (11):630–33.

5. Breslow, N. E., and Day, N. E. *Statistical Methods in Cancer Research*, Volume II. 1987. Oxford University Press, Oxford, UK.
6. Bithell, J. F., and Steward, M. A. (1975). Prenatal irradiation and childhood malignancy: A review of British data from the Oxford study. Brit. J. of Cancer (31):271–87.
7. Bross, I. D. J. (1960). How to use ridit analysis. Biometrics (14):18–38.
8. Conover, W. J. *Practical Nonparametric Statistics*. 1971. John Wiley and Sons, Inc., New York.
9. Selvin, S. (1977). A further note on the interpretation of ridit analysis. Am. J. Epid. (105):16–20.
10. Gail, M. Adjusting for covariates that have the same distribution in exposed and unexposed cohorts. *Modern Statistical Methods in Epidemiology*. Moolgavkar, S. H., and Prentice, R. L., eds. 1986. John Wiley and Sons, New York.
11. Kleinbaum, D. G., Kupper, L. L., and Morgenstern, H. *Epidemiologic Research: Principle and Methods*. 1982. Van Nostrand Reinhold Co., New York.
12. Simpson, E. H. (1951). The interpretation of interaction in contingency tables. J. Roy. Stat. Soc. B (13):238–41.

Chapter 7

1. Thomas, W. D. (1987). Statistical criteria in the interpretation of epidemiologic data. Am. J. Public Health (77):191–94.
2. Poole, C. (1987). Beyond the confidence interval. Am. J. Public Health (77):195–99.
3. Letters to the Editor. (1986). Am. J. Public Health (76):237 and (76):581.
4. Kahn, H. A., and Sempos, C. T. *An Introduction to Epidemiologic Methods*. 1989. Oxford University Press, New York.
5. Kleinbaum, D. G., Kupper, L. L., and Morgenstern, H. *Epidemiologic Research: Principle and Methods*. 1982. Van Nostrand Reinhold Co., New York.
6. Mantel, N., and Haenszel, W. (1959). Statistical aspects of the analysis of data from the retrospective studies of disease. J. National Cancer Inst. (22):719–48.
7. Cochran, W. G. (1954). Some methods of strengthening the common chi-square test. Biometrics (10):417–51.

Chapter 8

1. Draper, N. R., and Smith, H. *Applied Regression Analysis*. 1966. John Wiley and Sons, Inc., New York.
2. Hosmer, D. W., and Lemeshow, S. *Applied Logistic Regression*. 1989. John Wiley and Sons, Inc., New York.
3. Kleinbaum, D. G., Kupper, L. L., and Morgenstern, H. *Epidemiologic Research: Principle and Methods*. 1982. Van Nostrand Reinhold Co., New York.
4. Breslow, N. E., and Day, N. E. Statistical Methods in Cancer Research, Volume I. 1980. Oxford University Press, Oxford, UK.
5. Schlesselman, J. J. *Case-Control Studies*. 1982. Oxford University Press, New York.

Chapter 9

1. Kelsey, J. L., Thompson, W. D., and Evans, A. S. *Methods in Observational Epidemiology.* 1986. Oxford University Press. Oxford, UK.
2. Rothman, K. *Modern Epidemiology.* 1986. Little, Brown and Company, Boston.
3. Cochran, W. G. (1968). The effectiveness of adjustment by subclassification in removing bias in observational studies. Biometrics (24):295–313.
4. Kendall, M. G., and Stuart, A. *The Advanced Theory of Statistics,* Volume II. 1976. Charles Griffin and Co., London, UK.
5. Worcester, J. (1964). Matched samples in epidemiology. Biometrics (20):840–48.
6. Miettinen, O. (1969). Individual matching with multiple controls in the case of all-or-none responses. Biometrics (25):339–55.
7. Breslow, N. E., and Day, N. E. *Statistical Methods in Cancer Research,* Volume I. 1980. Oxford University Press, Oxford, UK.

Chapter 10

1. Chiang, C. L. *The Life Table and Its Applications.* 1984. Robert Krieger Co., Malabar, Florida.
2. Miller, R. *Survival Analysis.* 1981. John Wiley and Sons, Inc., New York.
3. Cutler, S. J., and Ederer, E. (1958). Maximum utilization of the life table in analysis of survival. J. Chronic Diseases (6):699–712.
4. National Center for Health Statistics: Ninth Revision International Classification of Diseases, 1978.
5. Berkson, J., and Elveback, L. (1960). Competing exponential risks, with particular reference to the study of smoking and lung cancer. J. Am. Stat. Soc. (55):415–28.
6. Hammond, E. C., and Horn, D. (1958). Smoking and death rates: Report on forty-four months of follow-up on 187,783 men. J. Am. Med. Assoc. (166):1294–1308.
7. Sheps, M. C. (1959). An examination of some methods of comparing several rates or proportions. Biometrics (15):87–97.

Chapter 11

1. Bartholomew, D. J. (1957). A problem in life testing. J. of Am. Stat. Assoc. (52):350–55.
2. Peto, R., Pike, M. C., Armitage, P., Breslow, N. E., Cox, D. R., Howard, S. V., Mantel, N., McPherson, K., Peto, J., and Smith, P. G. (1977). Design and analysis of randomized clinical trials requiring prolonged observation of each patient II. Analysis and examples. Br. J. Cancer (35):1–39.
3. Gross, A. J., and Clark, V. A. *Survival Distributions: Reliability Applications in the Biomedical Sciences.* 1975. John Wiley and Sons, Inc., New York.
4. Snedecor, G. W., and Cochran, W. G. *Statistical Methods.* 1974. The University of Iowa State Press, Ames, Iowa.
5. Elandt-Johnson, R. C., and Johnson, N. L. *Survival Models and Data Analysis.* 1980. John Wiley and Sons, Inc., New York.
6. Miller, R. *Survival Analysis.* 1981. John Wiley and Sons, Inc., New York.
7. Gehan, E. A. (1965). A generalized Wilcoxon test for comparing arbitrary simply-censored samples. Biometrika (52):457–81.

8. Owen, D. B. *Handbook of Statistical Tables*. 1962. Addison-Wesley Publishing Co., Reading, Mass.

Chapter 12

1. Kalbfleisch, J. D., and Prentice, R. L. *The Statistical Analysis of Failure Data*. 1980. John Wiley and Sons, Inc., New York.
2. Cox, D. R., and Oakes, D. *Analysis of Survival Data*. 1984. Chapman and Hall, New York.
3. Elandt-Johnson, R., and Johnson, N. L. *Survival Models and Data Analysis*. 1980. John Wiley and Sons, Inc., New York.
4. Miller, R. *Survival Analysis*. 1981. John Wiley and Sons, Inc., New York.
5. Anderson, R. E., Lang, W., Shiboski, S., et. al. (1990). Use of β_2-microglobulin level and CD4 lymphocyte count to predict development of acquired immunodeficiency syndrome in persons with human immunodeficiency virus infection. Arch. Inter. Med. (150):73–77.
6. Feigel, P., and Zelen, M. (1965). Estimation of exponential survival probabilities with concomitant information. Biometrics (21):826–38.
7. Glaser, M. (1967). Exponential survival with covariance. J. Am. Stat. Assoc. (82):561–68.
8. Prentice, R. L. (1973). Exponential survivals with censoring and explanatory variables. Biometrika (60):279–88.
9. SUGI Supplemental Library User's Guide. 1983 Edition. SAS Institute Inc., North Carolina.

Appendices

1. Rosenman, R. H., Brand, R. J., Jenkins, C. D., et. al. (1975). Coronary heart disease in the Western Collaborative Group Study. J. Am. Med. Assoc. (223):872–77.
2. Rosenman, R. H., Brand, R. J., Sholtz, R. I., and Friedmen, M. (1976). Multivariate prediction of coronary heart disease during 8.5 year follow-up in the Western Collaborative Group Study. Am. J. Cardiology (37):903–10.
3. Rosenman, R. H., Friedmen, M., Straus, R., et. al. (1970). Coronary heart disease in the Western Collaborative Group Study: A follow-up of 4.5 years. J. Chronic Diseases (23):173–90.
4. Ragland, D. R., and Brand, R. J. (1988). Coronary heart disease mortality in the Western Collaborative Group Study. Am. J. Epid. (1217):462–75.
5. Mosteller, F., Rourke, R. K., and Thomas, G. B. 1973. *Probability with Statistical Applications*. Addison-Wesley, Reading, Mass.
6. Lyon, J. L., Klauber, M. R., and Gardner, J. W., et. al. (1979). Childhood leukemia associated with fallout from nuclear testing. N. Eng. J. Med. 300:397–402.
7. Breslow, N. E., and Day, N. E. *Statistical Methods in Cancer Research*, Volume I. 1980. Oxford University Press, Oxford, UK.
8. Fleiss, J. *The Design and Analysis of Clinical Experiments*. 1986. John Wiley and Sons, Inc., New York.
9. Kahn, H. A., and Sempos, C. T. *An Introduction to Epidemiologic Methods*. 1989. Oxford University Press, New York.

10. Haldane, J. B. S. (1956). The estimation and significance of the logarithm of a ratio of frequencies. Annals of Human Genetics (20):309–11.
11. Jewell, N. J. (1986). On the bias of commonly used measures of association for 2 × 2 tables. Biometrics (42):351–58.
12. Kendall, M. G., and Stuart, A. *The Advanced Theory of Statistics*, Volume II. 1976. Charles Griffin and Co., London, UK.

Index